Atlas of Breast Reconstruction Following Mastectomy

Atlas of Breast Reconstruction Following Mastectomy

Edited by

Bernard M. McGibbon, M.D.

Assistant Professor, Division of Plastic Surgery
Johns Hopkins University
School of Medicine;
Chief, Division of Plastic Surgery
Greater Baltimore Medical Center;
Chief, Division of Plastic Surgery
Church Hospital
Baltimore, Maryland

Illustrated by Diane Abeloff, M.A., A.M.I.

Edward Arnold

University Park Press
International Publishers in Medicine and Human Services
300 North Charles Street
Baltimore, Maryland 21201

First Published 1984 by University Park Press,
300 North Charles Street, Baltimore, Maryland 21201.

First published in Great Britain by Edward Arnold (Publishers) Ltd.,
41 Bedford Square, London WC1B3DQ.

Sponsoring Editor: Ruby Richardson
Production Manager: Berta Steiner
Cover and text design: Caliber Design Planning, Inc.

Typeset by Kingsport Press
Manufactured in the United States of America by Halliday Lithograph

ISBN 0 7131 44467

Contents

Preface

This book is intended to document the most important plastic surgical techniques of breast reconstruction that exist today. On the premise that a picture is worth a thousand words an atlas format has been adopted. The beautiful plates and drawings were done by Diane Abeloff, who has been a tireless worker and an ardent supporter throughout the concept. I have been very fortunate to have as contributors men who are originators and acclaimed experts in their particular field of reconstruction. I am also indebted to them for the clinical slides that complimented their chapters. John Bostwick is a man whom I hold in high esteem and I have done my humble best to do justice to the topic of latissimus dorsi reconstruction, but he is a hard act to follow.

It has been fascinating to witness in a relatively short space of the last seven years, the tremendous advances in this field. This is the result of a series of stepping stones which has led to the state of the art as it exists today.

While not every woman who has had a mastectomy feels that she has the need for reconstruction, there are those who have been devastated by the operation. Today, with the techniques that are available, they can be offered a chance to restore their femininity. Hopefully, this will mean that dreaded lumps that strike terror will be reported earlier and will result in a better "cure rate."

No single reconstructive technique is suitable for every patient and an attempt has been made to show the various methods available today. The final choice is made after considering the patient's desires and her general health, the availability of local tissue and the surgeons personal preference.

I must acknowledge my debt to the many who have helped me in preparing this book. To my secretaries, Mrs. Eleanor King and Mrs. Iris Gwyer for their good humor and the willingness to type and retype the manuscript. To Betty Ann Howard for putting the text into readable prose. To Mr. Raymond E. Lund R.B.P., F.B.P.A. and his staff at the Johns Hopkins University Pathology Photography Department who have printed the many clinical slides. Again, a heartfelt thanks to Diane Abeloff who did a wonderful job depicting the various procedures, often complementing the clinical results. To Jennifer Phillips, B.F.A. for her fine photographic contribution to the cover. A special thanks to Ruby Richardson, Senior Medical Editor of University Park Press who stimulated me with the original idea, gave me great support and showed great patience during the project; and to Berta Steiner, Production Manager of University Park Press who has been very helpful during the final preparation and production. Finally, and by no means least, to my family for their long suffering patience and support, and particularly to my wife for her great help in the proofreading of the text.

Bernard M. McGibbon, M.D., F.A.C.S.
1205 York Road Suite 36
Lutherville, Baltimore, Maryland 21093

Acknowledgments

I would like to thank the following surgeons who kindly supplied photographs:

Dr. E.H. Courtiss of Newton Lower Falls, Massachusetts
Figures 10.32–10.35
Dr. C.E. Horton of Norfolk, Virginia, Figures 10.22, 10.23
Dr. J. Jarret of Eugene, Oregon, Figures 10.2–10.13
Dr. V. Pennisi of San Francisco, California, Figures 7.5(A and B)
Dr. L.O. Vasconez of San Francisco, California, Figures 2.11, 2.12

I would also like to acknowledge and thank Dr. L. Leonard of Salt Lake City, Utah, and Dr. N. Reisman of Houston, Texas who performed the microvascular anastomoses in the two cases shown in Figures 8.61–8.70.

I would finally like to thank the journal, *Plastic and Reconstructive Surgery* for permission to reproduce several photographs from the journal for inclusion in this volume.

B.M. McG.

Contributors

J. Michael Drever, M.D., F.R.C.S.
Chief, Division of Plastic Surgery
Etobicoke General Hospital
Toronto, Ontario, Canada

Alexander M. Guba, M.D.
Assistant Professor, Division of Plastic Surgery
Johns Hopkins University School of Medicine
615 North Wolfe Street
Baltimore, Maryland 21205

Carl R. Hartrampf, Jr., M.D.
Associate Clinical Professor, Division of Plastic Surgery
Emory University School of Medicine
1364 Clifton Road, NE
Atlanta, Georgia 30322

John E. Hoopes, M.D.
Professor and Chairman, Division of Plastic Surgery
Johns Hopkins University School of Medicine
615 North Wolfe Street
Baltimore, Maryland 21205

Charles E. Horton, M.D.
Professor and Chairman,
Department of Plastic Surgery
Eastern Virginia Medical School
Director, Eastern Virginia Graduate School of Medicine
P.O. Box 1980
Norfolk, Virginia 23501

Edward F. Lewison, M.D.
Associate Professor Surgery and Chief, Emeritus, Breast Clinic
Johns Hopkins Hospital
600 North Wolfe Street
Baltimore, Maryland 21205

Bernard M. McGibbon, M.D.
Assistant Professor
Division of Plastic Surgery
Johns Hopkins University
School of Medicine
615 North Wolfe Street
Baltimore, Maryland 21205,
Chief, Division of Plastic Surgery
Greater Baltimore Medical Center
6701 North Charles Street
Baltimore, Maryland 21204;

Chief, Division of Plastic Surgery
Church Hospital
100 North Broadway
Baltimore, Maryland 21231

Albert C.W. Montague, M.D.
Assistant Professor of Surgery
Johns Hopkins University School of Medicine
615 North Wolfe Street
Baltimore, Maryland 21205;
Director
Comprehensive Breast Care Clinic

Children's Hospital and Center for Reconstructive Surgery
3825 Greenspring Avenue
Baltimore, Maryland 21211

Raymond Morgan, M.D.
Assistant Professor of Plastic Surgery
University of Virginia School of Medicine
Morgantown, Virginia

Chedomir Radovan, M.D.
Encino, California 91436

Richard R. Roniger, M.D.
Clinical Faculty Tulane University Medical School and LSU Medical School
6823 Saint Charles Avenue
New Orleans, Louisiana 70118
Former Chief of Psychiatry–Union Memorial Hospital
201 East University Parkway
Baltimore, Maryland 21218

James J. Ryan, M.D.
Assistant Professor
Division of Plastic Surgery
Johns Hopkins University School of Medicine
615 North Wolfe Street
Baltimore, Maryland 21205

Luis O. Vasconez, M.D.
Professor of Surgery
Chief, Division of Plastic and Reconstructive Surgery
University of California
Extension Center
55 Laguna Street
San Francisco, California 94102

Introduction

Breast cancer is an all too common universal tragedy. Despite every-improving diagnostic methods and therapeutic skills, the breast remains the leading organ site of cancer incidence and of cancer deaths among women in our country. Seven percent of all American females develop this malignant and monstrously destructive disease at a rate of 100,000 each year.

The standard treatment for breast cancer today is the modified radical mastectomy or total mastectomy with or without an axillary dissection and complemented when necessary by chemotherapy and radiation therapy. However, more sophisticated techniques have resulted in finding smaller and smaller breast tumors, thereby favoring more conservative tissue sparing surgery, increasing the patient's life expectancy and facilitating reconstructive post-mastectomy procedures.

Reconstruction of the breast after mastectomy had its origin almost 100 year ago; yet it is only within the recent past that this important restorative procedure has gained public and professional acceptance. Refinements in the techniques of plastic surgery and the development of life-like silicone prostheses have brought excellent operative results and helped to foster a more supportive public attitude.

The symbolic significance of the breast as a focal point of the female image, as well as a key to feminine attractiveness, body allure, sexuality and the psychologic emotions of the liberated woman are among the many important human values for restoring and enhancing the post-mastectomy patient's quality of life. If women are made fully aware of the possibility of reconstructive surgery following mastectomy they may not delay seeking treatment because of fear of permanent disfigurement.

This book by Dr. Bernard McGibbon and his distinguished co-authors is a major contribution to the literature of breast reconstruction.

Edward F. Lewison, M.D.
Chief, Breast Clinic, Emeritus
Johns Hopkins Hospital
Baltimore, Maryland

Foreword

The most common major cancer affecting women develops within the breast tissue. Removal of the female breast unquestionably causes sadness and may even be perceived as a loss of femininity. In addition the patient must live with the uncertainty of whether or not she has truly been "cured."

Current developments in medicine now allow plastic surgeons to work with general surgeons in alleviating some of the emotional trauma stemming from breast cancer therapy. Using implants, myocutaneous flaps, tissue expanders or grafts, the plastic surgeon is frequently able to reconstruct the breast.

Fifteen years ago breast reconstruction was seldom attempted. General surgeons usually counselled the patient that she could resume normal life if she "kept a stiff upper lip and did not let the loss of a simple thing like a breast change her life." Physicians are now much more sensitive to the deep grief that many women sustain with the loss of breast contour and appreciate that restoring the breast often improves the quality of the patient's life.

The timing for the evolution of breast reconstruction as part of the total treatment for mastectomy patients has been particularly fortuitous. Conscientious general surgeons had begun to evaluate scientifically the necessity in every case for radical operations routinely performed for all breast cancer patients. As the need for radical surgery diminished and was frequently replaced by less drastic techniques, surgical reconstruction became more applicable. The discovery of inert materials which could be retained in the body, the use of myocutaneous flaps, the refinement of plastic surgery techniques, and the willingness of general surgeons and plastic surgeons to work together have all contributed to the growing acceptance of breast reconstruction.

Although the general surgeon remains responsible for the comprehensive management of the mastectomy patient, the plastic surgeon must choose and provide the reconstructive technique appropriate to each woman. Working together, physicians can assure patients who have breast cancer that they need no longer fear disfigurement; hopefully, this will encourage women to seek earlier therapy which may in turn produce more cures.

Dr. McGibbon and his co-authors have attempted to present breast reconstruction as it exists today. They show the conscientious general surgeon and plastic surgeon working together for the benefit of the patient, accomplishing an end of which all can be proud. The results of today are vastly improved over those ten years ago; ten years from now they will be even better if we can continue our efforts of unselfish cooperation toward scientific advancement. This book is a timely, well illustrated, pertinent attempt to disseminate knowledge of this ever-emerging new field which affects such a large percentage of our population.

Charles E. Horton, M.D.
Professor and Chairman
Department of Plastic Surgery
Eastern Virginia Medical School;
Director, Eastern Virginia Graduate School of Medicine
Norfolk, Virginia

1

Philosophy of Breast Reconstruction

John E. Hoopes

Although breast surgery has been performed since antiquity and breast reconstruction has been executed since the latter part of the nineteenth century, it must be emphasized that reconstruction of the breast following mastectomy for cancer is an entirely new field of surgical endeavor. During the last decade, however, few areas within surgery have provoked such an explosion of interest. In the past, a number of theoretical arguments have opposed postmastectomy reconstruction. Reactivation of the cancer, concealment of recurrence, and interference with the immune mechanism secondary to reconstructive intervention have all been cited as potential risks of the procedure. Moreover, the aesthetic results obtainable with earlier operations did not convince either the oncologic surgeons or the patients that reconstruction was a worthwhile pursuit.

More recently, a number of trends have encouraged reconstruction: 1) There are no studies to support the aforementioned theoretical objections, and recent data indicate that reconstruction of the breast does not influence the course of the disease (4). 2) Vastly improved cosmetic results have been obtained, and public awareness and acceptance of available reconstructive techniques are increasing. 3) Plastic surgeons are becoming increasingly interested in body image problems. 4) Oncologic surgeons have gained greater understanding of the biology and natural history of breast cancer, which has led them away from "supraradical" procedures and inclined them toward the modified radical mastectomy (8,12). They are beginning to think in terms of reconstruction.

The trends encouraging reconstruction resulted in a publication by Hueston and McKenzie in 1970 (6). Subsequently, Snyderman and Guthrie presented their experience with a limited group of postmastectomy reconstruction patients at the Annual Meeting of The American Society of Plastic and Reconstructive Surgeons (11). The interest generated by their presentation resulted in a combined conference of oncologic and plastic surgeons convened at the Memorial Hospital for Cancer and Allied Disease (10). The current texts by Gant and Vasconez, and more recently by Bostwick, summarize in excellent fashion the state of the art concerning postmastectomy reconstruction (2,3). Currently available techniques and materials render possible the conceptualization and application of operative procedures which could not reasonably be considered as recently as 10 years ago. Oncologic and reconstructive surgeons alike have completely embraced the concept of immediate reconstruction following ablation of head and neck cancer; and it is likely that postmastectomy reconstruction occupies the evolutionary status of head and neck cancer surgery 10–15 years ago.

Who is a candidate for breast reconstruction? Clearly, a psychological need on the part of the patient is the primary motivating factor. It is well understood that, in general, an external prosthesis cannot be incorporated psychologically into one's body image concept. It is evident, however, that a maximum of only 8–10% of patients undergoing mastectomy eventually seek reconstruction; we must attempt to understand the differences between patients seeking reconstruction and those who seem to accept the postmastectomy deformity.

When should postmastectomy reconstruction be performed? The considerations relate to wound healing, other modalities of treatment, and the aggressiveness of the cancer. At the present time the majority of patients undergo reconstruction on a delayed basis. Increasingly, oncologic surgeons and plastic surgeons are considering both premastectomy reconstructive surgery consultation and immediate reconstruction (4,5,7,9,11). It is anticipated that both of these concepts will receive progressively widespread acceptance. In terms of wound healing, a fundamental surgical principle dictates that a period of 3–6 months is required for wound maturation, and that this period of time should elapse prior to entertaining the possibility of secondary procedures. It is also agreed that elective surgery should not be undertaken in patients undergoing chemotherapy and/or radiation therapy. It must be noted, however, that reconstruction does not preclude subsequent chemotherapy and/or radiation therapy, nor do these two treatment forms preclude subsequent reconstruction. It is only the patients who demonstrate inflammatory carcinoma who are perceived not to be reasonable candidates for reconstruction.

How should postmastectomy reconstruction be performed? This issue relates to the selection of alloplastic materials (silicone) versus autogenous tissue. The revolutionary development of musculocutaneous flaps has perhaps resulted in an excessive trend toward the utilization of autogenous tissue. At the present time a good percentage of patients undergoing a modified radical mastectomy can be reconstructed satisfactorily by means of simple insertion of an internal prosthesis. In others, however, more extensive reconstruction using a flap technique is required.

A major unresolved philosophical question pertains to management of the contralateral breast. The considerations relate to both symmetry and pathology. It is well documented that 10–12% of patients with breast cancer will develop cancer in the contralateral breast, and of the survivors living 20 years 20% will develop cancer in the contralateral breast. There is no question that surgery on the contralateral breast impairs both clinical and mammographic evaluation. Currently, there are no data to support the "prophylactic" value of subcutaneous mastectomy; and the question must be resolved as to whether any surgical procedure on the contralateral breast (other than mastectomy) is acceptable. Increasing experience will result in a clarified perception of the appropriateness of various procedures.

Plastic surgeons, in general, are not qualified to assume responsibility for the management of breast pathology and have little interest in doing so. However, they are concerned with body image concepts and the possibility of eliminating a "sense of deformity" on the part of the patient. Currently, all patients undergoing mastectomy for breast cancer (with the exception of those demonstrating inflammatory carcinoma) may be considered potential candidates for breast reconstruction.

References

1. Asken MJ, 1975: Psychoemotional aspects of mastectomy: a review of recent literature. Am J Psychiatry 132:56–59.
2. Bostwick J III, 1983: Aesthetic and Reconstructive Breast Surgery. Mosby, St. Louis.
3. Gant TD, Vasconez LO, 1981: Post-mastectomy Reconstruction. Williams & Wilkins, Baltimore.
4. Georgiade GS, Siegler HF, Fergeson BJ, McCarty KS, and Georgiade NG, 1983: Immediate reconstruction of the breast following mastectomy for cancer. Ann Surg (in press).
5. Horton CE, Rosato FA, McCraw JB, and Dowden RV, 1979: Immediate reconstruction following mastectomy for cancer. Clin Plast Surg 6:37–46.
6. Hueston J, McKenzie GA, 1970: Breast reconstruction after radical mastectomy. Aust NZ J Surg 39:367–370.
7. Noone RB, Frazier TG, Haywood CZ, and Skiles MS, 1982: Patient acceptance of immediate reconstruction following mastectomy. Plast Reconstr Surg 69:632–638.
8. Serafin FA, 1979: Reconstruction of the breast: rationale, prognosis, and timing. In: Breast Reconstruction Following Mastectomy, edited by NG Georgiade, p 131. Mosby, St. Louis.
9. Snyderman RK, Guthrie RH, 1971: Reconstruction of the female breast following radical mastectomy. Plast Reconstr Surg 47:565–567.
10. Snyderman RK, 1973: Symposium on Neoplastic and Reconstructive Problems of the Female Breast. Mosby, St. Louis.
11. Patey DH, Dyson WH, 1948: The prognosis of carcinoma of the breast in relation to the type of operation performed. Br J Cancer 2:7–13.
12. Urban JA, 1970: Bilateral breast cancer. In: Breast Cancer, Early and Late. Yearbook Medical Publishers, Chicago.

2

Evolution of Breast Reconstruction

Alexander M. Guba

The evolution of breast reconstruction must begin with the era of breast ablation. Before the late nineteenth century carcinoma of the breast was considered to be a hopeless affliction, not amenable to surgical therapy. Consequently, the disease ran its course unchecked and was uniformly fatal until the techniques of Halsted, Meyers, and others demonstrated that certain patients could be treated successfully by surgery.

Prior to the adoption of Halsted's principles by most surgeons, there were scattered reports in the literature of simultaneous breast ablation and reconstruction for benign disease. Most of these were published in European journals before 1920.

As early as 1877 Verneuil described the closure of a mastectomy site by means of a pedicled portion of the remaining breast (51). Tansini, working in Italy during the late nineteenth century, believed that the only way to allow maximal breast gland and skin excision was to use a large skin flap to reconstruct the wide defect overlying the anterior chest (48). Tansini described several large skin flaps that he used for closing mastectomy sites during the primary procedure. As Maxwell pointed out, Tansini's procedure was the first use of the latissimus dorsi flap for breast reconstruction and was quite popular in Europe until 1920 (31). Tansini initially used a skin flap that necrosed distally. His subsequent anatomic studies allowed him to describe and utilize a true musculocutaneous flap, the cutaneous portion of which consistently lived (Figure 2.1).

Most early reports of breast reconstruction were concerned with the procedure done after resection for benign disease and were based on the use of free fat grafts. Goldwyn reported that Gustav Neuber initially used free fat grafts in 1893 in a patient with a facial deformity (14). Czerny described a case of breast reconstruction in 1895 in which he removed an adenofibroma from a patient's breast and used a lipoma from the lumbar region as a free graft to the breast to restore volume and symmetry. From Czerny's description, the fat graft liquefied postoperatively and resulted in a "somewhat smaller and firmer" breast (10).

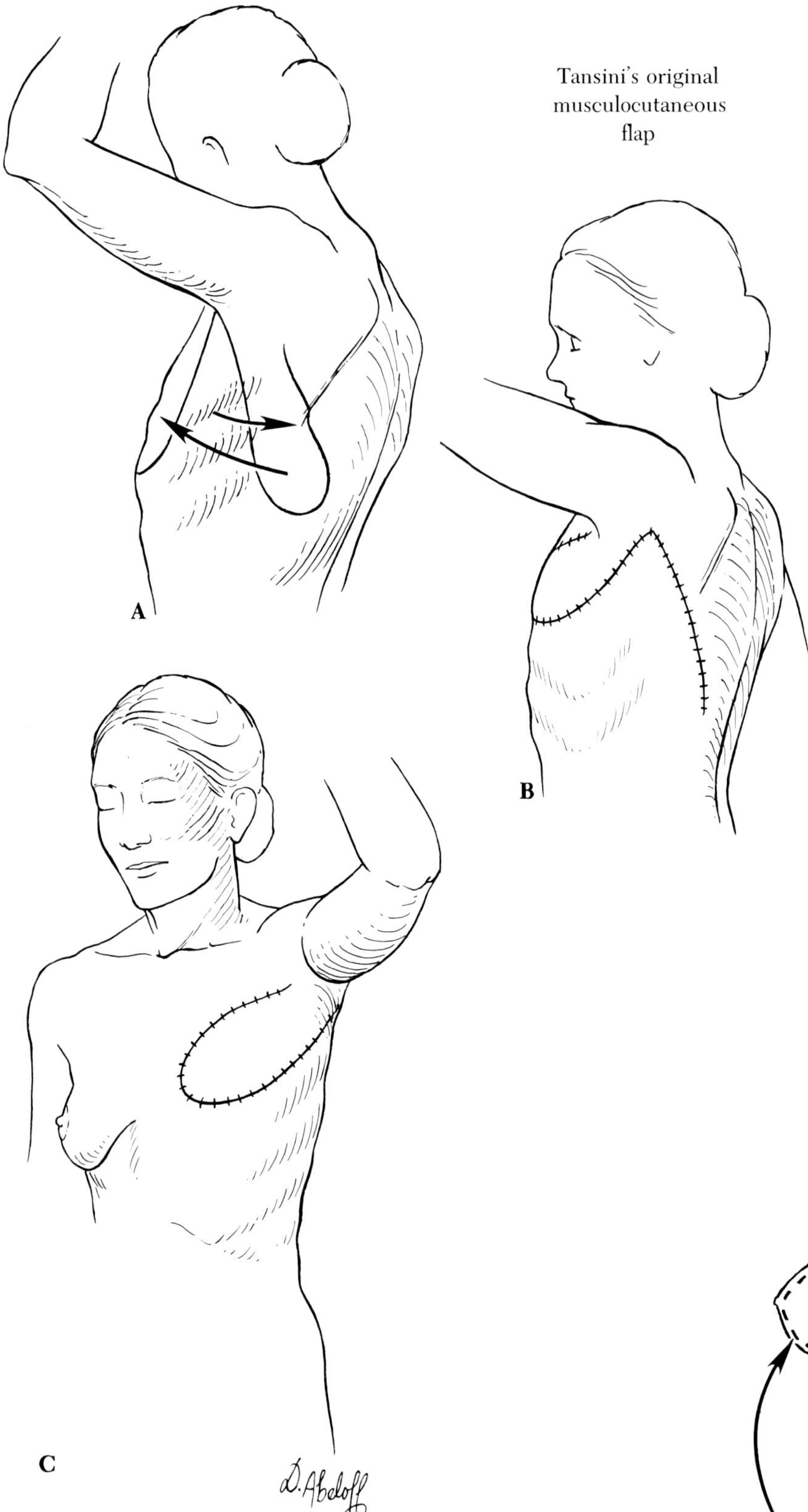

Figure 2.1 Original latissimus dorsi musculocutaneous flap as described by Tansini.

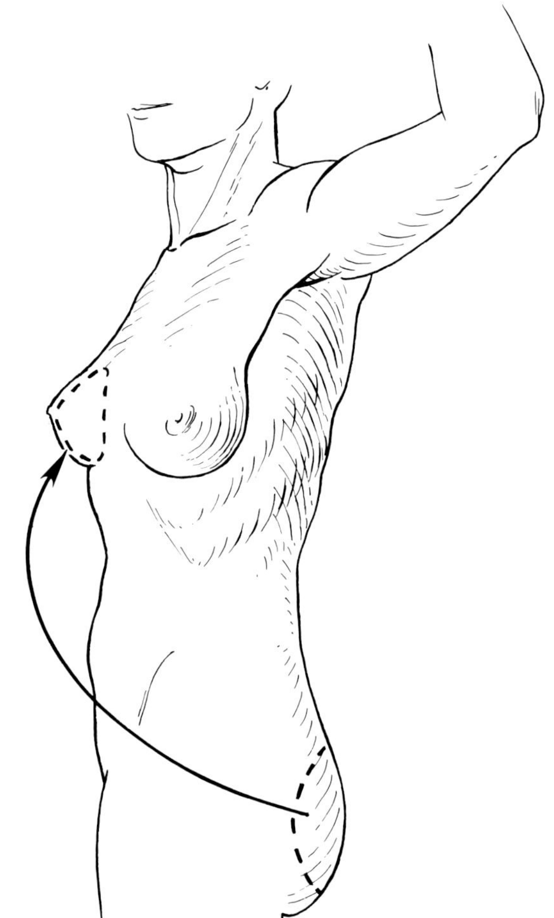

Figure 2.2 Free adipose tissue grafts.

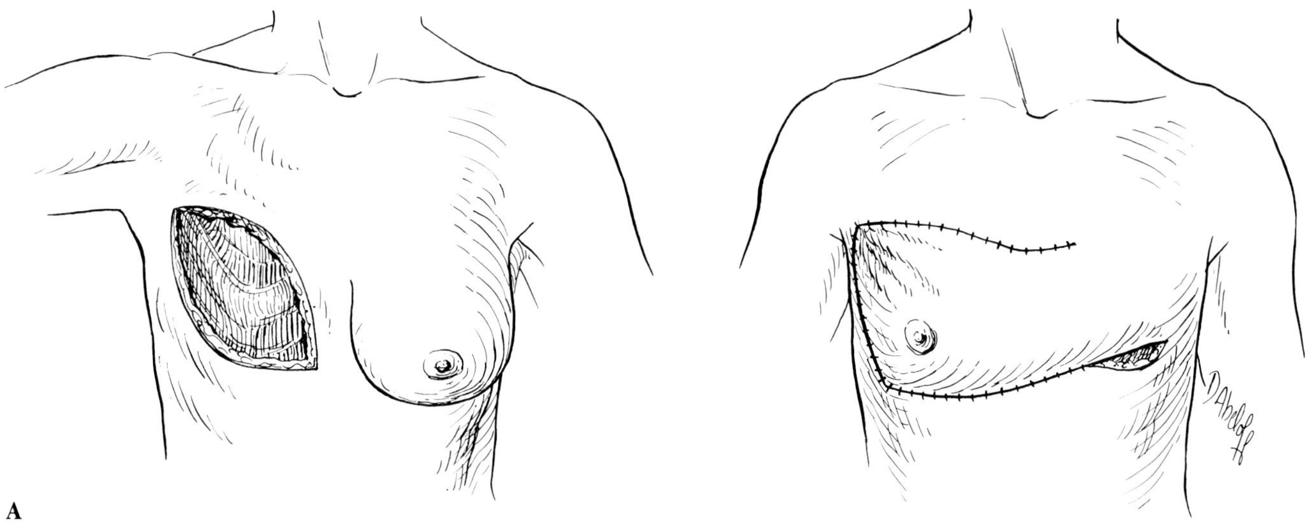

A

Figure 2.3 Transposition breast flap. **B**

Free fat grafts continued to be popular in the early 1900s. Bartlett published a report in 1917 in which he described shelling out a "precancerous" breast lesion and replacing the breast volume with free adipose tissue from the abdomen or buttocks (4) (Figure 2.2). He recommended using 50% greater fat volume than breast tissue removed to allow for graft "shrinkage." Lexer published a similar report (27).

The enthusiasm for free fat grafts eventually declined, and multiple skin flaps were utilized for breast reconstruction. Heidenhain (20), writing in 1911, used a large abdominal flap not unlike that later described by Baroudi et al. in 1978 (3) to cover a defect caused by mastectomy for carcinoma. In 1924 Kleinschmidt utilized an oblique thoracoabdominal flap to cover a similar defect (23).

Legue is credited with being one of the first surgeons to use the opposite breast to reconstruct a breast removed for benign disease (24), and Asaki described the operation in 1900 (2). Morestin reported a breast-halving procedure in 1903 (34), and Reinhardt published a similar technique in 1932 (41). Sauerbruch transposed the remaining breast to close a chest wall defect after an extensive resection for carcinoma of the breast in 1925 (44) (Figure 2.3).

By the 1920s the Halstedian philosophy of breast carcinoma and its management had become thoroughly adopted by the surgical world. It was universally accepted that cancer metastasized by regional lymphatic progression and that hematologic metastases occurred rarely if ever. It was therefore believed that wider resection offered the best chance for cure.

Halsted credits Follis with the statement, "the operator whose duty it is to close the wound should not be entrusted with the planning of the skin incision" (16). Moreover, Halsted himself believed that "to attempt to close the breast wound more or less regularly by any plastic method is hazardous, and, in my opinion, to be vigorously discountenanced." These concepts have dominated surgical thought for most of the twentieth century and have only recently been challenged.

Although several other surgeons described early "plastic" closures of mastectomy sites, the ultimate dominance of Halsted's philosophy laid these techniques to rest. Indeed, Purpura's defense of the "Tansini method" in *The Lancet* in 1908 was repeatedly critized by Handley in an interesting interchange of "Letters to the Editor" in that journal that year (17,38,39). The majority of subsequently published reports of breast reconstruction usually presented patients with nonmalignant diagnoses. Patients who had mastectomies for carcinoma were deemed fortunate to be alive and were not candidates for breast mound reconstruction.

One of the first English language reports to discuss reconstruction after mastectomy was that of Gillies in 1945 (13). He reported the use of a tubed abdominal flap, including the umbilicus, to reconstruct the breast after mastec-

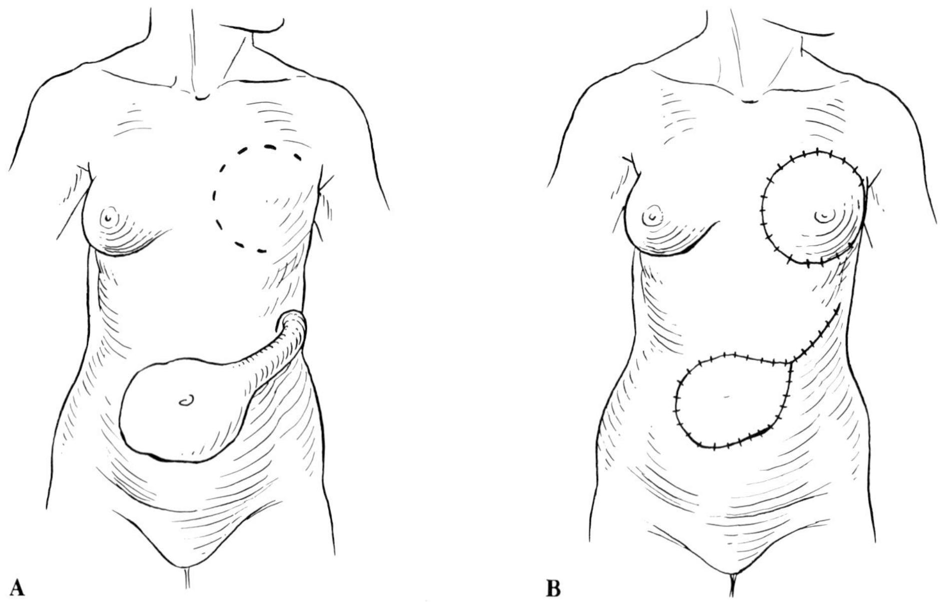

A B

Figure 2.4 Tubed abdominal flap.

tomy (13) (Figure 2.4). Millard updated this technique in 1976 using a tubed flap of the tissue usually discarded during an abdominal lipectomy (33). Harris (18) and Alexander and Block (1) published additional uses of tubed flaps for breast reconstruction. Ortichochea used the buttock on an arm carrier for breast mound reconstruction (35) (Figure 2.5).

Holdsworth in 1956 used a portion of the contralateral breast as a tubed flap (21), and Pontes in 1973 described an opposite breast splitting procedure

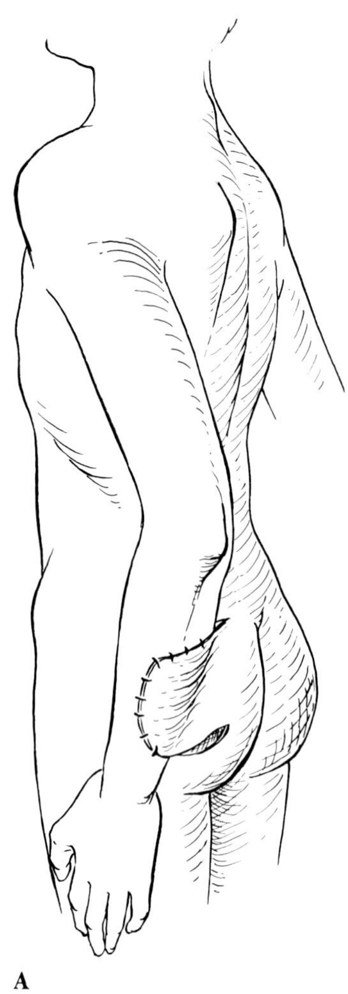

A

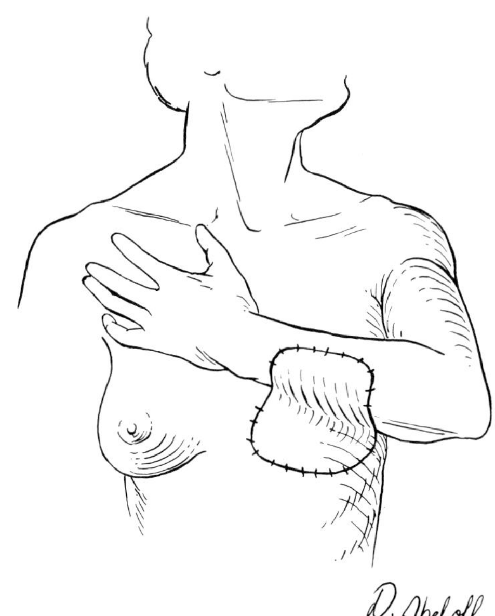

B

Figure 2.5 Buttock composite graft with the arm as carrier.

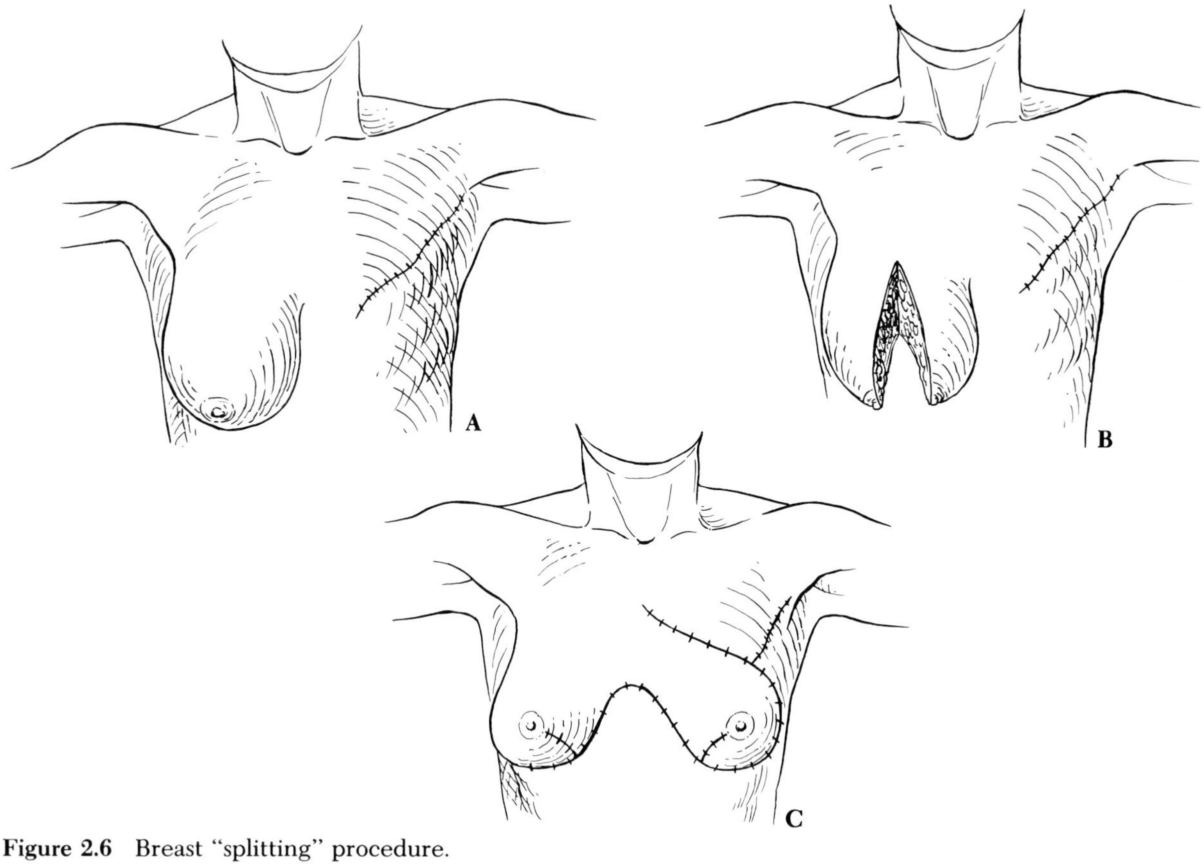

Figure 2.6 Breast "splitting" procedure.

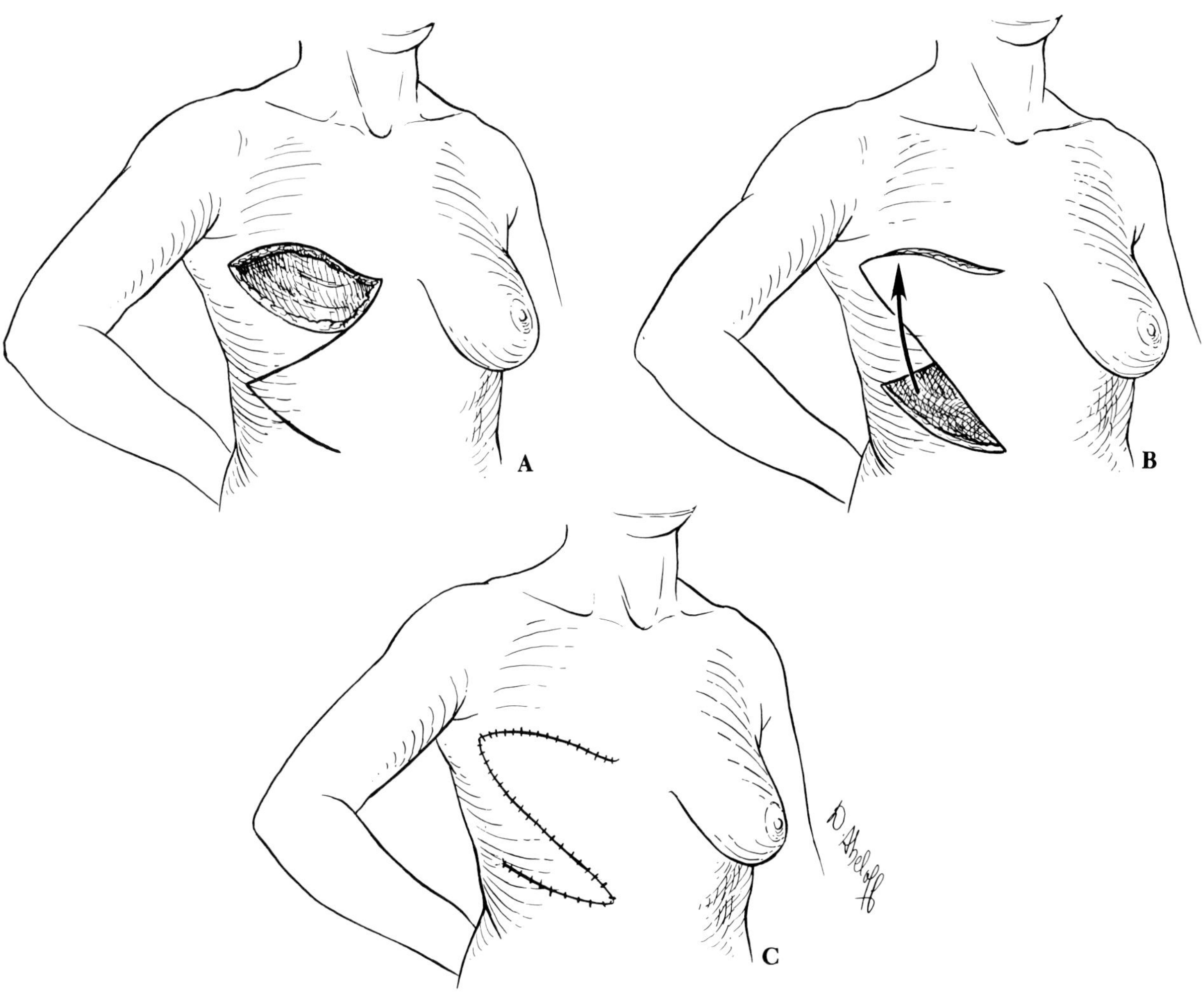

Figure 2.7 Local dermafat flaps.

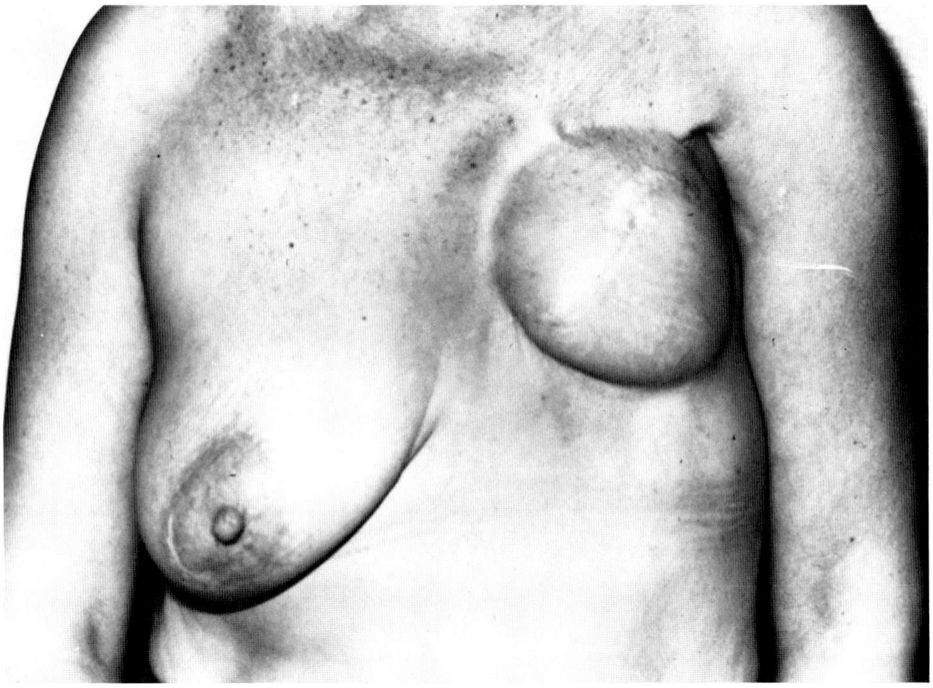

Figure 2.8 Post left radical mastectomy reconstruction performed 10 years ago with a subcutaneous silicone implant showing an unsatisfactory result.

to reconstruct a breast after mastectomy (37) (Figure 2.6). However, the use of the contralateral breast has been controversial both for cosmetic reasons and because of the risk of developing metachronous lesions in the remaining breast. A number of surgeons have described the use of various local dermafat flaps to improve the volume of tissue on the side of a breast resected for benign disease (5,11,25,28–30) (Figure 2.7).

The next significant addition to reconstructive techniques was the application of Cronin's silicone breast implant to the mastectomized breast, as reported by Guthrie and Snyderman in 1969 (15,46). Although the initial results of this technique were less than optimal (Figure 2.8), multiple reports since this study have established the role of silicone prostheses in reconstruction of the breast. Other authors, e.g., Birnbaum and Olsen (6), reported that the use of "custom" silicone prostheses gives excellent results (Figure 2.9). Lewis recommended upward advancement of the abdominal wall to provide skin to shape a breast mound (26). Pennisi (36) and later Ryan (43) amplified this

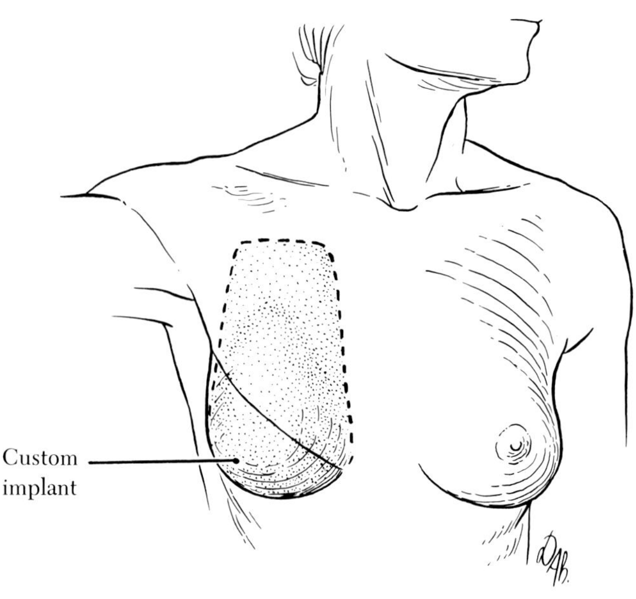

Figure 2.9 "Custom" silicone implant.

technique and added the development of the inframammary fold. Recently Radovan demonstrated the applicability of tissue expansion (40).

In 1970 Hueston and McKenzie published the first account of silicone implant reconstruction performed within several days of mastectomy (22). In 1977, when Cronin combined the use of thoracoepigastric flaps and silicone implants, the plastic surgical world applauded, and it was thought that this must be the definitive way to reconstruct the breast (9) (Figures 2.10–2.12).

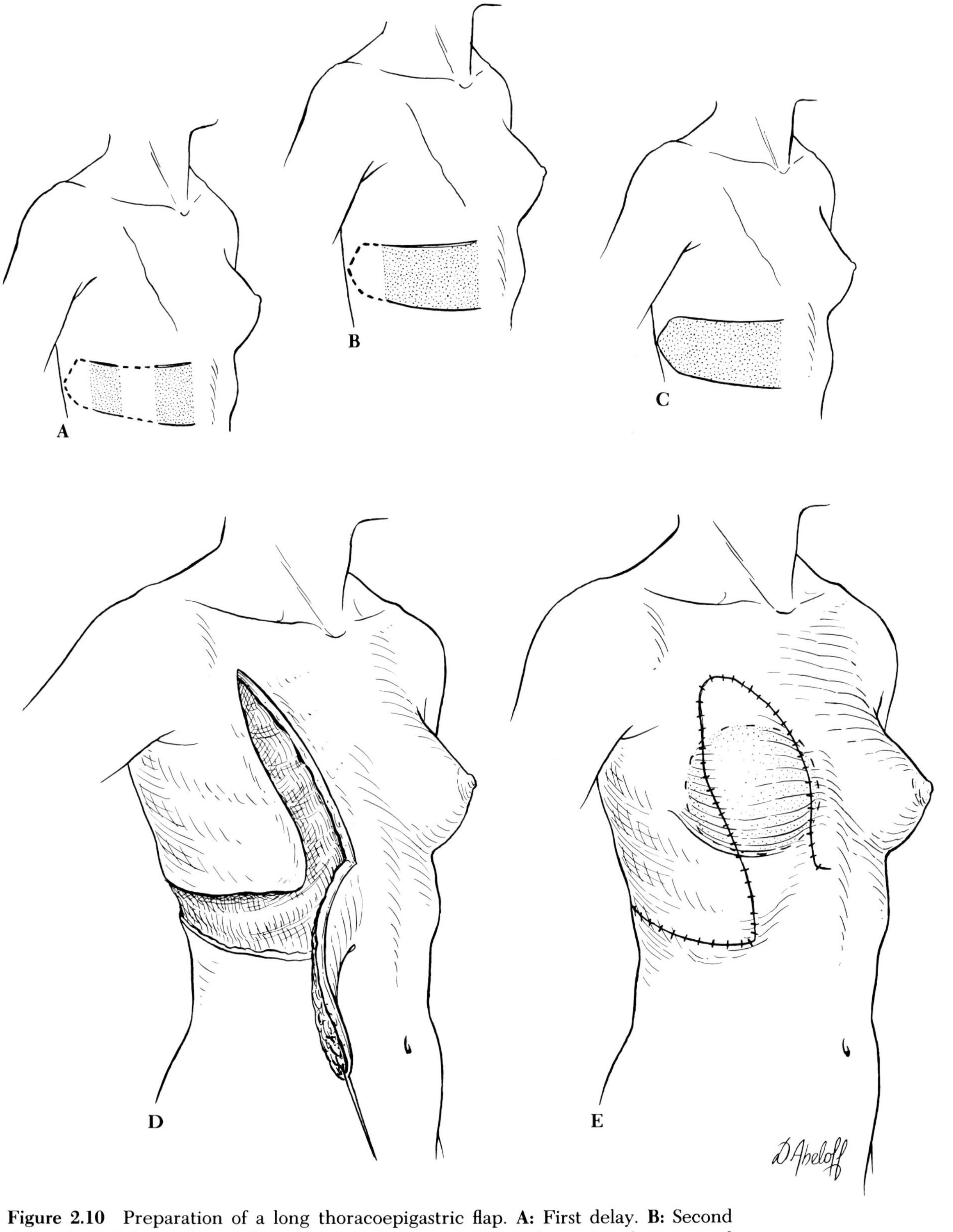

Figure 2.10 Preparation of a long thoracoepigastric flap. **A:** First delay. **B:** Second delay, 1 week later. **C:** Third delay, 2 weeks later. **D:** Flap elevated and transposed at the fourth week. **E:** The implant may be inserted when the flap is transposed if flap viability is good, or it may be done some weeks afterward.

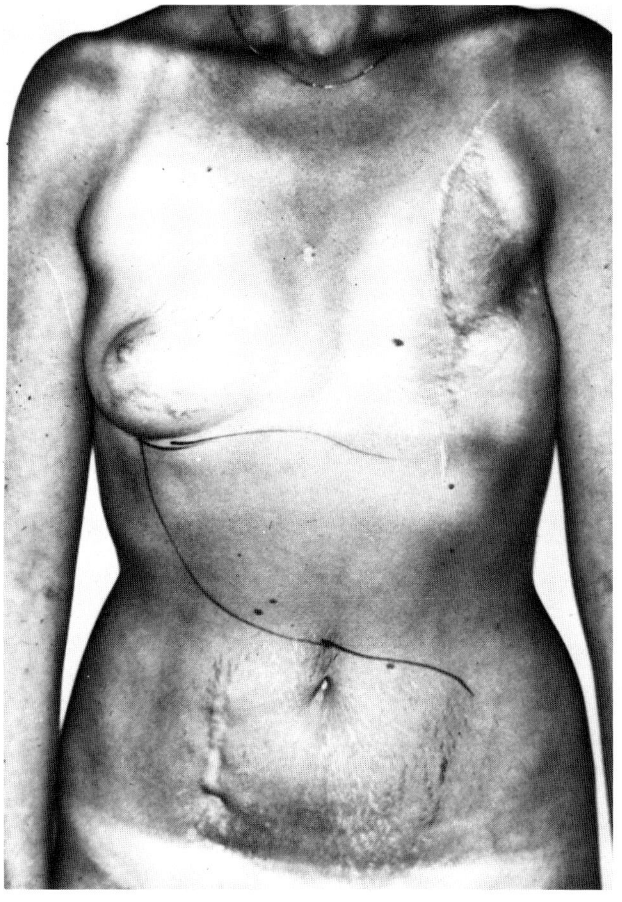

Figure 2.11 Left post radical mastectomy defect marked for a Baroudi flap. This was not done because the right lower abdominal scar would prevent upward advancement of the abdominal wall.

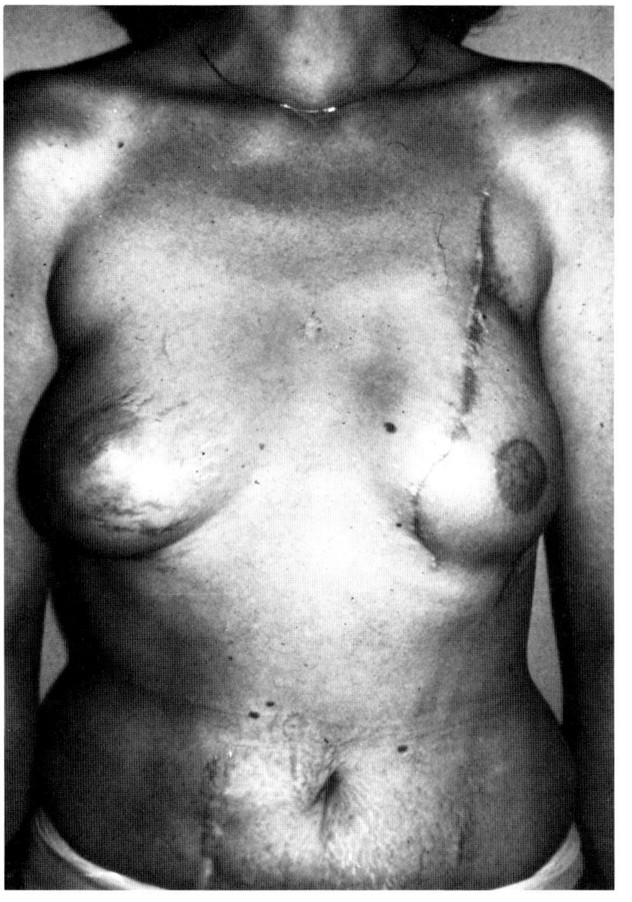

Figure 2.12 Left breast reconstruction using a thoraco-epigastric flap in the same patient as in Figure 2.11, postoperatively. (Photographs of this patient were kindly supplied by L. O. Vasconez, MD.)

Thorek described Tansini's forgotten latissimus dorsi flap in 1942 (49). Following the work by McCraw and Dibbell in 1977 on musculocutaneous flaps (32), Schneider et al. (45) and Bostwick et al. (7) rediscovered the latissimus flap and demonstrated its versatility. This flap has become the workhorse of breast reconstruction today. Still more advances were spawning, and the rectus abdominis musculocutaneous flaps were added to the breast surgeon's armamentarium. Robbins (42) and Drever (12) used the vertical island rectus flap often without an implant. Utilizing work by Tai and Hasegawa (47) in 1974 and Brown et al. (8) in 1975, Vasconez developed the contralateral inframammary rectus flap (50). More recently, Hartrampf et al. constructed a breast of adequate size and projection without the need of an implant; they used a large transverse abdominal island flap based on the rectus muscle (19).

References

1. Alexander JE, Block LI, 1967: Breast reconstruction following radical mastectomy. Plast Reconstr Surg 40:175–179.
2. Asaki, 1900: Praetimer I:85.
3. Baroudi R, Pinotti JA, Keppke EM, 1978: A transverse thoracoabdominal flap for closure after radical mastectomy. Plast Reconstr Surg 61:547–554.
4. Bartlett W, 1917: An anatomic substitute for the female breast. Ann Surg 66:208–211.
5. Berson MI, 1944: Derma-fat-fascia transplants used in building up breasts. Surgery 15:451–456.
6. Birnbaum L, Olsen JA, 1978: Breast reconstruction following radical mastectomy using custom designed implants. Plast Reconstr Surg 61:355–363.

7. Bostwick J III, Vasconez LO, Jurkiewicz MJ, 1978: Breast reconstruction after a radical mastectomy. Plast Reconstr Surg 61:682–693.
8. Brown RG, Vasconez LO, Jurkiewicz MJ, 1975: Transverse abdominal flap and the deep epigastric arcade. Plast Reconstr Surg 55:416–424.
9. Cronin TD, Upton J, McDonough JM, 1977: Reconstruction of the breast after mastectomy. Plast Reconstr Surg 59:1–14.
10. Czerny V, 1895: Plastischer Erastz der Brustdruse durch ein Lip. Zentralbl Chir 27:72.
11. DeCholonoky T, 1958: Mastectomies with simultaneous reconstruction of breasts. Surgery 44:689–697.
12. Drever JM, 1981: Total breast reconstruction. Ann Plast Surg 7:54–61.
13. Gillies H, 1945: Operative replacement of the mammary prominence. Br J Surg 32:477–479.
14. Goldwyn RM, 1978: Vincenz Czerny and the beginnings of breast reconstruction. Plast Reconstr Surg 61:673–681.
15. Guthrie RH Jr, 1976: Breast reconstruction after radical mastectomy. Plast Reconstr Surg 57:14–22.
16. Halsted WS, 1907: The results of radical operations for the cure of carcinoma of the breast. Ann Surg 26:1–19.
17. Handley WS, 1908: Tansini method for the cure of cancer of the breast (letter to the editor). Lancet 1:967.
18. Harris HI, 1949: Automammaplasty. J Int Coll Surg 12:827–839.
19. Hartrampf CR, Scheffan M, Black PW, 1982: Breast reconstruction with a transverse abdominal island flap. Plast Reconstr Surg 69:216–225.
20. Heidenhain L, 1911: Ueber Deckung grosser Defekten der Brushaut. Dtsch Ztschr Chir 108.
21. Holdsworth WG, 1956: A method of reconstructing the breast. Br J Plast Surg 9:161–162.
22. Hueston J, McKenzie G, 1970: Breast reconstruction after radical mastectomy. Aust NZ J Surg 39:367–370.
23. Kleinschmidt O, 1924: Uber Mammo-Plastik. Zentrabl Chir 51:488–493 (cited by Thorek, ref. 49).
24. Legue, 1898: De l'Autoplastie par Gilssmement Du Sein. Congress Francaise Chirurgie.
25. Letterman GS, Schurter M, 1955: Total mammary gland excision with immediate breast reconstruction. Am Surg 21:835–844.
26. Lewis JR, 1979: Use of a sliding flap from the abdomen to provide cover in breast reconstructions. Plast Reconstr Surg 64:491–497.
27. Lexer E, 1919: Die Frien En Transplantationen. Ferindand Enke, Stuttgart.
28. Longacre JJ, 1954: Correction of the hypoplastic breast with special reference to reconstruction of the nipple type breast with local dermo-fat pedicle flaps. Plast Reconstr Surg 14:431–441.
29. Maliniac JW, 1950: Breast Deformities and Their Repair. Waverly Press, Baltimore.
30. Marino H, 1952: Glandular mastectomy: immediate reconstruction. Plast Reconstr Surg 10:204–208.
31. Maxwell GP, 1980: Iginio Tansini and the origin of the latissimus dorsi musculocutateous flap. Plast Reconstr Surg 65:686–692.
32. McCraw JB, Dibbell DG, Carraway JH, 1977: Clinical definitions of independent myocutaneous vascular territories. Plast Reconstr Surg 60:341–352.
33. Millard DR, 1976: Breast reconstruction after a radical mastectomy. Plast Reconstr Surg 58:283–291.
34. Morestin J, 1903: Arch Gen De Med 43.
35. Ortichochea M, 1973: Use of the buttock to reconstruct the breast. Br J Plast Surg 26:304–309.
36. Pennisi VR, 1979: Making a definite inframammary fold under a reconstructed breast. Plast Reconstr Surg 60:523–525.
37. Pontes R, 1973: Single stage reconstruction of the missing breast. Br J Plast Surg 26:377–380.
38. Purpura F, 1908: Tansini method for the cure of cancer of the breast (letter to the editor). Lancet 1:634.
39. Purpura F, 1908: Tansini method for the cure of cancer of the breast (letter to the editor). Lancet 1:1715.
40. Radovan C, 1982: Breast reconstruction after mastectomy using the temporary expander. Plast Reconstr Surg 69:195–208.
41. Reinhart W, 1932: Z Chir, (cited by Thorek, ref. 49).

42. Robbins TH, 1979: Rectus abdominis myocutaneous flap for breast reconstruction. Aust NZ J Surg 49:527–530.
43. Ryan JJ, 1982: A lower thoracic advancement flap in breast reconstruction after mastectomy. Plast Reconstr Surg 70:153–158.
44. Sauerbruch, 1925: Surgery of the Chest, 3rd ed (cited by Thorek, ref. 49).
45. Schneider WJ, Hill HL Jr, Brown RG, 1977: Latissimus dorsi myocutaneous flap for breast reconstruction. Br J Plast Surg 30:277–281.
46. Snyderman RK, Guthrie RH Jr, 1971: Reconstruction of the female breast following radical mastectomy. Plast Reconstr Surg 47:565.
47. Tai Y, Hasegawa H, 1974: A transverse abdominal flap for reconstruction after radical operation for recurrent breast cancer. Plast Reconstr Surg 53:52–54.
48. Tansini I, 1846: Nuovo processo per l'amputazione della mammaela per cancre. Reforma Med 12:3.
49. Thorek M, 1942: Plastic Surgery of the Breast and Abdominal Wall. Charles C Thomas, Springfield, IL.
50. Vasconez LO, 1983: Construction of the breast using the contralateral upper rectus abdominis flap. Plast Reconstr Surg 71:668–675.
51. Verneuil A, 1887: Memoires de Chirurgie, Vols 1–5. Masson, Paris.

3

Psychiatric Considerations of Breast Reconstruction

Richard R. Roniger

The female breast is significant not only on a personal level but on family and social levels as well. Therefore when breast cancer occurs and must be surgically treated, not only the patient but also the members of her family and the people around her experience a psychological reaction.

A woman normally perceives her breasts as being outward manifestations of her femininity. From early teenage years when the first signs of breast development appear, through young adulthood when "bust" size and contour are related to a sense of attractiveness, through child-bearing years when the ability to nurse babies frequently makes a woman feel more "motherly," through the mature years when the individual seeks to maintain and perhaps enhance a sense of well-being, a woman's breasts give her both a characteristic physical shape and an emotional sense of womanliness. These "secondary sexual" organs clearly separate women from men. In fact, because of their visibility, they frequently carry greater significance than the primary sexual organs.

Little girls become young women in the eyes of the family when breast development takes place. Moreover, a woman's physical attractiveness, although seen in the composite, is frequently broken down into component parts by society. For example, references are made to "good legs," a "beautiful face," and an "attractive bosom."

Throughout a woman's life, her breasts play a major role in sexual behavior. The nipple, particularly, is replete with sensory nerve endings which render it sensitive to touch and afford pleasure to both sexual participants. Moreover, if a woman becomes a mother, she is aware of her breasts as a gratifying source of food for her baby.

Even in her mature years, the woman who desires to keep herself attractive pays attention to physical fitness and feminine form. Manufacturers of women's clothing are prolific in their endeavors to display the breast of women in ways thought to be unique and desirable.

The threat of mastectomy precipitates a variety of psychological reactions (2). Detection of a breast lump or mass, usually by the woman herself, is accompanied by fear that the lump may be due to the worse possible cause—cancer! If she seeks a medical consultation and her physician refers her to a surgeon for a possible biopsy, her anxiety increases, not only because of the threat of cancer but also because of the uncertainty of the outcome of the biopsy. If a patient gives preoperative consent to a radical or modified radical surgical procedure and if the biopsy is positive, she may emerge from anesthesia to discover that a vital part of her is missing. She must make the emotional transition from not really knowing if she has a disease to accepting the fact that she does indeed have cancer and that her breast has been removed. The patient frequently enters into a state of shock, disbelief, and denial. However, had she agreed to only a biopsy she would have been faced with a prolonged period of anxiety before definite treatment could be undertaken.

The psychological recovery from breast surgery does not always keep pace with the physical recovery. The patient frequently feels "less like a woman" and finds it difficult to wear suitable clothes. There is a feeling of imbalance, asymmetry, and awkwardness if one breast is removed. The breast prosthesis may be difficult to manage and may be an embarrassment.

The patient may feel extreme anger. This may be directed toward herself or even toward her parents or grandparents if there is a family history of cancer. It may be directed toward the spouse or even the medical team. The anger may be taken out on the manufacturer of external breast prostheses or on the prosthesis itself. The patient's self-esteem may deteriorate, and she may experience clinical depression characterized by an inability to experience pleasure of any kind, as well as psychomotor retardation and a decreased appetite. A spouse may be quite supportive but may also have feelings of disbelief and may not want to look at his wife without clothing. He too may become depressed.

Above all, lurking in the background, are other questions. Has the cancer been fully removed? Has it spread? Is the patient's life threatened?

However, in time, without the recurrence of illness, a resolution takes place. There is an acceptance of severe illness, its treatment, and the price one has to pay. Often a woman who has had cancer and has had a successful treatment experiences a greater sense of self. She has grown emotionally and is now more in touch with the basic needs of life.

Breast reconstruction often hastens the resolution process. It allows a woman to leave her existence as a "patient" and to return to her life as a "woman." When coupled with a positive attitude on the part of the physician, early discussion of reconstruction, and, in fact, integrating the procedure into the overall treatment plan when possible help the patient see past the illness.

After successful reconstruction, the patient has the feeling of "I'm me again." In a miraculous sense she may almost feel as if nothing really happened. This mental mechanism is not a pathologic denial but rather a firming up of the resolution stage of the psychological processes following severe loss (1).

References

1. Berkowitch S, 1980: Psychological results of reconstructed patients. Acta Chir Belg 79:165–167.
2. Goin MK, 1982: Psychological reaction to surgery of the breast. Clin Plast Surg 9(3):347–366.

4

Role of the General Surgeon

Albert C.W. Montague

During the past decade the philosophy of curative breast surgery has undergone a major change as it has gradually become apparent that the cure rate among patients who have undergone a radical mastectomy is no higher than that of patients who have had a modified radical operation. It is now clear that in many cases breast cancer is a disseminated disease that requires measures in addition to surgery for its control. As a result of these findings, surgeons are performing fewer radical procedures; the modified radical mastectomy or total mastectomy with appropriate lymph node dissection has become the standard treatment for most breast cancers. The effectiveness of these operations is reinforced in patients in whom dissemination is either proved or suspected by chemotherapy and radiation therapy (2,6,9).

Along with this new approach to the management of breast cancer has come a subtle change in the patient's attitude toward surgery. As a result of increased feminist awareness and rising consumer expectations, there has been a growing demand for improvement in the patient's physical appearance after mastectomy. The request for cosmetic adjustment, present for over 20 years in the area of head and neck surgery where reconstruction is considered an integral part of surgical extirpation, has now reached the field of breast surgery (4,5,8).

There are many mastectomy patients who may be candidates for reconstructive surgery. Although their eligibility cannot be finally determined until after the cancer operation has been performed and the extent of their disease evaluated, the general surgeon should be aware of the fact that the mastectomy patient may one day desire reconstruction and so take this into consideration when planning the operative technique. There are several ways in which the general surgeon can facilitate the process of reconstruction, beginning with the type of incision he chooses for the initial cancer operation.

Although the Halsted and Stewart incisions (Figure 4.1A,B) are commonly used for mastectomy, an oblique elliptical incision (Figure 4.1C) has been found to be equally effective and to result in a scar that is more adaptive to reconstruction. In selected patients with minimal disease, a skin envelope saving incision, similar to that used in reduction mammoplasty, may be useful

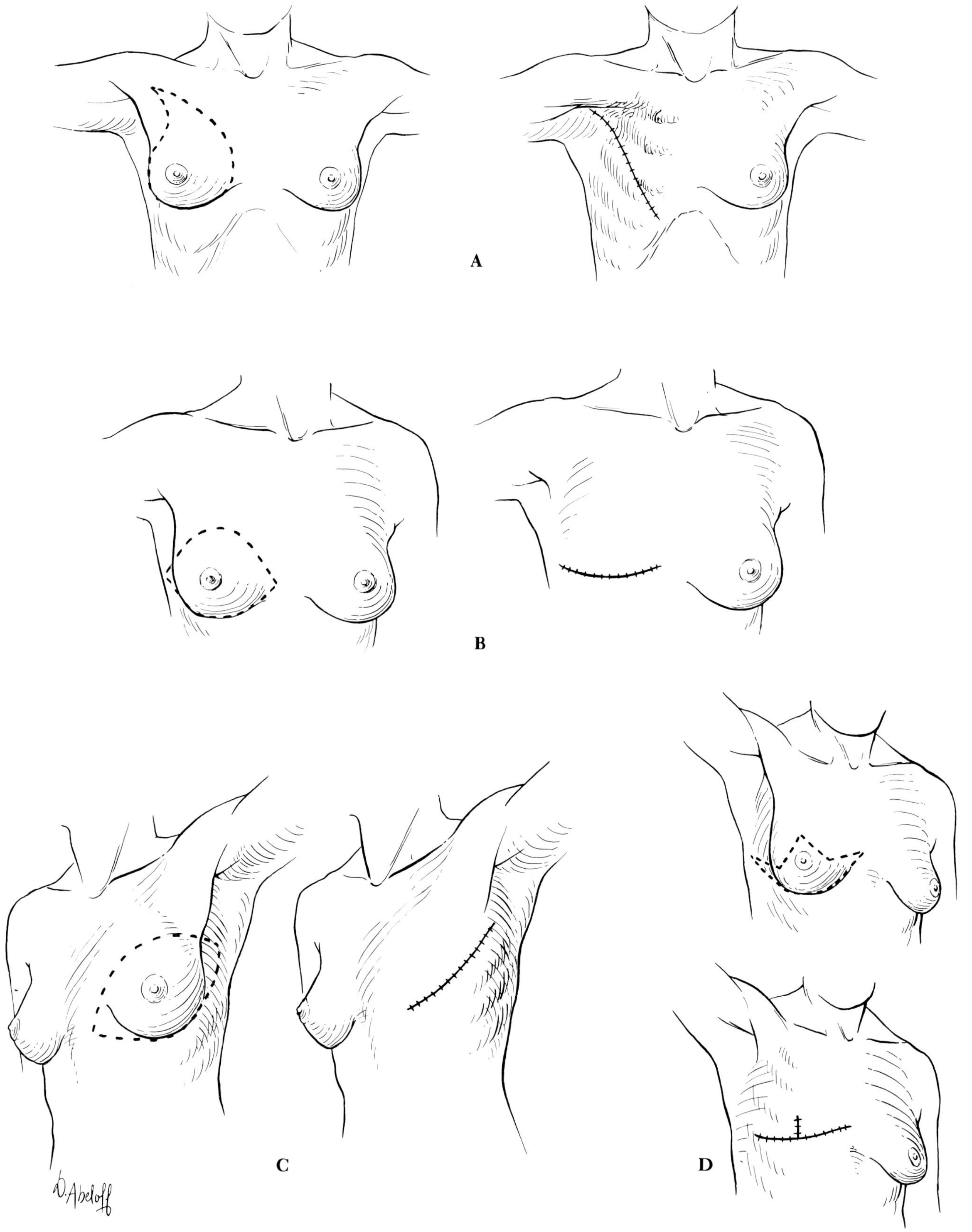

Figure 4.1 **A:** The classic Halsted incision, also showing the postoperative deformity. **B:** Stewart incision. **C:** Modified Stewart incision as used by the author. **D:** Skin envelope saving incision.

(Figure 4.1D). This incision is quite easy to perform using a "keyhole" pattern and is cosmetically good when reconstruction is performed.

During recent years the techniques of reconstruction have changed significantly. The general surgeon should be familiar with current procedures and aware of how they relate to the anatomy of the patient. For example, the

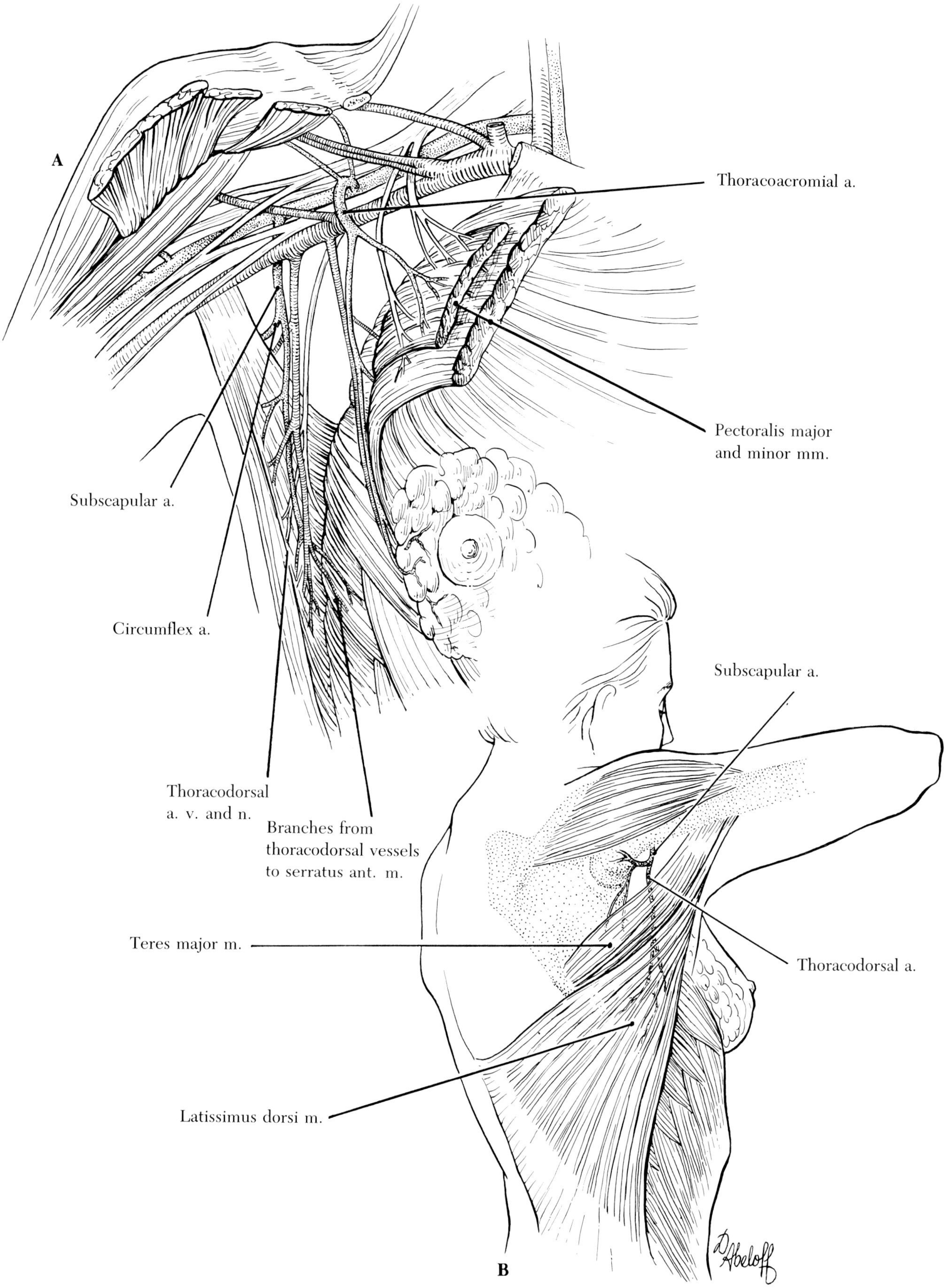

Figure 4.2 Innervation and blood supply to the latissimus dorsi and pectoralis muscles.

method of reconstruction most frequently used at present is based on the use of the latissimus dorsi musculocutaneous flap. The surgeon should therefore, when possible, seek to preserve both the innervation and the vascular pedicle to the latissimus dorsi muscle (Figures 4.2).

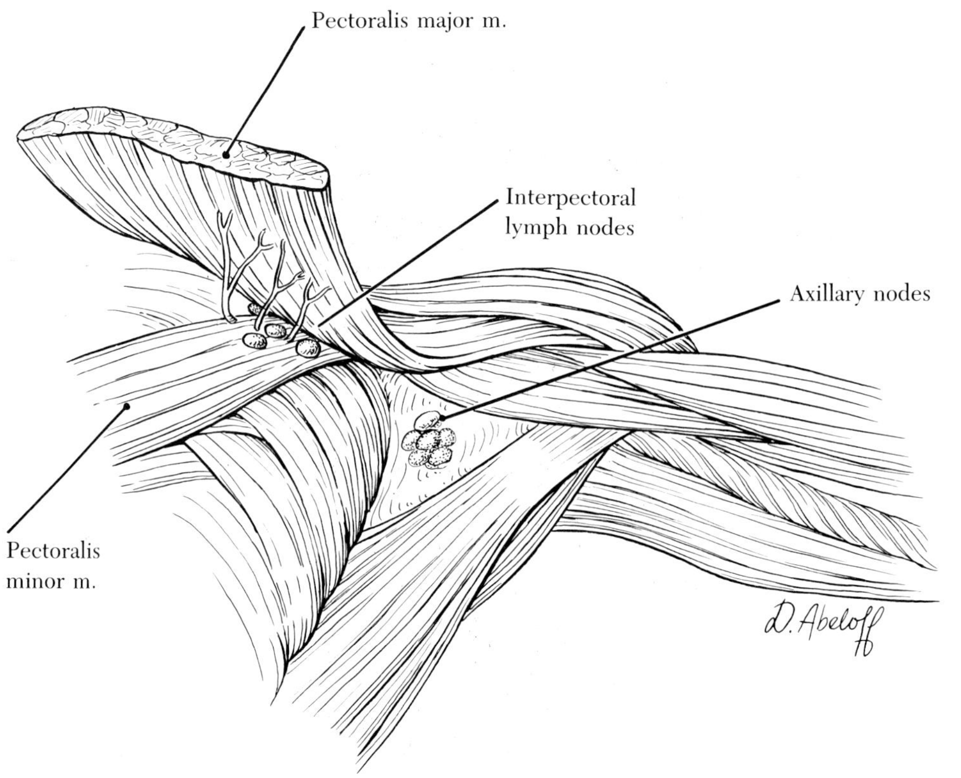

Figure 4.3 Details of the interpectoral nerves and nodes.

The cancer surgeon should also realize that if reconstruction is performed the area of the interpectoral nodes will become inaccessible after insertion of the prosthesis. Therefore this area should be thoroughly examined at surgery. During this part of the dissection it is important not to injure the blood and nerve supply to the pectoralis major muscle (Figure 4.3) because of the danger of subsequent atrophy.

It is hoped that from the outset the general surgeon will be sensitive to the psychological needs of the patient. Although not all women desire reconstruction, it is often comforting to the patient to realize that this option is available as the final stage of her treatment. In cases where patients do elect reconstruction, the general surgeon should maintain a working relationship with the plastic surgeon in making a decision on the patient's eligibility for further surgery and the optimum time for this to be performed (1,3,7,10).

References

1. Cronin TD, Upton J, McDonogh JM, 1977: Reconstruction of the breast after mastectomy. Plast Reconstr Surg 59:1–14.
2. Donegan WL, Perez-Merea CM, Watson FR, 1966: A biostatistical study of locally recurrent breast carcinoma. Surg Gynecol Obstet 122:529–540.
3. Horton CE, Rosato FA, McCraw JB, et al, 1979: Immediate reconstruction following mastectomy for cancer. Clin Plast Surg 6:37–46.
4. Hueston J, McKenzie G, 1970: Breast reconstruction after mastectomy. Aust NZ J Surg 39:367–370.
5. Miller S, Graham WD III, 1975: Breast reconstruction after mastectomy. Am Family Physician 11:97–101.
6. Montague AC, Brones M, 1978: Comparison of incidence of local recurrences of breast cancer treated by modified radical versus radical mastectomy. Paper presented at the 12th International Congress on Breast Cancer, Bueno Aires.
7. Rosato FD, Fink PJ, Horton CE, et al, 1976: Immediate post-mastectomy reconstruction. J Surg Oncol 8:277–280.
8. Rubin LR, 1979: Foreward: reconstruction of breast after mastectomy. Clin Plastic Surg 6:1–3.
9. Seidman H, 1979: Statistical and epidemiological data on cancer of the breast. American Cancer Society Publication No. 50.
10. Snyderman RK, 1976: On breast reconstruction after mastectomy (editorial). Plast Reconstr Surg 57:224–226.

5

Preoperative Evaluation and Planning

Bernard M. McGibbon

The time of the initial meeting between the plastic surgeon and the mastectomy patient varies from case to case. In circumstances where reconstruction of the breast is considered at the outset to be part of the total treatment, the general surgeon may arrange a brief meeting between the patient and the reconstructive surgeon before the cancer operation. Such an encounter, followed by a visit from the plastic surgeon after the mastectomy, is frequently psychologically reassuring to the patient. In other cases, however, the patient may not be in contact with a plastic surgeon until months, even years, after her operation.

When postmastectomy consultation for breast reconstruction is requested, two meetings are scheduled at the plastic surgeon's office. If the patient is married, it is ideal if the husband can be present on these occasions, as his support is very beneficial.

First Consultation

At the first consultation a thorough history is taken and a physical examination performed. Reconstruction should not be attempted in the presence of severe systemic illness. The general body habitus is noted regarding whether the patient is tall or short, lean or stocky, obese or thin. Information about the mastectomy is obtained, and the history is documented regarding breast cancer in first-order relatives, i.e., mother, sister, and maternal aunt (8). If breast cancer has occurred in these relatives, it is important to know whether it arose pre- or postmenopausally.

Attention is given to the mastectomy scar—its direction and quality of healing, the mobility of the surrounding skin and subcutaneous tissue, and the presence or absence of the pectoralis muscle (Figures 5.1–5.3). Pectoralis muscle function is demonstrated by asking the patient to adduct the arm against resistance. Palpation at this time reveals either a well developed or a deficient muscle. The lower half of the pectoralis muscle may have atrophied

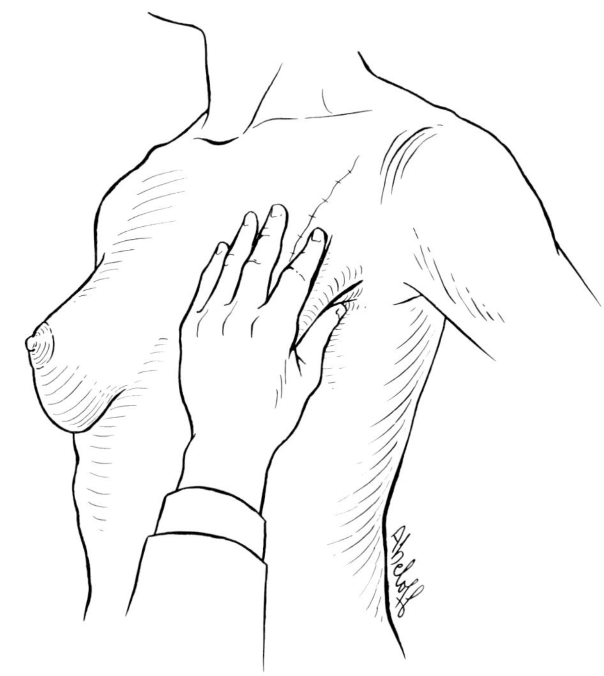

Figure 5.1 Testing the mobility of the mastectomy scar and surrounding skin.

because of inadverent transection of the medial and lateral pectoral nerves during the mastectomy. The location and size of any skin grafts are noted (Figure 5.4). If the patient has undergone radiation therapy, the area of irradiation is observed and the presence or absence of skin changes is recorded (Figure 5.5).

The function of the ipsilateral latissimus dorsi muscle is evaluated by asking the patient to forcibly extend her arm backward against pressure. A functioning latissimus dorsi muscle stands out and can easily be seen and felt by palpation (Figure 5.6). The presence and direction of lower abdominal scars as well as the looseness of the abdominal wall is noted.

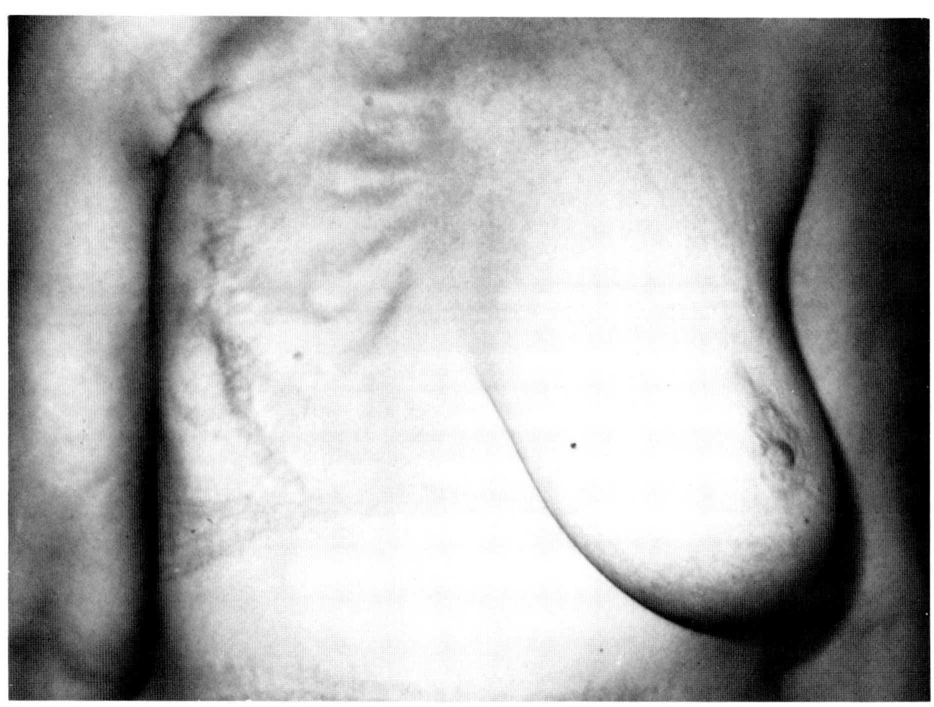

Figure 5.2 Radical mastectomy defect.

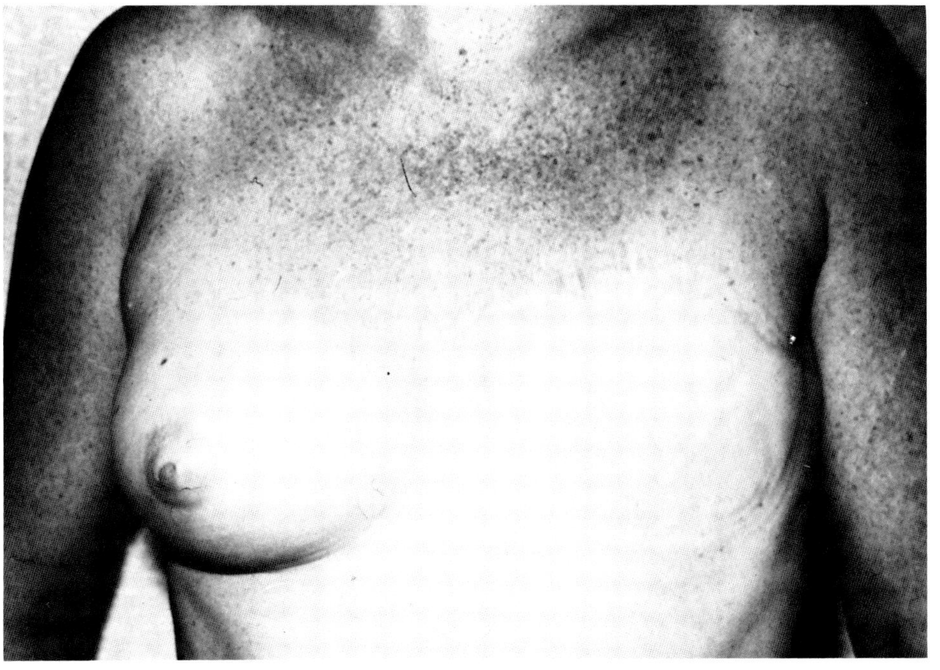

Figure 5.3 Modified radical mastectomy defect.

The contralateral normal breast is examined, and measurements are made from the jugular notch or the midclavicular region to the nipple in order to determine the presence or absence of ptosis. The premastectomy brassiere size is recorded.

Information on Available Techniques

If it is thought that the patient is a suitable candidate, she should be given as much information as possible about breast reconstruction at the initial consultation (5). Some women are well informed about the various operations through the popular press, women's magazines, and television. Others, however, are quite ignorant of the techniques available. Occasionally, women have a precon-

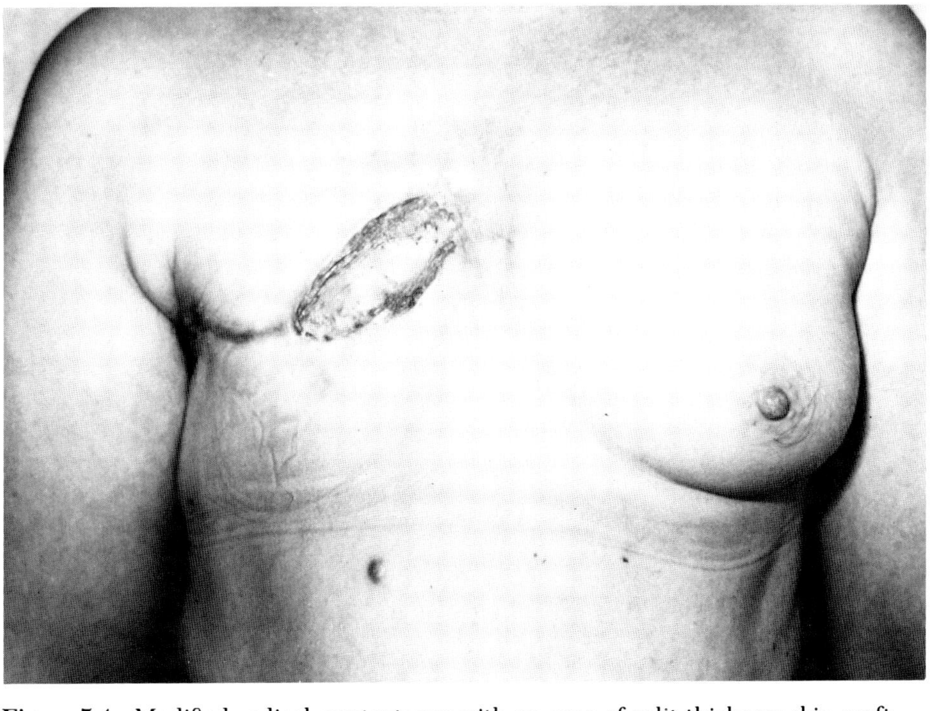

Figure 5.4 Modified radical mastectomy with an area of split-thickness skin graft.

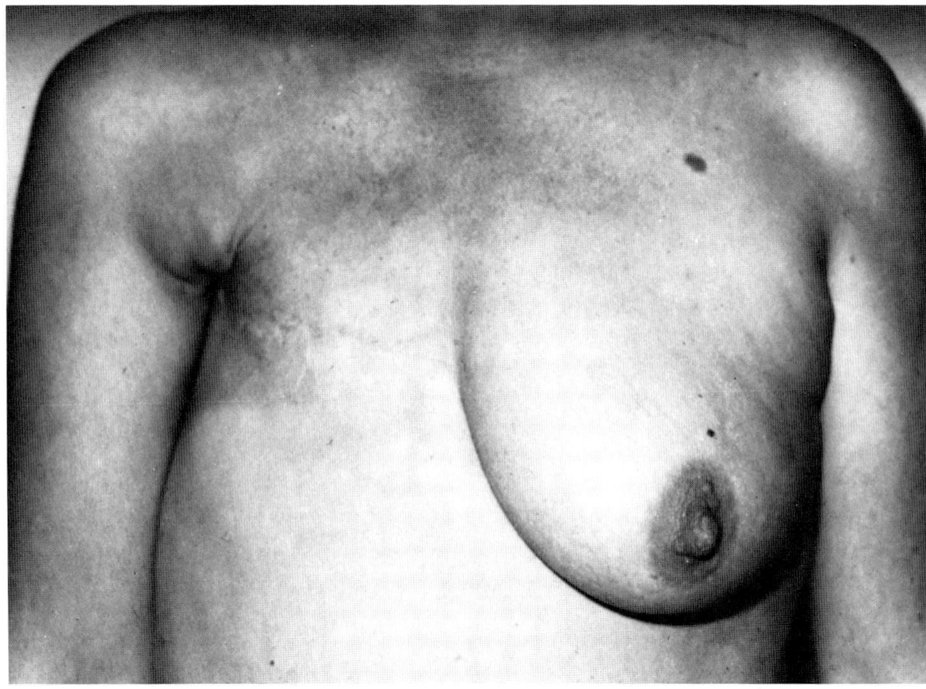

Figure 5.5 Area of skin change from irradiation.

ceived idea of the method of reconstruction they desire; others have an open mind.

The advantages and disadvantages of the various techniques should be described and the method most applicable to the patient's case recommended. Drawings of the various reconstructive techniques can be very useful at this stage. The patient is shown and allowed to handle a sample silicone gel breast prosthesis. It is important that she be asked what her desires are regarding reconstruction: whether she wishes a simple breast mound or a complete recon-

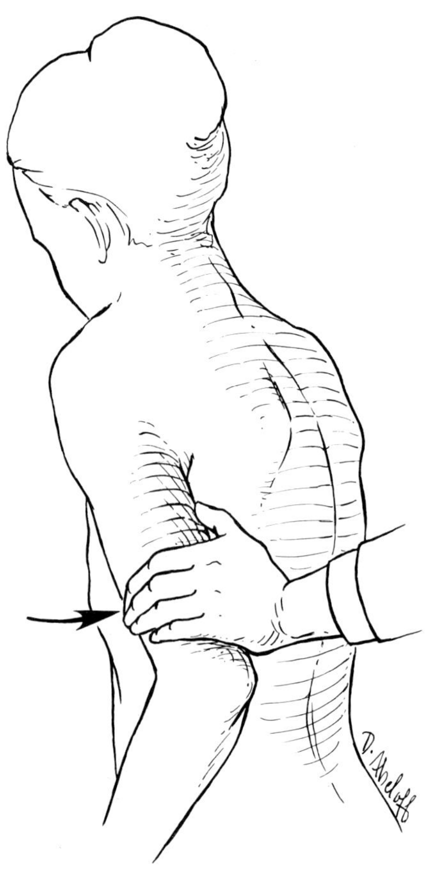

Figure 5.6 Testing for function of the latissimus dorsi muscle.

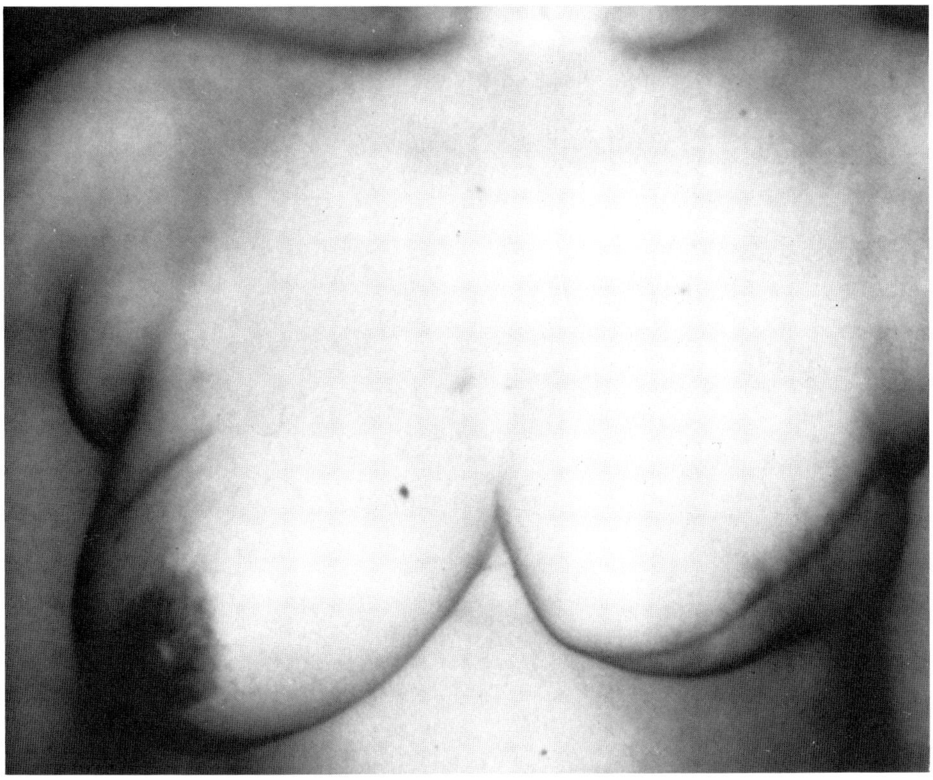

A

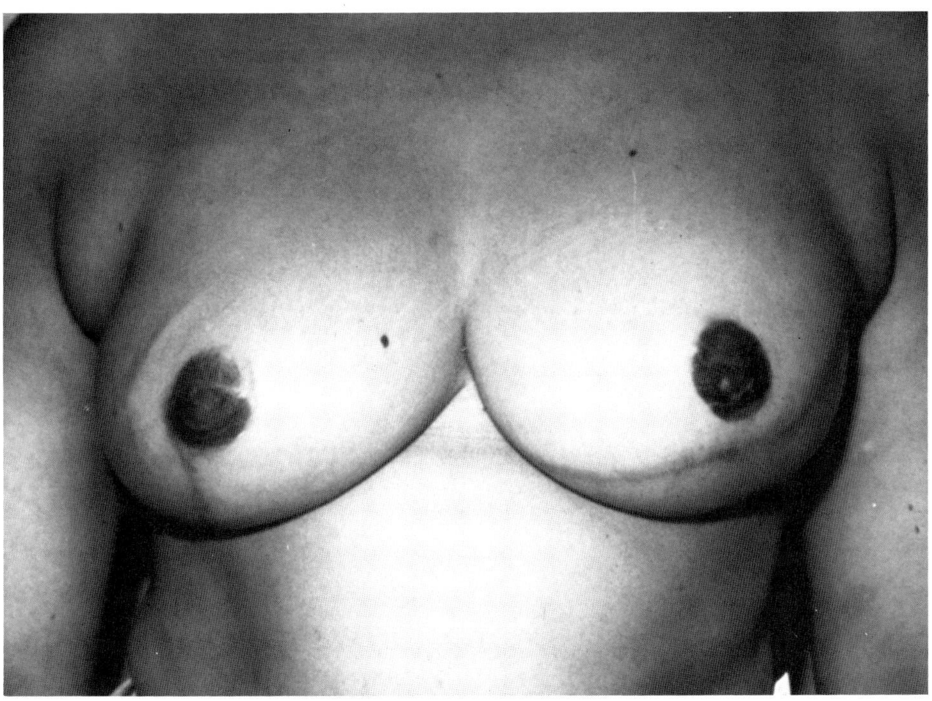

B

Figure 5.7 Top: Left mastectomy scar with an abundance of soft tissue remaining. Ptotic right breast with biopsy scar. **Bottom:** Left breast reconstruction with submuscular insertion of a silicone gel implant. Nipple was reconstructed by the sharing technique from the right side. The right breast underwent reduction mammoplasty and free nipple graft with the sharing technique to produce an areola from the left side.

struction with nipple and areola; whether she can accept a scar on the back or abdomen in addition to a chest scar, or a scar on the chest alone. In the discussion with the patient, the surgeon gives her an overview of the methods of reconstruction (9,23,28). It is important to emphasize that although reconstruction is possible a cosmetic triumph is never obtained (24,25).

Local Tissue Techniques

If a modified mastectomy has been done and the above-mentioned chest wall factors are favorable, reconstruction techniques using local tissue can be considered (Figure 5.7). The original mastectomy scar can be "opened," and by

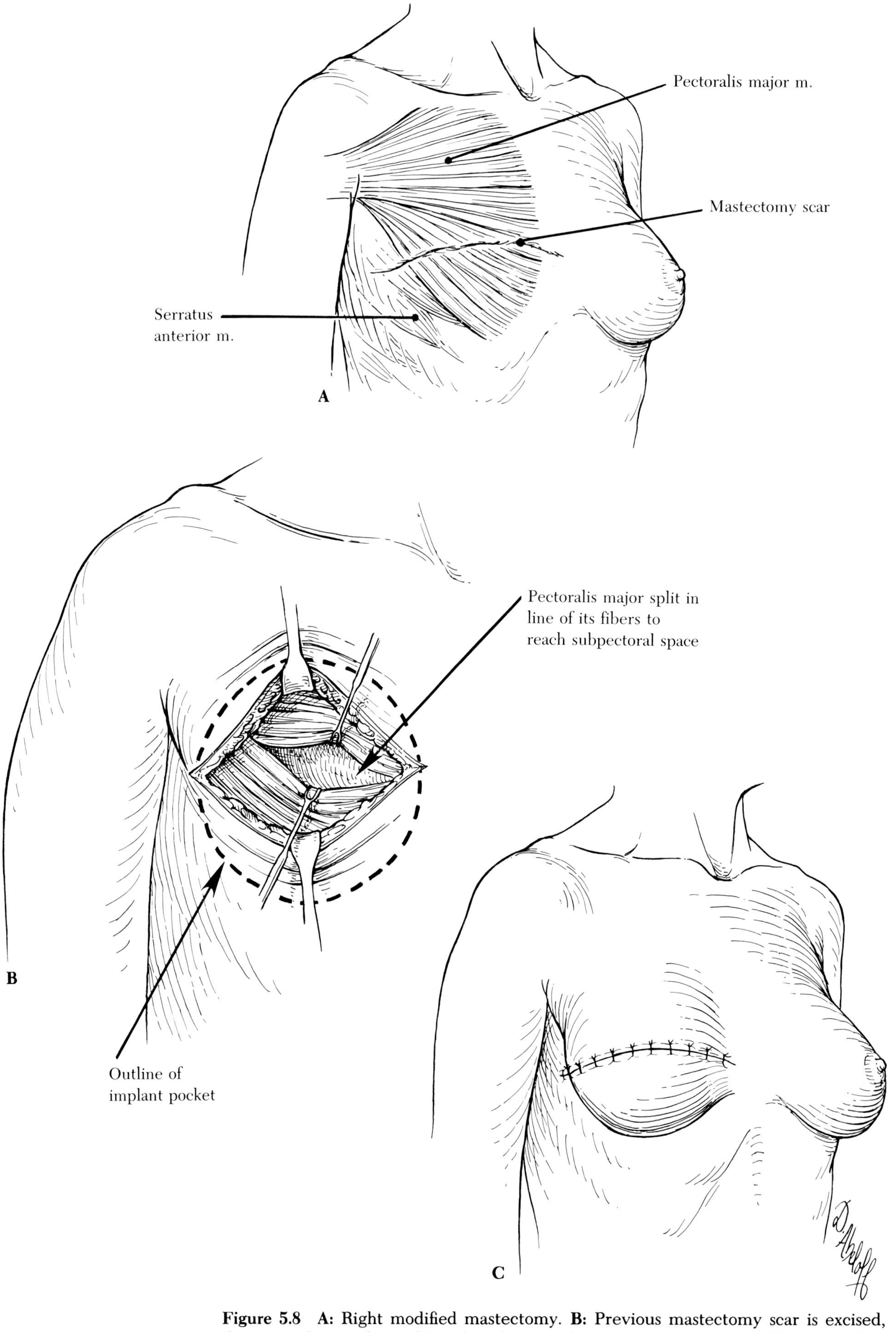

Figure 5.8 **A:** Right modified mastectomy. **B:** Previous mastectomy scar is excised, the pectoralis muscle is split, and a subpectoral pocket is developed. **C:** Silicone implant inserted subpectorally.

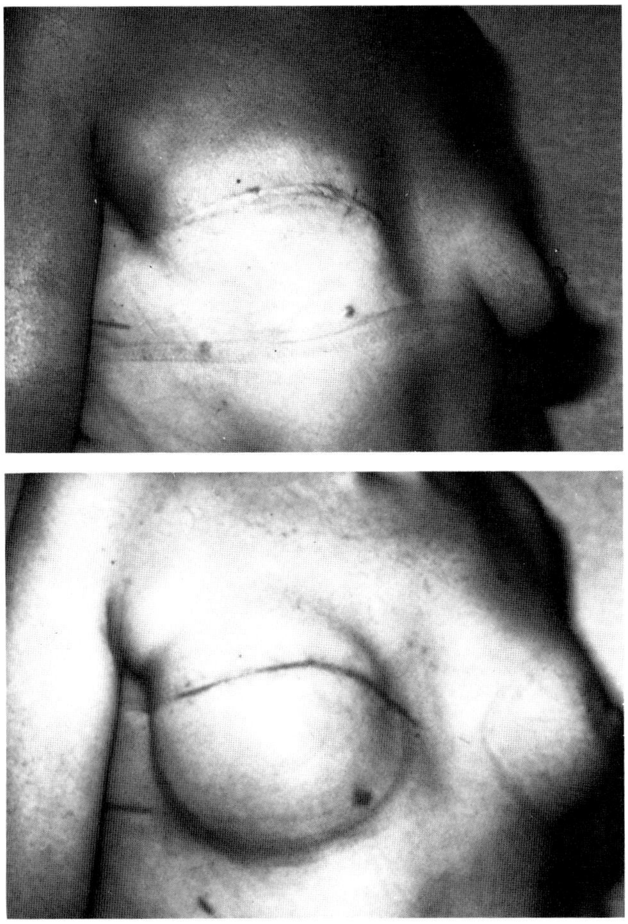

Figure 5.9 **Top:** Right modified radical mastectomy scar with adequate soft tissue and a small ptotic left breast with fibrocystic disease. **Bottom:** Right subpectoral prosthestic implantation after excising the mastectomy scar, producing a satisfactory breast mound but little evidence of an inframammary crease. A subcutaneous mastectomy was performed on the left breast with subpectoral implantation.

splitting the pectoralis muscle in the direction of its fibers a submuscular pocket (subpectoral and subserratus) can be developed (Figures 5.8 and 5.9). An adequate-sized prosthesis can be inserted, producing a satisfactory breast mound, although the inframammary fold is difficult to establish, and usually little ptosis can be obtained (1,11,15,17,22,29). However, Birnbaum has produced excellent results using a custom-designed compartmented prosthesis (3). If local tissue is available but scant, subcutaneous reconstruction using a temporary expander may be performed. This method is described by Radovan (20) in Chapter 6. A third method which gives a well-defined inframammary fold is the lower thoracic advancement flap, described by Ryan in Chapter 7.

Flap Techniques

If local factors are unfavorable—with thin tight skin flaps, little subcutaneous fat, adherent scars, and absent or atrophied pectoralis muscle—flap techniques are suitable. Three methods of flap reconstruction are currently utilized: the thoracoepigastric cutaneous flap, the latissimus dorsi musculocutaneous flap (Chapter 8), and the various rectus flaps (Chapter 9), which are combinations of random cutaneous and musculocutaneous flaps.

The thoracoepigastric flap is very useful for introducing additional skin where needed. Cronin et al. popularized this technique and used it to produce spectacular results, as noted in Chapter 2 (Figures 2.10–2.12) (4). However, it is of limited use in correcting a radical mastectomy infraclavicular defect and an absent anterior axillary fold.

A second method, the latissimus dorsi musculocutaneous flap, is extremely versatile and can be used in any situation, except when a posterior thoracotomy scar is present on the same side as the mastectomy or when the patient objects to a scar on her back. A functioning latissimus dorsi muscle is preferable. The thoracodorsal artery and nerve are in close proximity, and a functioning muscle suggests that the artery is intact and has not been interfered with

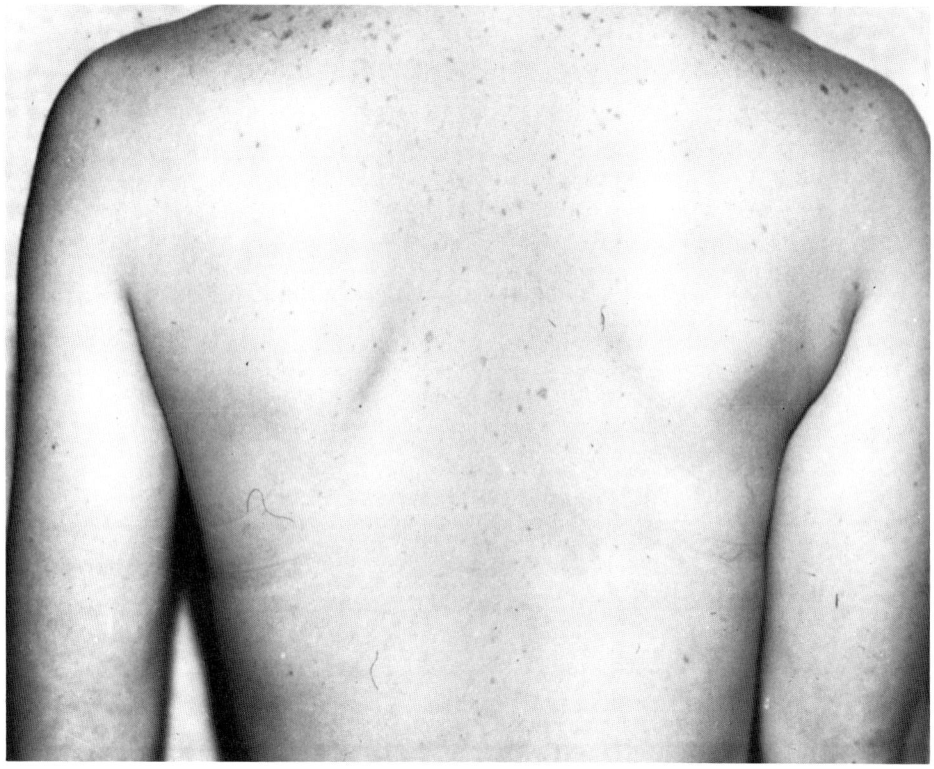

Figure 5.10 Patient standing erect with arms by her side. Note the depression caused by an atrophic latissimus dorsi muscle. Review of the mastectomy operative record confirmed that the thoracodorsal nerve had been transected.

by the mastectomy procedure. However, studies by Maxwell et al. show that the latissimus dorsi musculocutaneous flap can be mobilized even if the thoracodorsal artery has been ligated (16). The absence of an active latissimus dorsi muscle is suggested by a depression in the anatomic area (Figure 5.10). In this situation angiographic studies to determine if the thoracodorsal artery is patent may be indicated (21).

A third method, using the rectus muscle, involves three distinct techniques, as described in Chapter 9. These all rely on the presence of a patent superior epigastric artery; therefore upper abdominal scars, which may indicate a transected artery, should be noted. The rectus flaps have the advantage of avoiding a scar on the back; moreover, a silicone prosthesis is often not necessary. The main disadvantages of these techniques are a long abdominal scar and the potential weakness for hernia.

In summary the selection of the method of reconstruction depends on the availability of local tissue (Figure 5.11).

Oncology Evaluation

Arrangements are made for the patient to have an oncology evaluation. This should include a mammogram of the contralateral breast, an alkaline phosphatase assay, a bone scan, and a liver scan when necessary.

Counseling

Patients are advised at the first consultation that it is often helpful to speak to others who have already undergone the operation (2,19). This can be arranged through counseling groups, e.g., A.W.E.A.R. (A Woman Educating About Reconstruction) and A.F.T.E.R. (Ask a Friend to Explain Reconstruction), or with individual patients. In some regions the American Cancer Society is using reconstructed patients as its volunteers.

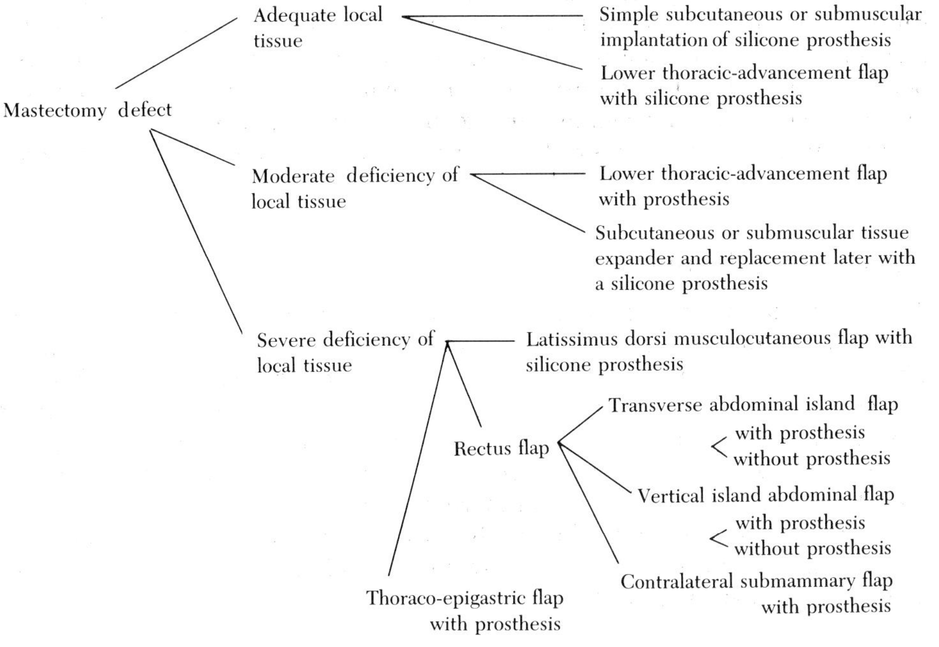

Figure 5.11 Selection of the method of reconstruction depends on the availability of local tissue.

At the end of the first consultation, the patient is given appropriate literature to take home and peruse. The pamphlet *Breast Reconstruction Following Carcinoma* produced by the American Society of Plastic and Reconstructive Surgeons is very suitable.

Financial Planning

The patient is advised of the approximate cost of the operation at the first meeting. Although most insurance companies recognize that breast reconstruction is not a cosmetic procedure, it is wise for preauthorization to be obtained in writing before surgery is scheduled (6).

Second Consultation

The second consultation is held some weeks after the first meeting. During the interim the patient has had time to digest the information she received at the first meeting and to contact a counseling group if she desired to do so. The surgeon has by now received the results of the patient's tests and oncology evaluation and has hopefully had an opportunity to confer with the patient's primary surgeon regarding the proposed reconstruction.

At the second meeting all the relevant information is reviewed. Questions are encouraged and answered, hopefully allaying fears and apprehensions and clearing up areas of misunderstanding. The oncology studies and mammograms are explained, and reference is made to the mastectomy operative note and the pathology report.

A further examination of the chest wall deformity is performed to reevaluate the mobility of the scar, the laxity and thickness of the surrounding skin and subcutaneous tissue, and the presence or absence of a functioning pectoralis major muscle.

If the patient is considered eligible for breast reconstruction, a decision must be made about the kind of procedure to be performed (Figure 5.11), when it should be scheduled, and if the surgery should include any operation on the contralateral breast (10,13). Surgeons differ in their views regarding the optimum time for reconstruction. Some advocate immediate reconstruction, whereas others prefer waiting some months (12,18). Because local recurrences have been seen to develop most often within the first 6–9 months following mastectomy, it is recommended that this period of time should elapse before definite plans for reconstruction are finalized. The scar and surrounding tissues become soft and mobile during this interval (22). If chemotherapy or irradiation is being considered, a further postponement is recommended (14,26).

Sizing of the Implant

As most reconstructive procedures (except those with certain rectus flaps) involve a silicone gel prosthesis, accurate sizing of the implant is essential. This can be done by various methods at the second consultation after the procedure has been chosen. One way is to measure the external prosthesis the patient is currently using by volumetric displacement. Another is to replace the external prosthesis, usually worn in the brassiere, with a sample size of the silicone gel prosthesis and compare the appearance with the other side when the brassiere is worn. The width of the contralateral breast can be measured, and this also can be a guide to the size of the prosthesis. Sometimes mammometers are helpful (27).

Complications

The patient should be given detailed information on the possible complications which may attend her surgery—including skin slough, infection, hematoma or seroma, hypertrophic and keloid scar formation, and widening of the scars. She should also be warned that it is difficult to get a symmetrical effect after the first operation and that surgical revisions are sometimes necessary to achieve the optimal result (7).

Women are anxious to know the length of time they will be in the hospital and the period of convalesence afterward. If the reconstruction is to be undertaken in two stages—i.e., breast mound reconstruction first and nipple-areola reconstruction second—the time frame regarding both operations and periods of recovery should be decided. This depends on the types of procedure involved and if surgery of the contralateral breast is indicated (Chapter 10).

References

1. Apfelberg DB, Laub DR, Maser MR, et al, 1981: Submuscular breast reconstruction—indications and techniques. Ann Plast Surg 7:213–221.
2. Berkowitch S, 1980: Psychological results of reconstructed patients. Acta Chir Belg 79(2):165–167.
3. Birnbaum L, 1981: Breast reconstruction utilizing custom implants. In: Post-Mastectomy Reconstruction, edited by TD Gant, LO Vasconez, pp 37–67. Williams & Wilkins, Baltimore.
4. Cronin TD, Upton J, McDonough JM, 1977: Reconstruction of the breast after mastectomy. Plast Reconstr Surg 59:1–14.
5. Dowden RV, Horton CE, McGraw JB, 1979: Advising the mastectomy patient about reconstruction. Am Fam Physician 19:103–106.
6. Dowden RV, McGraw JB, Dibbel, DG, 1979: The breast reconstruction patient and her health insurance carrier. JAMA 24:2779–2782.
7. Freeman BS, Wiemer DR, 1979: Untoward results and complications following reconstruction after mastectomy. Clin Plast Surg 6:93–105.
8. Furnival C, 1979: The surgical pathology of breast cancer in relation to reconstruction after mastectomy. Aust NZ J Surg 49:561–564.
9. Gibson EW, 1976: Reconstruction of the breast after mastectomy for cancer. Clin Plast Surg 3:371–378.
10. Goin JM, Kern WH, 1979: Multicentric ductal and lobular atypia and occult carci-

noma in prophylactic subcutaneous mastectomies: a preliminary report. Ann Plast Surg 2:121–127.
11. Gruber RP, et al, 1981: Breast reconstruction following mastectomy: a comparison of submuscular and subcutaneous techniques. Plast Reconstr Surg 67:312–317.
12. Horton CE, et al, 1979: Immediate reconstruction following mastectomy for cancer. Clin Plast Surg 6(1):37–46.
13. Lejour M, Gregoire JP, 1979: The management of the remaining breast in reconstruction. Acta Chir Belg 79(2):145–146.
14. Logan H, 1980: The insertion of prostheses at mastectomy for carcinoma of the breast: a preliminary report. 67(1):69–70.
15. Lynch JB, Madden JJ Jr, Franklin JD, 1978: Breast reconstruction following mastectomy for cancer. Ann Surg 187(5):490–501.
16. Maxwell GP, McGibbon BM, Hoopes JE, 1979: Vascular considerations in the use of the latissimus dorsi myocutaneous flap after mastectomy with an axillary dissection. Plast Reconstr Surg 64(6):771–780.
17. McShane RH, Omotunde O, Weatherly-White RCA, 1981: Individualized muscle coverage of implants in breast reconstruction. Plast Reconstr Surg 67:318–327.
18. Pennisi VR, 1979: Timing of breast reconstruction after mastectomy. Clin Plast Surg 6(1):31–36.
19. Pettavel J, Maillard GF, Wuliemier F, et al, 1980: Surgery and psychology of breast reconstruction after mastectomy for cancer. Acta Chir Belg 79(2):161–164.
20. Radovan C, 1982: Breast reconstruction after mastectomy using the temporary expander. Plast Reconstr Surg 69(2):195–206.
21. Rubinstein J, Shafter R, Tsur H, 1979: The value of angiography prior to the use of the latissimus dorsi musculocutaneous flap. Plast Reconstr Surg 63:374.
22. Ruetschi MS, Jovachev D, Kinne DW, et al, 1980: Breast reconstruction after mastectomy. I. Reconstruction with no additional skin or muscle flaps. Clin Bull 10:53–61.
23. Scheflan MD, Dinner M, Dowden RV, et al, 1982: Advances in breast reconstruction following mastectomy. Contemp Surg 21:49–60.
24. Snyderman RK, 1976: On breast reconstruction after cancer (editorial). Plast Reconstr Surg 57(2):224–226.
25. Snyderman RK, 1980: Alternatives in reconstructive surgery after mastectomy. Cancer (Suppl) 46:1053–1058.
26. Stabile RJ, Santoro E, Dispaltro F, et al, 1980: Reconstructive breast surgery following mastectomy and adjunctive radiation therapy. Cancer 45(11):2738–2743.
27. Tegtmier RE, 1978: A quick, accurate mammometer. Ann Plast Surg 1(6):625–626.
28. Wolf LE, Biggs TM, 1979: Breast reconstruction after mastectomy. Am J Surg 138(6):777–782.
29. Woods JE, Irons GB Jr, Arnold PG, 1980: The case for submuscular implantation of prosthesis in reconstructive breast surgery. Ann Plast Surg 5:115–122.

6

Breast Reconstruction Using the Temporary Expander

Chedomir Radovan

Breast reconstruction using the temporary expander involves a procedure which makes use of the ability of the chest skin to be expanded in order to recover skin lost during radical mastectomy. The postmastectomy chest skin with its scar is intermittently and gradually expanded, providing the skin envelope needed for the new breast. Various postmastectomy deformities may be reconstructed by this technique, but it is especially applicable to the defect that occurs after a modified radical mastectomy.

The reconstruction is performed under local or general anesthesia, and patients are advised to maintain their normal physical activities during the expansion process. A temporary expander is initially inserted, and chest expansion is achieved by a series of injections beginning with 100–150 cc of normal saline, increasing this by 50 cc at each office visit. Injections are administered at 3- to 5-day intervals over a 3- to 4-week period. The average breast is expanded up to 600 cc. The temporary expander is then replaced by a mammary prosthesis of slighter size, creating a smaller breast mound within the larger skin envelope. This has the appearance of a natural breast with a forward teardrop projection (1–4). The procedure is attractive to patients even though it is performed in two stages, because neither stage involves a major surgical operation.

Stage I

A small (5 cm) subaxillary incision is made either through the lateral tail of the old mastectomy scar or through a new oblique incision. The inferior level of the pocket is placed on the same line as the inframammary crease of the opposite breast. When the inframammary crease is formed and the skin is expanded to a large envelope, the breast is given a natural fold when the implant is finally placed in the pocket (Figure 6.1A).

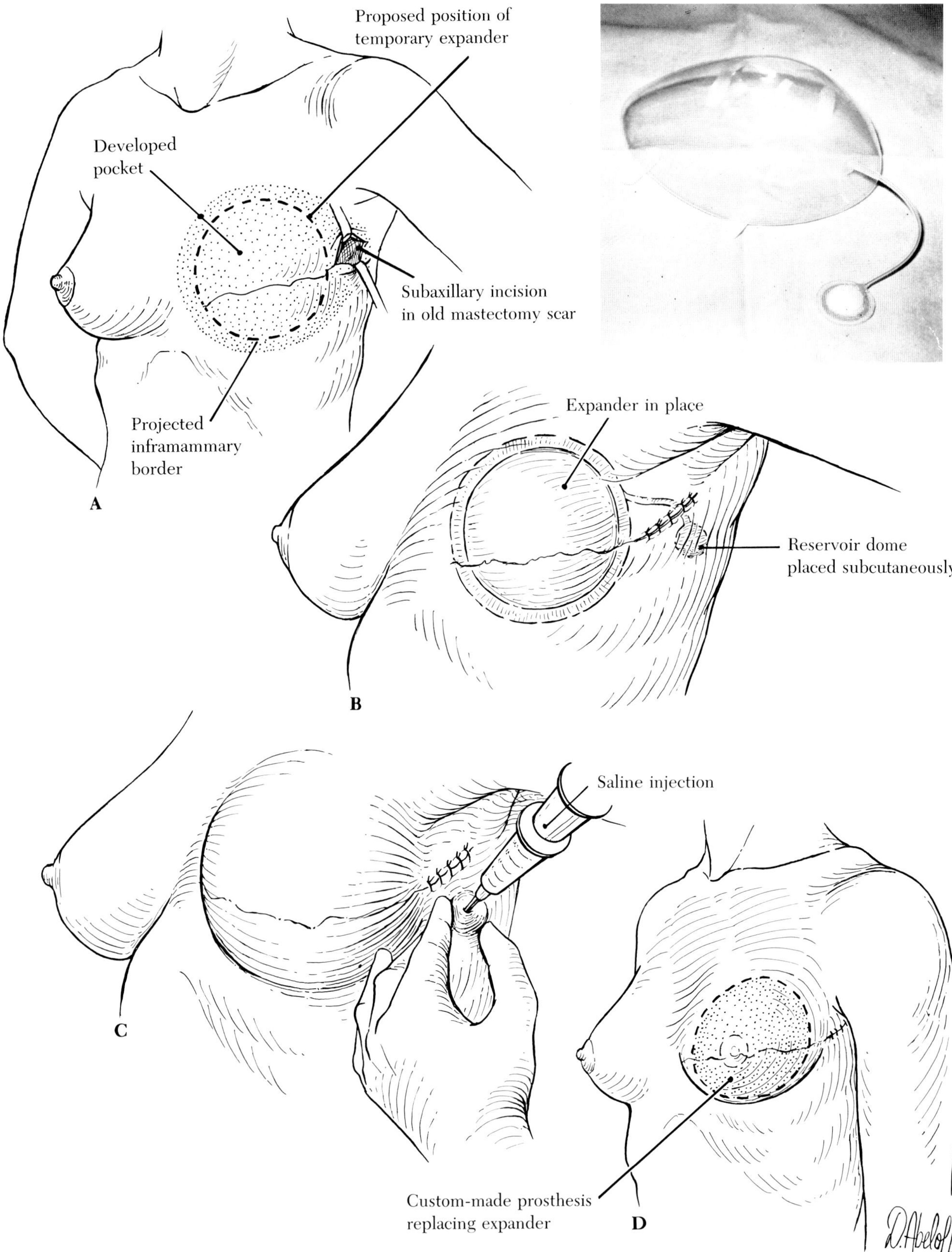

Figure 6.1 Steps of the operative technique. **A:** A subcutaneous pocket is developed through a small subaxillary incision. The inferior level of the pocket is on the same horizontal line as the opposite inframammary crease. **B:** The temporary expander is in place, containing 50–100 cc of normal saline. The subcutaneous tissue space between the reservoir and the expander is closed with sutures. **C:** The subcutaneous reservoir is grasped between the index finger and thumb. Using syringe and a No. 22 or 25 needle, the skin and the dome of the reservoir are pierced. After the needle makes contact with the metal base, it should be retracted 1–2 mm before the normal saline is injected. **D:** After 3–4 weeks the pocket has been expanded more than the desired size of the implant. The saline is withdrawn by syringe, and the expander is removed through the same subaxillary incision. A smaller silicone gel prosthesis of the desired size is then inserted.

The pocket is developed by blunt-scissor or finger dissection and is preferably about 3 cm wider in circumference than the base of the expander. A small subcutaneous pocket is developed posterior to the incision for placement of the reservoir dome (Figure 6.1B).

Initially, the expander is filled with 100 to 150 cc of normal saline through the connecting tube. The tube should be shortened to the appropriate length and the expander then attached to the reservoir dome. The subcutaneous tissue between the expander and the reservoir is approximated with sutures to prevent sliding of the reservoir toward the expander.

Further normal saline injections of approximately 50 cc, or less if the skin becomes tight, are administered in the office at a minimum of 3-day intervals. The patient experiences only minor discomfort. The reservoir dome is palpated and then held between the fingers while a No. 22 or 25 needle is inserted through the skin and into the dome (Figure 6.1C).

Stage II

The expander and the reservoir are removed through the same subaxillary approach. The amount of normal saline in the expander is calculated, and a smaller implant is replaced in the pocket, allowing mobility and flexibility of the reconstructed breast. The incision is then closed in layers (Figure 6.1D). Clinical examples are shown in Figures 6.2–6.5.

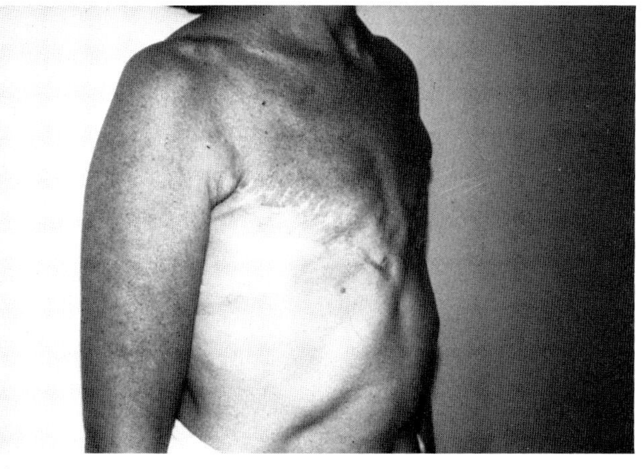

A

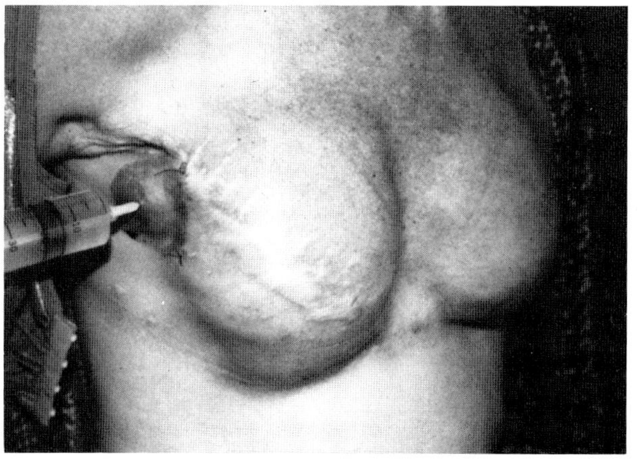

B

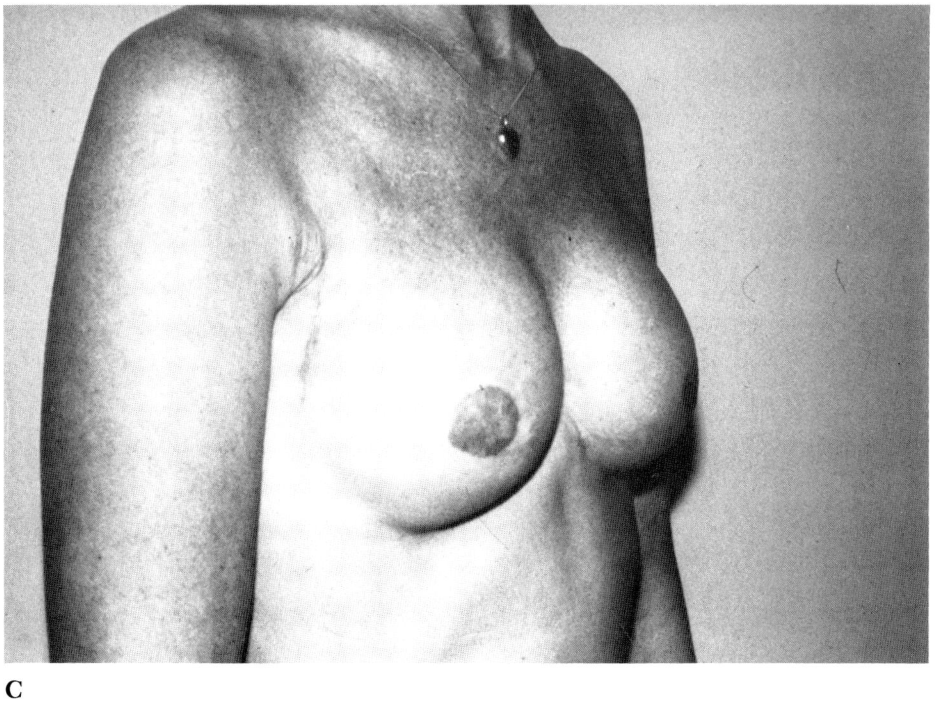

C

Figure 6.2 **A:** A 42-year-old woman 1 year after a bilateral modified radical mastectomy. At the initial insertion of the expanders, extremely tight chest skin would allow only 100 cc of normal saline in each expander. **B:** Expanders were injected to a total of 600 cc and were then replaced with 450-cc mammary implants. **C:** Labial grafts were used for nipple reconstruction. The degree of natural folding of the breast at the inframammary line was very satisfactory.

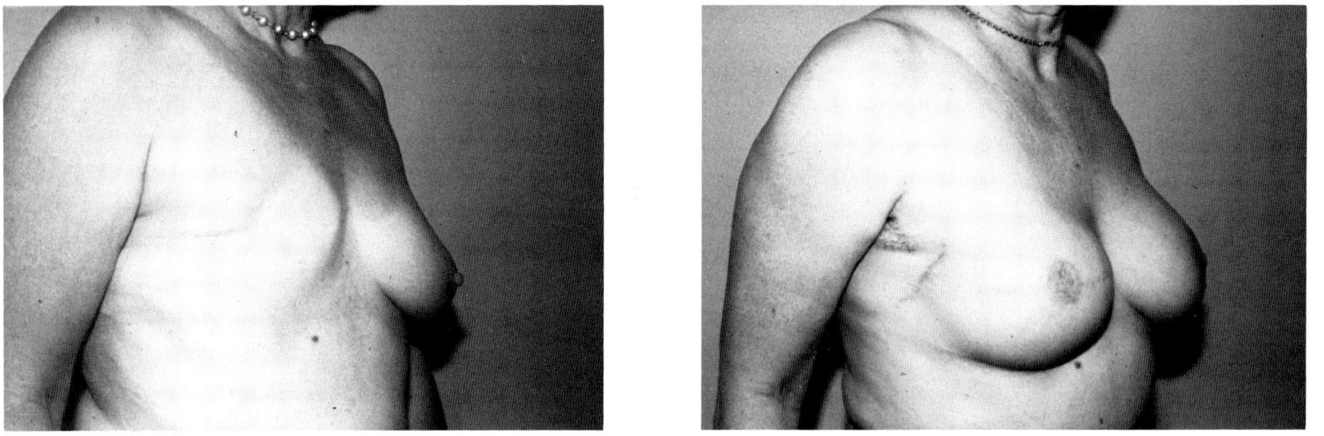

A B

Figure 6.3 **A:** A 45-year-old woman 2 years after modified radical mastectomy of the right breast. **B:** The chest skin was expanded up to 650 cc and the expander then replaced with a 450-cc mammary implant. Left breast round dermal mastopexy was performed combined with augmentation by a 200-cc mammary implant. Right nipple reconstruction was performed using the outer ring of the left areola.

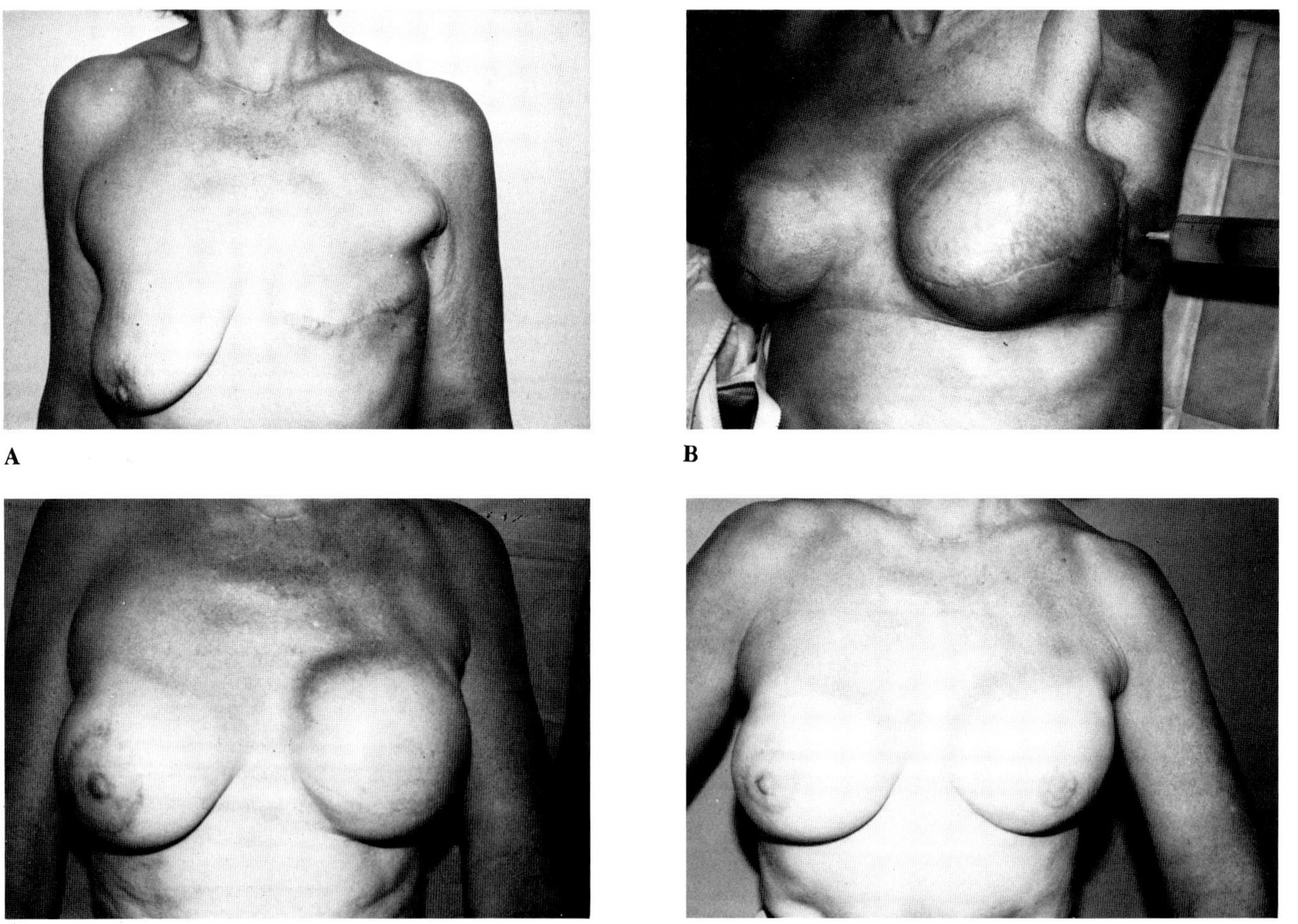

A B

C D

Figure 6.4 **A:** This 62-year-old patient with very tight chest skin was started with only 100 cc of normal saline in the expander 4 months after left modified radical mastectomy. **B:** The left breast was gradually expanded to 650 cc. **C:** Right subcutaneous mastectomy was performed through the round dermal mastopexy, and a nipple enlargement procedure was done with immediate reconstruction using a 450-cc implant. **D:** The left temporary expander with 650 cc was replaced with a 450-cc implant, and the nipple-areola was reconstructed with the outer ring of the initially enlarged right areola.

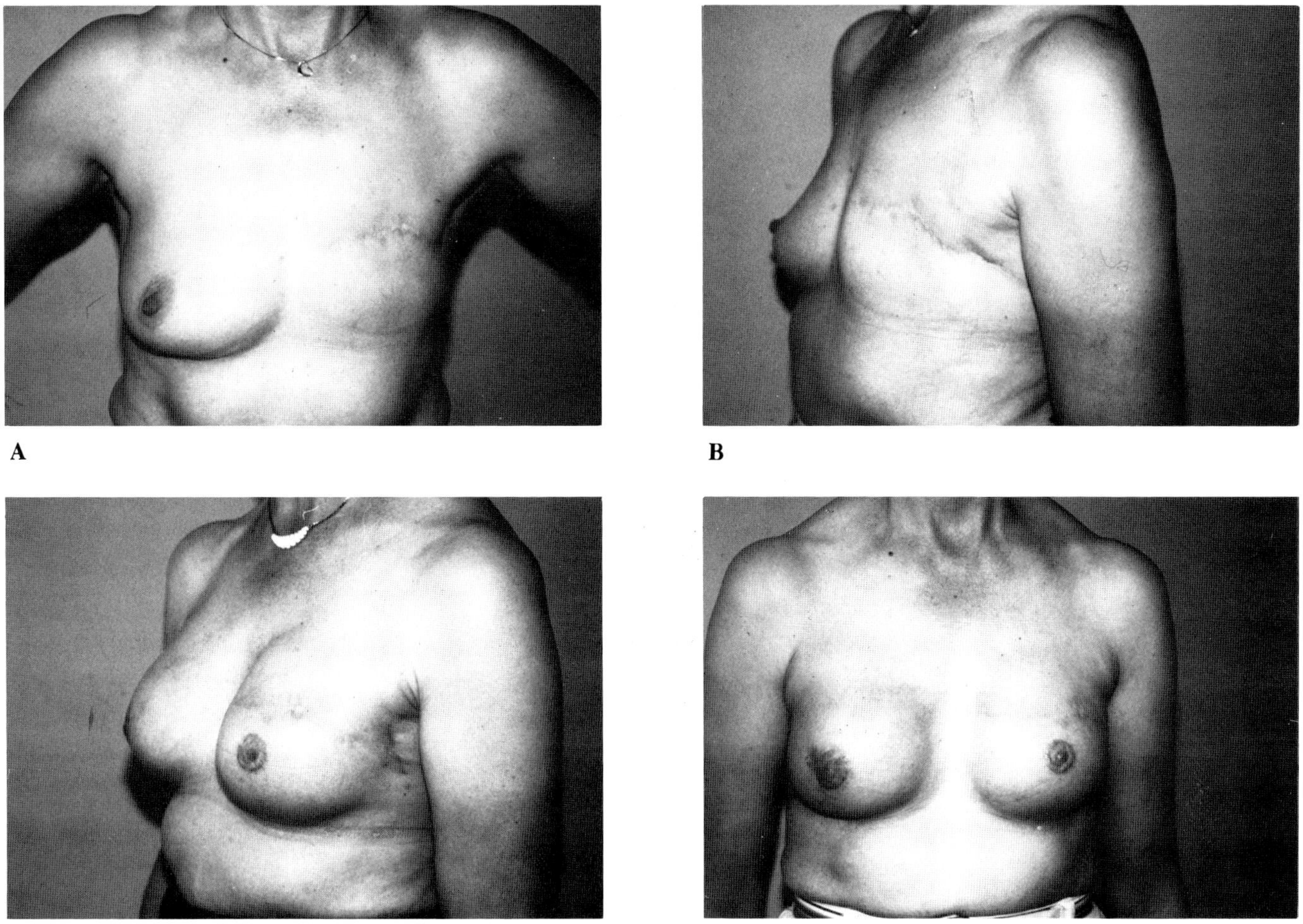

A B C D

Figure 6.5 **A, B:** This is a 52 year-old woman with a left modified radical mastectomy. **C:** After expanding the chest skin up to 650 cc, the temporary expander was replaced with a 400-cc mammary implant. **D:** Right breast subcutaneous mastectomy was performed through a round dermal mastopexy, and a nipple enlargement procedure was done with immediate reconstruction using a 400-cc mammary implant. The right nipple was shared for reconstruction of the left nipple.

Postoperative Complications

Hematoma

If a hematoma occurs, the expander should be removed, the hematoma evacuated, and hemostasis established.

Infection

Infection should be treated with antibiotics and drainage. It may be necessary to remove the expander and reinsert it at a later date.

Necrosis

The ability of the expander to be deflated when necrosis is pending has proved to be a great advantage in reconstruction.

Capsular Contracture

The fact that the initial pocket is 150 to 200 cc larger than the size of the permanent implant seems to reduce the incidence of contracture in breasts reconstructed by the temporary expander method.

EDITORS NOTE: Successful results have been obtained with the temporary expander being used beneath the pectoralis and serratus muscle.

Comment

Breast reconstruction cannot be considered successful unless acceptable symmetry with the opposite breast is achieved. Use of the expander facilitates reconstruction of large breasts, thereby usually avoiding the necessity for reduction of the good opposite breast.

References

1. Radovan C, 1978: Reconstruction of the breast after radical mastectomy using temporary expander. ASPRS Plast Surg Forum 1:41.
2. Radovan C, 1979: Development of adjacent flaps using a temporary expander. ASPRS Plast Surg Forum 2:62.
3. Radovan C, 1980: Advantages and complications of breast reconstruction using temporary expander. ASPRS Plast Surg Forum 3:63.
4. Radovan C, 1982: Breast reconstruction after mastectomy using the temporary expander. Plast Reconstr Surg 69:195–206.

7

Lower Thoracic Advancement Flap

James J. Ryan

Patients who have undergone modified or radical mastectomy have a loss of prethoracic skin. In some women this may prohibit placement and proper shaping of an implant equal in size to the remaining breast, but it may not be so great as to necessitate the use of a myocutaneous flap. Reconstruction of the breast using the lower thoracic advancement flap is the procedure of choice under these circumstances and/or when the patient objects to the donor site scar of the latissimus flap or to the various rectus flaps. It is a modification of the sliding flap from the abdomen of Lewis (1) (Figure 7.1). It allows an increase of some 2–5 cm in the central portion of the skin covering the implant, and it establishes a firm, fixed, well-defined inframammary fold (4).

It is very important for the surgeon to carefully study the body habitus and mobility of the lower lateral thoracic skin in patients considered for this technique (3). In general, the most suitable candidates for this operation are women with loose skin on a broad, rather than long torso because these conditions facilitate recruitment and movement of the skin. In contrast, the very tall, thin, tight-skinned individual seldom has enough excess skin for recruitment skin in this manner. This technique is recommended when the transverse diameter of the remaining breast is less than 18 cm, when there is a need for moderate skin enhancement (up to 5 cm at the most), and when the initial implant measures less than 450 cc. Secondary planned implant expansion of up to 725 cc may be successfully carried out at a later date.

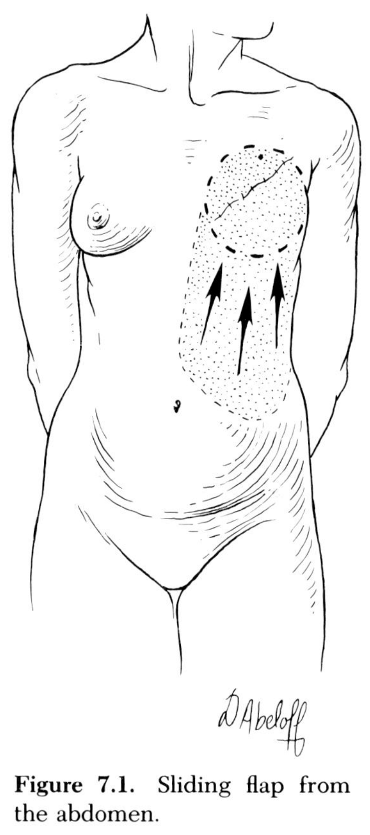

Figure 7.1. Sliding flap from the abdomen.

Operative Technique

The actual drawing and measurement of the breast to be reconstructed is carried out with the patient in a sitting position. The patient places her external prosthesis and brassiere in a comfortable position, and the outline of the margins of the external prosthesis is marked on the skin as well as the inferior extension of the brassiere at the line of maximal pressure (Figure 7.2A). This

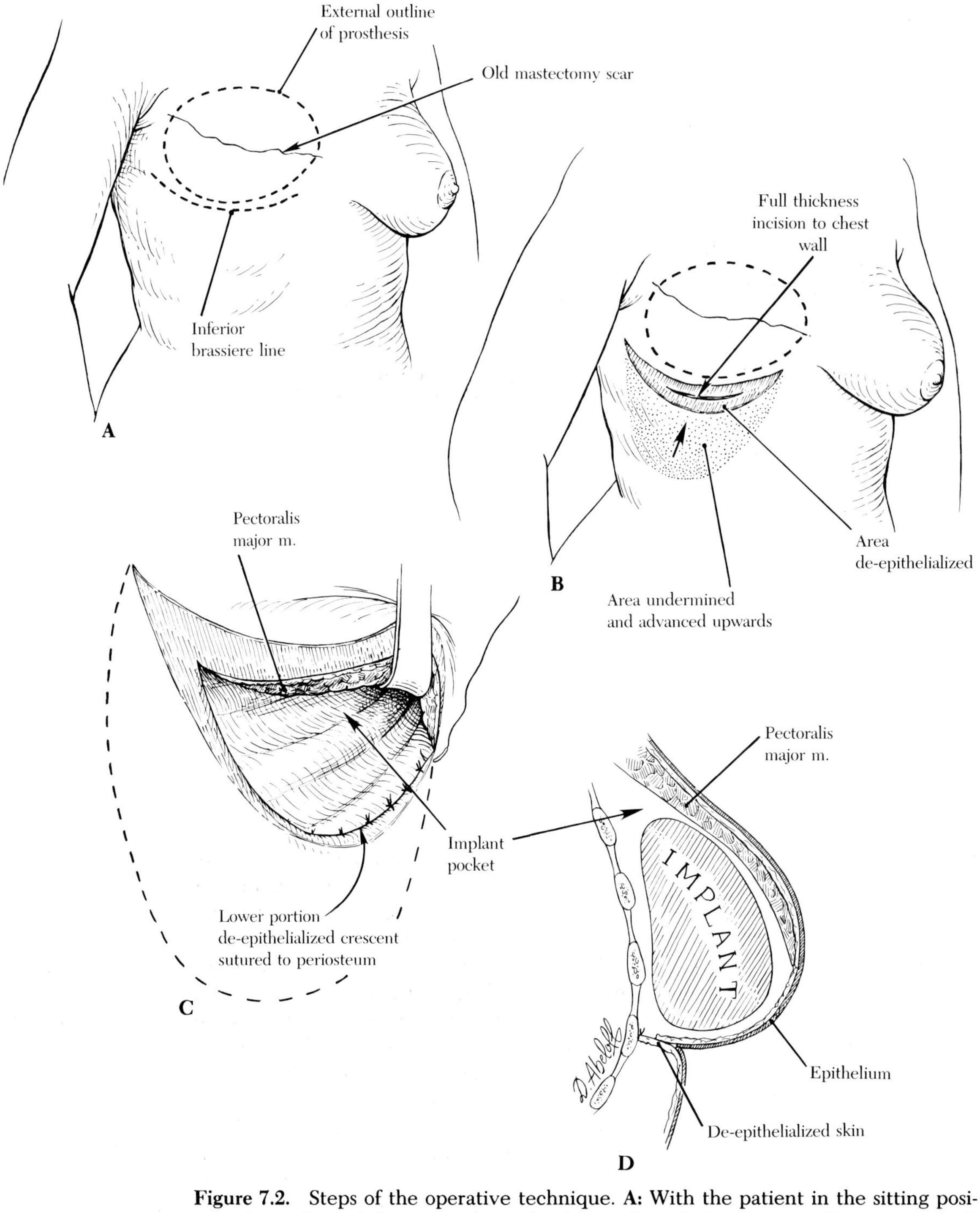

Figure 7.2. Steps of the operative technique. **A:** With the patient in the sitting position, the outline of the external prosthesis and the inferior brassiere line are marked. **B:** Note the crescentic area to be deepithelialized, the full-thickness incision, and the inferior flap to be undermined. **C:** The advanced inferior flap with its deepithelialized edge is sutured to the chest wall and rib cage. **D:** The implant is inserted, and the edge of the deepithelialized superior flap is sutured to the inferior flap.

is compared to the inframammary fold of the opposite breast. Below this a line is drawn forming a crescent, lowered 2–5 cm at its widest mid-point. The medial extent of this crescent is at a point level with the medial limit of the inframammary fold on the opposite breast. This allows the development of a good shape following insertion of the largest implant that can be accommodated by the initial pocket. Over a period of several months, with relaxation and stretching of skin, the implant can be replaced by a larger one if desired. The crescentic area is deepithelialized. Thus the deepithelialized crescent is approximately 1 cm in its central width and narrows toward each end (Figure 7.2B). An area of inferior undermining is frequently marked below the crescent. The inframammary fold on the opposite breast is marked at the presternal and xiphoid level, on the lateral thorax, and on the arm to provide reference points when the patient is reclining. The volume of the external prosthesis worn to give symmetry is usually determined by volumetric displacement, and its transverse dimension also serves to correlate the implant volume selected.

The crescent area is deepithelialized. A full-thickness skin incision 7–8 cm long is made approximately half way between the upper and lower borders of the crescent and is carried down on the chest wall to the preserratus fascial plane. If the full-thickness incision is too long, there is a danger of devitalizing an area of tissue between it and the mastectomy scar. Dissection then continues superiorly to the edge of the pectoralis muscle where the retropectoral plane is entered. The lower costal origins of the pectoralis major are carefully detached, and a pocket of maximal volume is created which does not extend laterally beyond the anterior axillary line. Prior to final implant placement, the inferior edge of the deepithelialized pocket is elevated and dissection carried inferiorly (usually 12–15 cm) external to the muscle layer. This is sufficient to allow advancement of the midportion of the flap to the level of the inframammary fold. The inferior deepithelialized edge of the flap is then affixed to the perichondrium and periosteum of the rib and the intercostal tissues with a large-caliber (i.e., 2–0) absorbable suture (Figure 7.2C). Assistance is required to take tension off the flap until a number of sutures are placed. It is useful to tailor the flap from both ends toward the center in order to prevent "dog ears." These are objectionable when they occur medially and laterally. After the implant is inserted, the edge of the deepithelialized superior flap is affixed to the deepithelialized inferior flap with smaller absorbable sutures and a running intradermal absorbable suture. Occasionally everting nylon completes the closure (2) (Figure 7.2D).

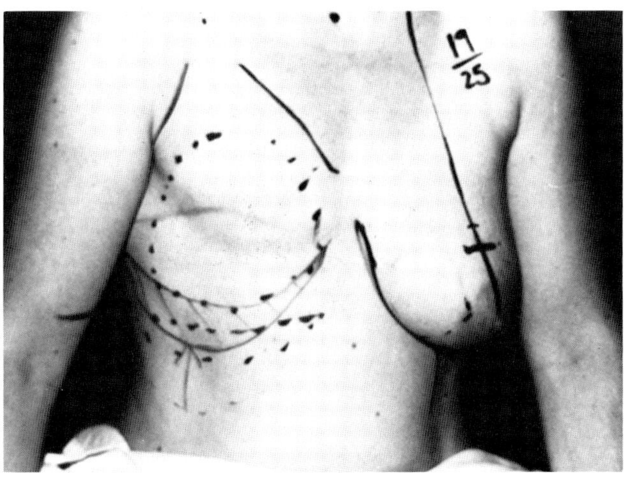

A

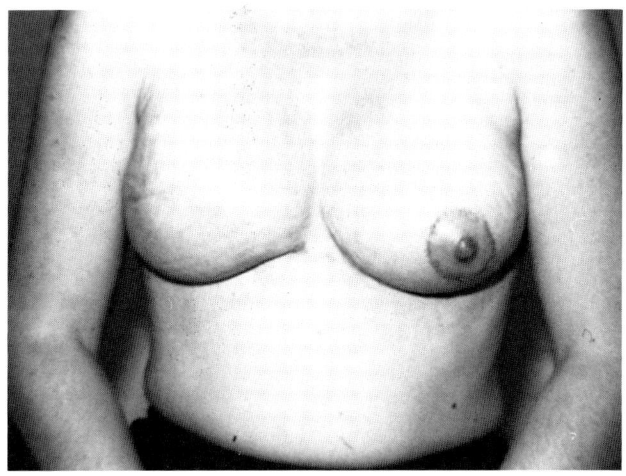

B

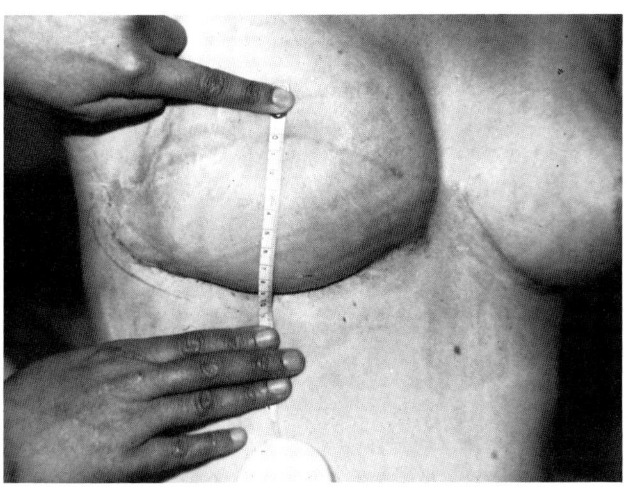

C

Figure 7.3. **A:** This is a 32-year-old woman after a right modified mastectomy. She is marked for reduction of a ptotic left breast and the first stage of reconstruction of the right breast by a lower thoracic flap with buried dermal inframammary fold formation and a right subpectoral implant. **B:** The 3-month postoperative result, before nipple reconstruction. **C:** Note the definition of the inframammary fold and the increased distance from the mastectomy incision to the inframammary fold from the preoperative state.

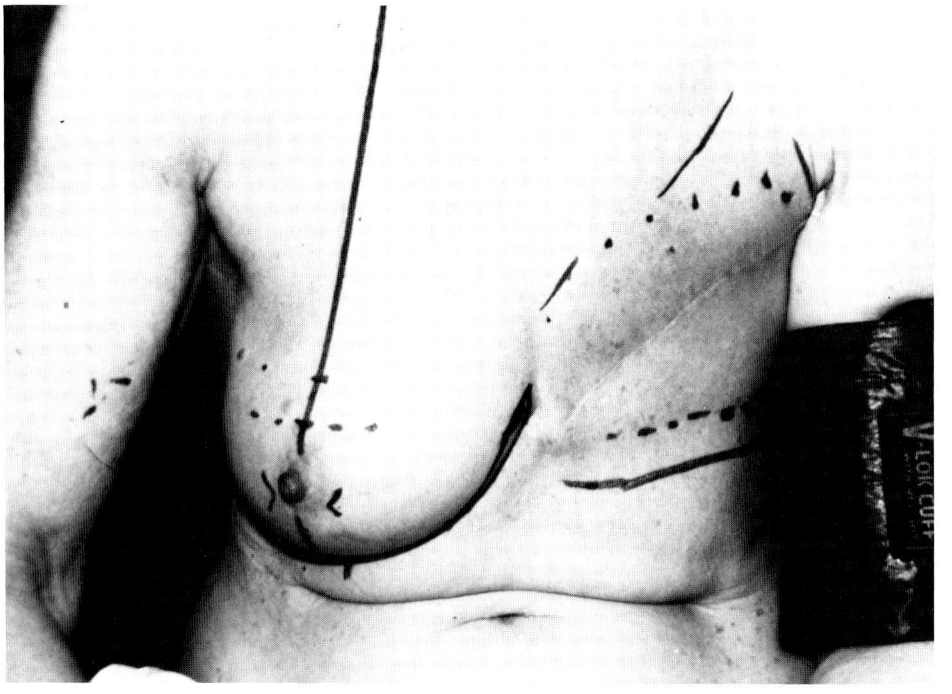

A

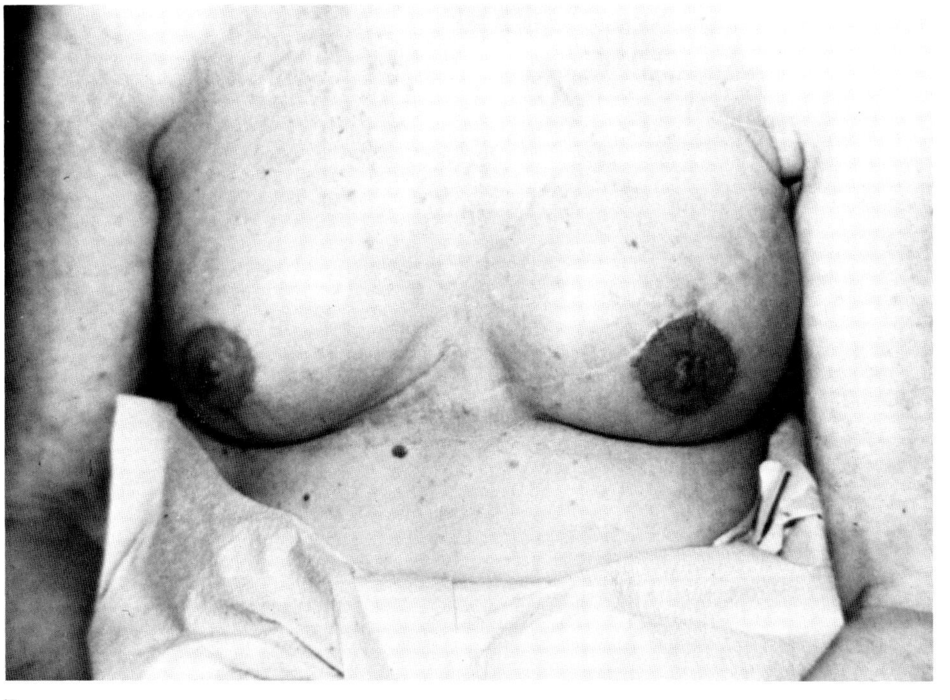

B

Figure 7.4. **A:** Patient after left modified mastectomy and biopsy-proved lobular carcinoma in situ. The left side is marked for the first stage of reconstruction with a lower thoracic advancement flap, buried dermal flap inframammary fold formation, and subpectoral implant placement. The right side is marked for subcutaneous mastectomy with simultaneous nipple areolar transposition and breast skin reduction (a right reduction mammoplasty with extended glandular resection). **B:** Six months after the second-stage procedures of right breast implant and left nipple areolar reconstruction.

Postoperative Complications

No major postoperative complications have been reported with this procedure. Most patients experience discomfort and a feeling of tightness during the first few days, but these complaints subside. Seroma has been a rare occurrence as has hypertrophic scarring.

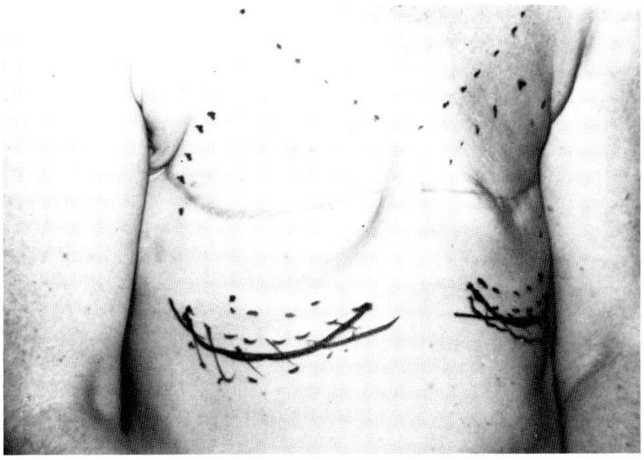

A

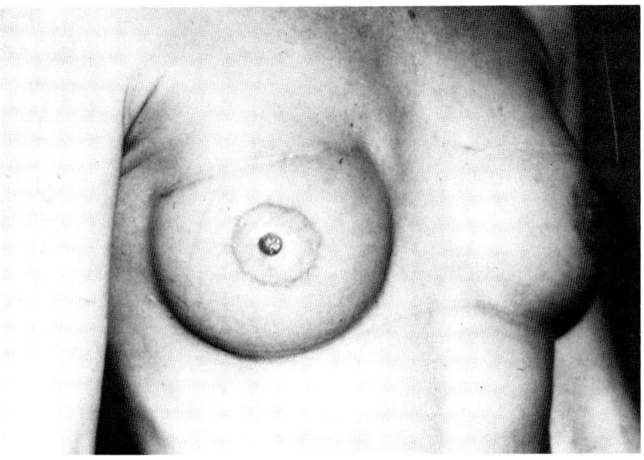

B

Figure 7.5. **A:** Patient having undergone bilateral modified mastectomy. **Top:** With markings for first stage reconstruction by lower thoracic advancement flap and submuscular implant placement. **Bottom:** Results one year later with a second stage nipple-areola reconstruction by thigh graft and labial nipple graft.

Results

Figures 7.3–7.6 illustrate the effectiveness of this operation. Among the great benefits of the technique is the fact that the scar is hidden in the depths of the inframammary fold and is usually fairly inconspicuous (Figure 7.4). A key landmark of the breast, the inframammary fold, is reestablished. The technique increases the prethoracic skin coverage to a moderate degree, but this expands

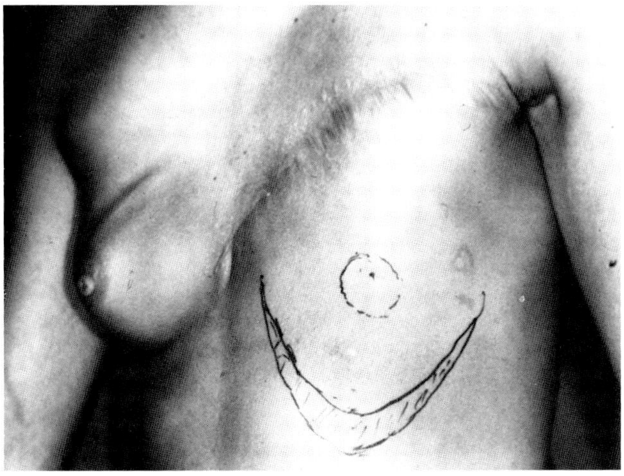

A

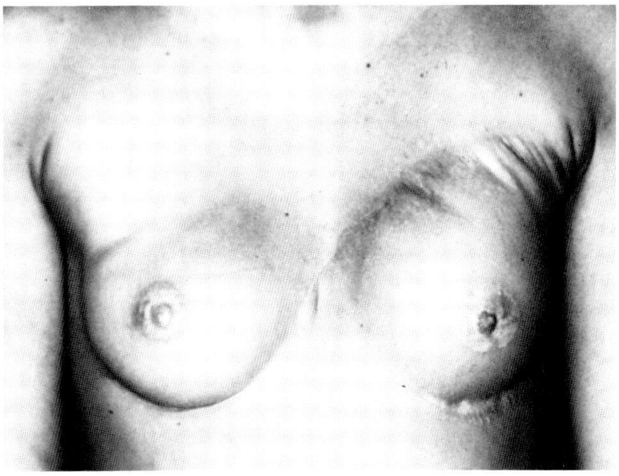

B

Figure 7.6. **A:** Patient following left modified mastectomy with preoperative marking. **B:** Postoperative view of patient. (Photographs in Figures 7.6A,B were kindly supplied by Dr. V. Pennisi, San Francisco.)

postoperatively to nearly 50% above the actual measurement at the time of surgery (Figure 7.3C). Thus the central part which measured 5 cm at the initial planning expands to 9–10 cm within a 6-month interval. This gives an increasingly natural and becoming breast shape. Lastly, the execution is appealingly easy, particularly when bilateral breast surgery has been performed.

References

1. Lewis JR, 1979: Use of a sliding flap from the abdomen to provide cover in breast reconstruction. Plast Reconstr Surg 64:491–497.
2. Pennisi VR, 1979: Making a definite inframammary fold under a reconstructed breast. Plast Reconstr Surg 60:523–525.
3. Ryan JJ, 1981: The planning of breast reconstruction after mastectomy. In: Diagnosis and Treatment of Breast Cancer, edited by EF Lewison, ACW Montague, pp 255–287. Williams & Wilkins, Baltimore.
4. Ryan JJ, 1982: A lower thoracic advancement flap in breast reconstruction after mastectomy. Plast Reconstr Surg 70:153–158.

8

Latissimus Dorsi Musculocutaneous Flap

Bernard M. McGibbon

The adaption of musculocutaneous flaps for use in reconstructive surgery has had a profound impact on the field of breast reconstruction. Procedures are performed today that could not have been considered 10 years ago (8,10,11).

The latissimus dorsi musculocutaneous flap has become the "workhorse" of breast reconstruction and can be used for most mastectomy defects. It is particularly applicable when there is a deficiency of soft tissue coverage of the chest wall, with partial or complete loss of the pectoralis muscle, and a tightness of the mastectomy scar which prevents reconstruction with local tissue alone (1,2,7) (Figure 8.1).

Anatomy

Anatomically, the latissimus dorsi muscle is flat and triangular. It is situated below the scapula, arising posteriorly by tendinous fibers from the lower thoracic spines and the fascia of the upper lumbar spines and by muscle fibers from the iliac crest, inserting into the humerus (Figure 8.3). Its blood supply comes from the thoracodorsal artery, a branch of the subscapular artery, which arises from the subclavian artery. As the thoracodorsal artery descends toward the muscle, it gives off a branch to the serratus anterior muscle. The nerve supply arises from the posterior cord of the brachial plexus and runs closely with the artery.

The shape and position of the latissimus dorsi muscle is almost a "mirror image" of the anteriorly placed pectoralis major muscle. This anatomic similarity permits use of the transposed latissimus dorsi musculocutaneous flap in breast reconstruction following radical mastectomy (Figure 8.2).

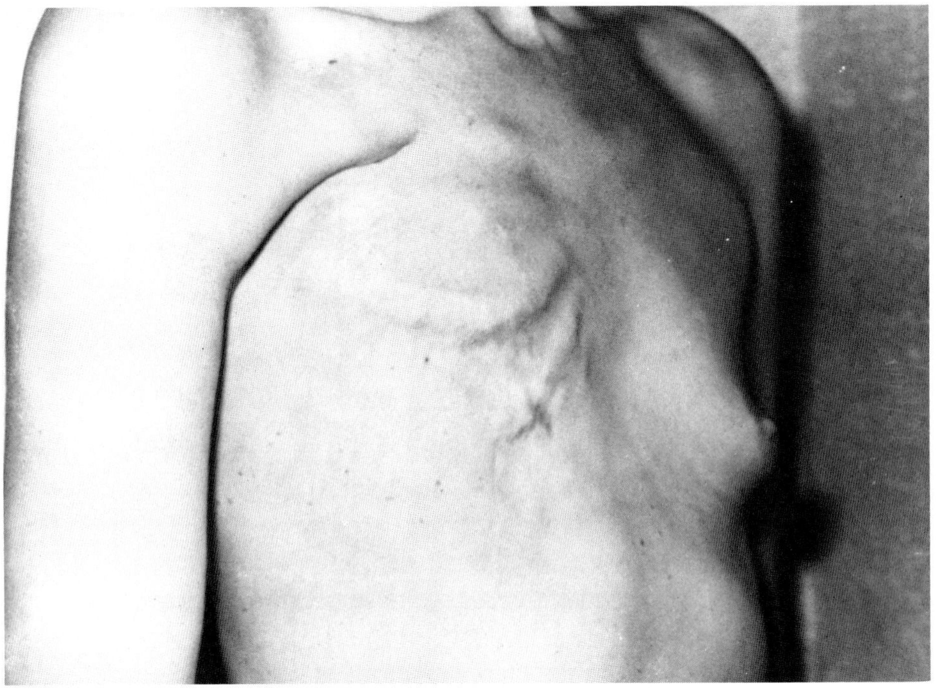

Figure 8.1. Right radical mastectomy defect.

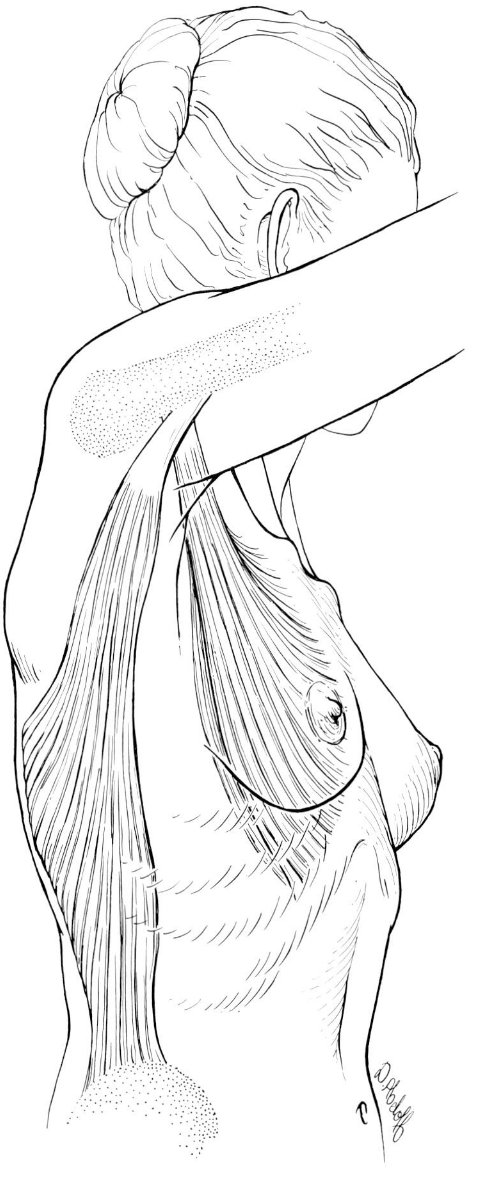

Figure 8.2. The latissimus dorsi muscle posteriorly is almost a "mirror image" of the anteriorly placed pectoralis major muscle.

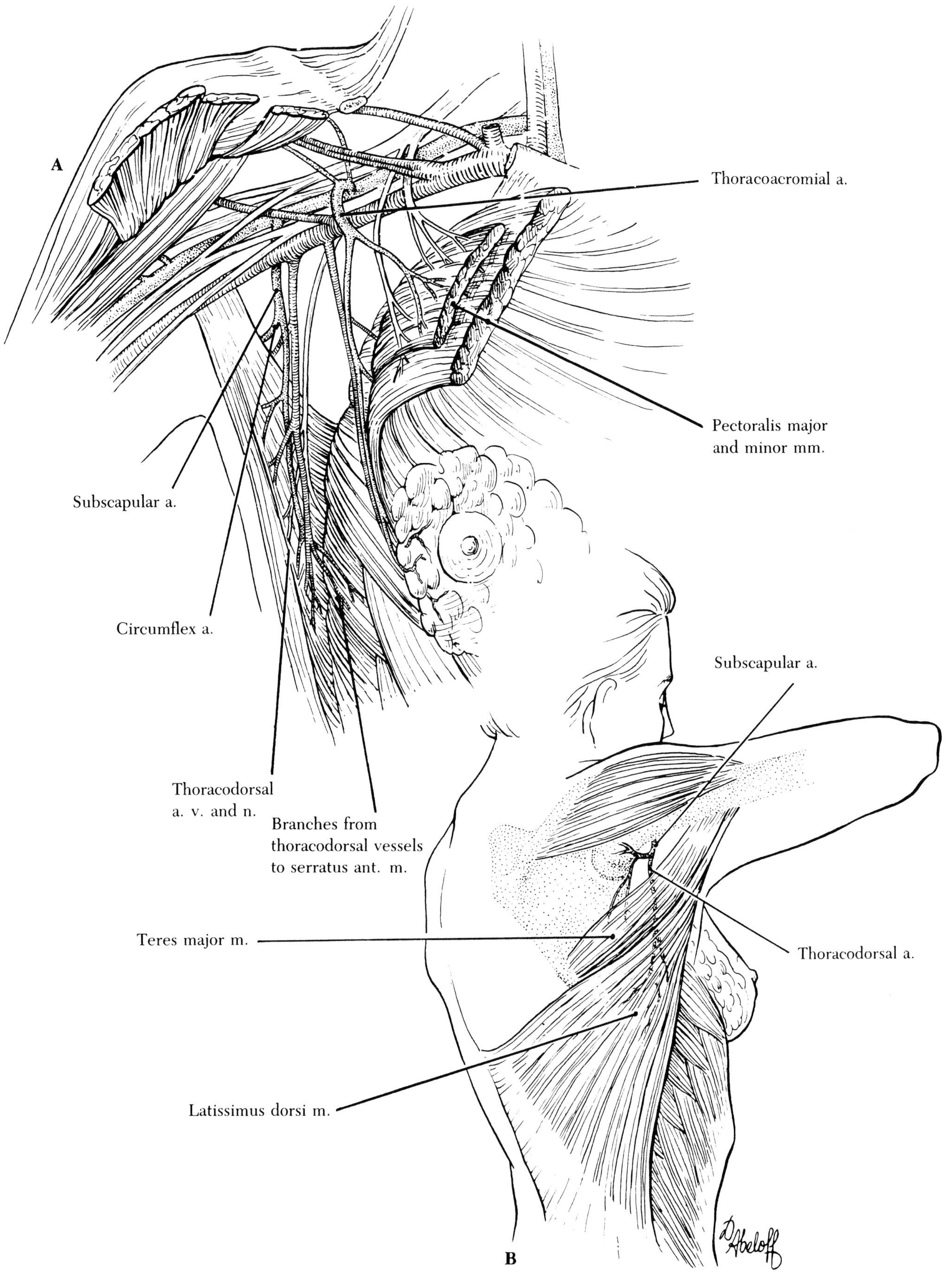

Figure 8.3. Anatomy of the latissimus dorsi muscle.

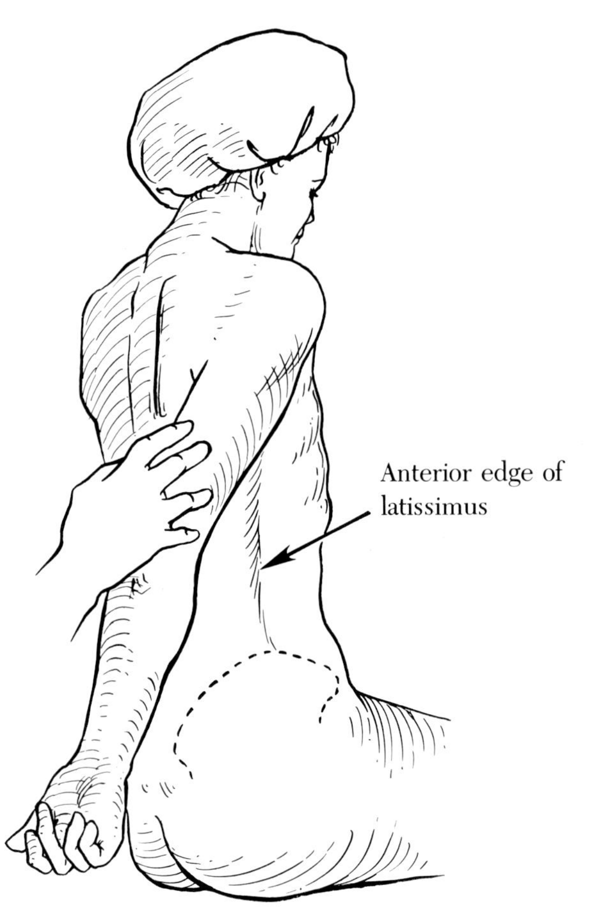

Figure 8.4. If the nerve supply is intact, the anterior edge of the latissimus muscle can be felt when the patient extends her arm backward against resistance.

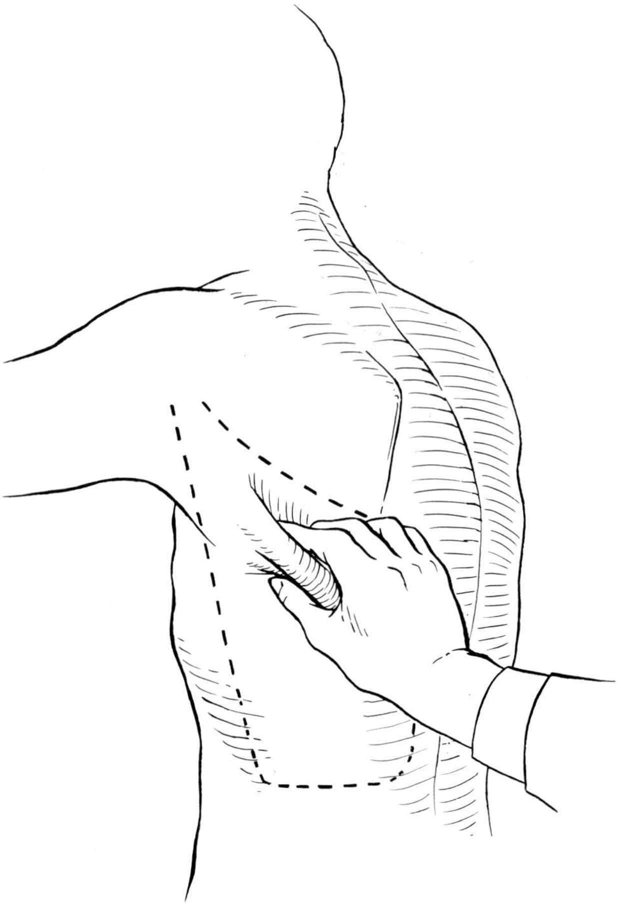

Figure 8.5. The muscle is outlined with a marking pen. The width of the skin paddle is estimated to allow for primary closure of the back wound.

Operative Technique

Immediately before surgery the patient is placed in a sitting position and the proposed inframammary crease is marked. The anterior edge of the latissimus muscle can usually be felt by digital examination if the patient extends her arm backward against resistance; the inferior spine of the scapula is also palpated (Figure 8.4). The muscle is outlined on the skin with a marking pen, and the width of the skin paddle is estimated to allow for primary closure of the back wound (Figure 8.5).

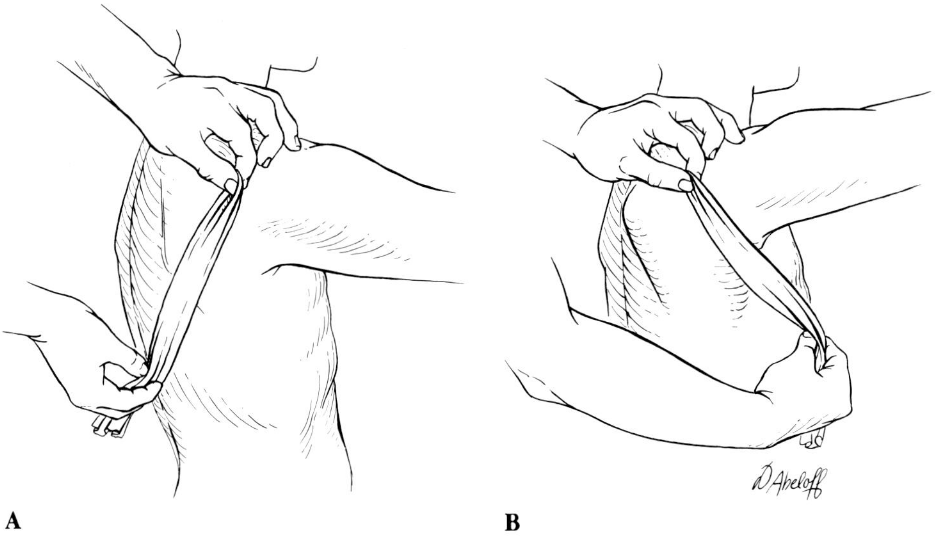

Figure 8.6. Estimating the length of the skin paddle and of the pedicle to allow easy transposition.

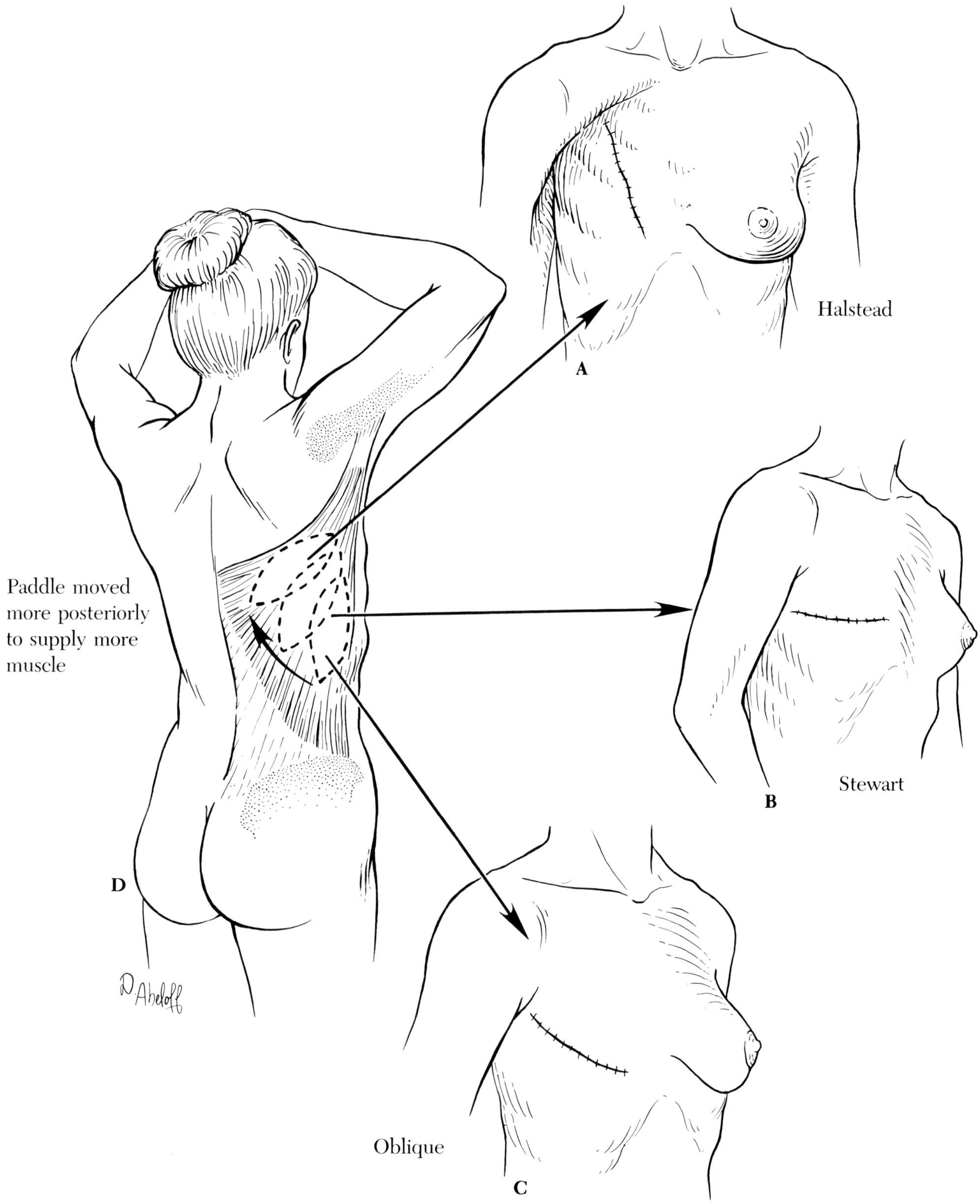

Figure 8.7. Variations in the position of the skin paddle. **A:** Typical radical mastectomy defect requiring a large amount of latissimus muscle. **B** and **C:** Modified radical mastectomy defects, with the paddle placed anteriorly. **D:** The skin paddle can be moved posteriorly to satisfy the requirements of the latissimus muscle on the anterior chest wall.

Position of the Skin Paddle and Measuring the Length of the Flap

The position of the skin paddle on the latissimus dorsi muscle must provide a pedicle long enough for easy transposition. If the humeral attachment is regarded as the axis of rotation, the paddle should be placed low enough on the muscle so that when transposed its inferior end reaches the most medial point of the breast to be reconstructed. An easy way to determine this is shown in Figure 8.6.

With the radical mastectomy, the skin paddle should be located posteriorly so that a large amount of anterior muscle can be used for reconstruction of the chest wall defect where the pectoralis muscle is absent (Figure 8.7A). With the modified radical mastectomy (Figure 8.7B,C), the skin paddle can usually be located much more anteriorly because less muscle is required on the anterior chest and the latissimus muscle is sutured to the lower edge of the pectoralis muscle. If there is a well-developed pectoralis muscle, less latissimus dorsi muscle is needed. Location of the skin paddle near the midlateral chest wall where the skin is thin, as opposed to more posteriorly where the skin is much thicker, allows "blending in" of the skin with the anterior chest skin. If the pectoralis muscle has atrophied and is reduced, however, more latissimus muscle is needed and the paddle is moved more posteriorly (Figure 8.7D).

Shaping the Skin Paddle

The most desirable breast reconstruction recreates the slight ptosis of the natural breast. It has been suggested by Vasconez (*personal communication*) that an arc- or crescent-shaped flap is more likely to give this result (Figure 8.8). The convex edge is inserted close to the inframammary crease (Figure 8.9). The resulting breast develops ptosis but may not have the projection that is desired. To achieve greater projection, the flap can be designed in a "wide pie wedge" as suggested by Millard (12) (Figure 8.10). However, the shape of the skin paddle is not limited to an ellipse or a crescent. There are

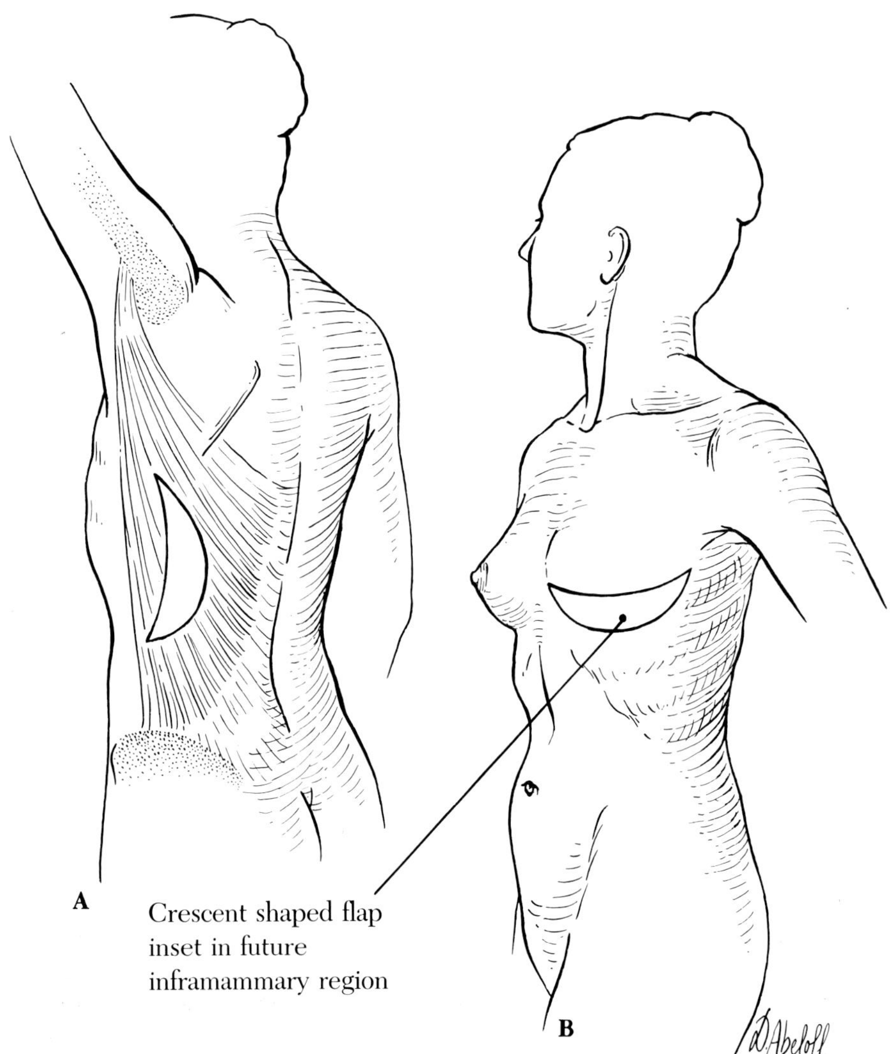

Figure 8.8. An arc- or crescent-shaped flap, when placed on the inframammary line, tends to produce ptosis.

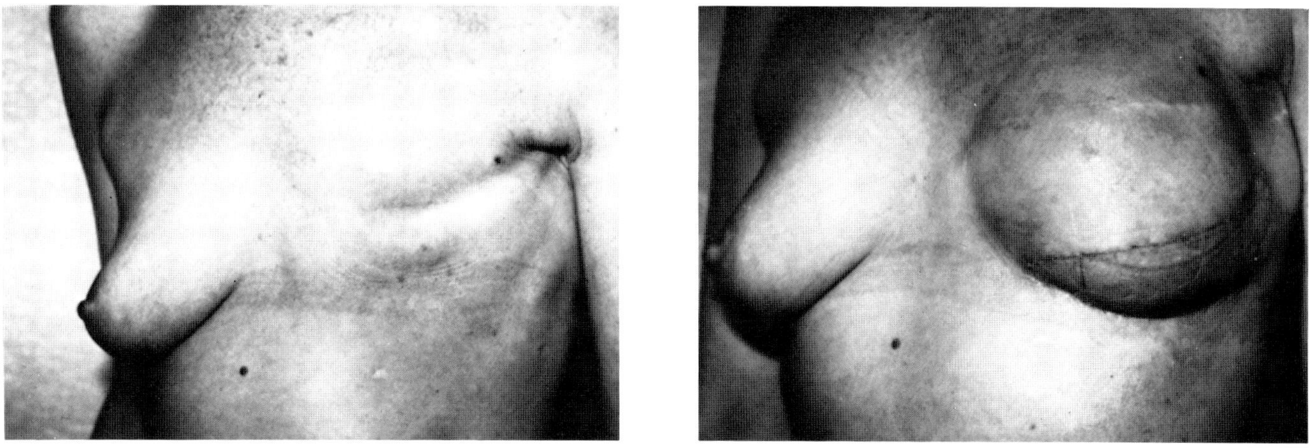

Figure 8.9. **Left:** Modified radical mastectomy with a transverse scar. **Right:** Crescent-shaped flap inset in the inframammary lines gives a ptotic effect but does not produce much projection.

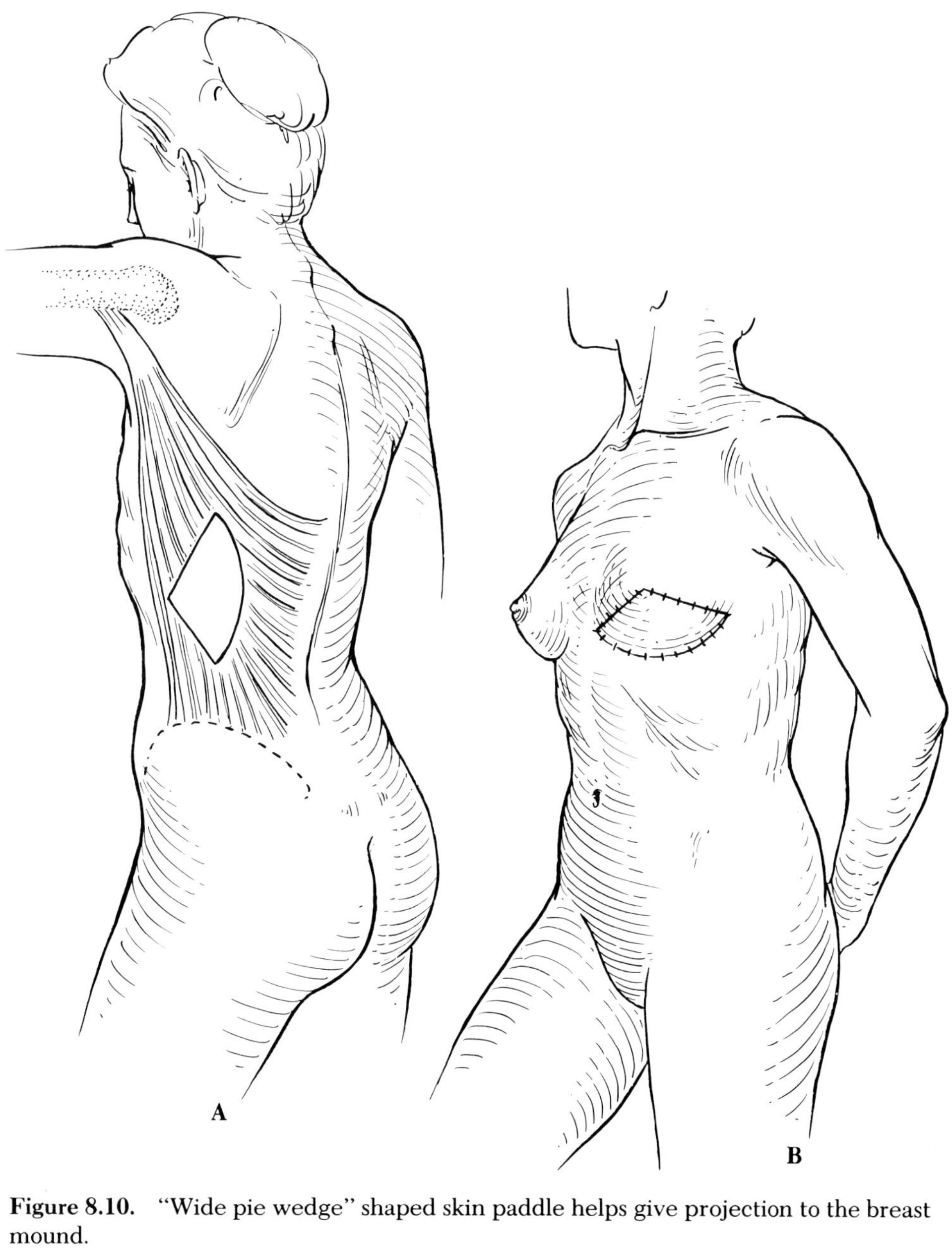

Figure 8.10. "Wide pie wedge" shaped skin paddle helps give projection to the breast mound.

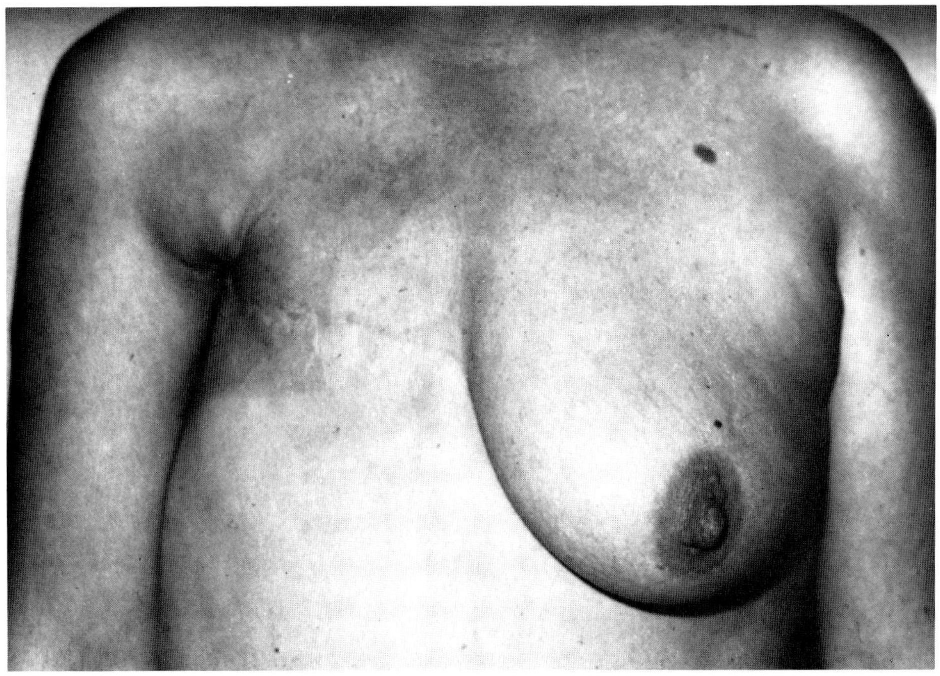

Figure 8.11. Right radical mastectomy scar with radiation changes in the anterior axillary region.

situations where darts can be added to the paddles, superiorly or inferiorly (12). These darts are used either to increase relaxation of the anterior chest wall skin at a particular site or to allow excision of an area of unsuitable skin. The following examples demonstrate these points:

1. With a right radical mastectomy deformity, the chest wall skin is very tight and adherent and there are radiation changes near the anterior axillary region (Figures 8.11 and 8.12A). The skin paddle is designed with superior and inferior darts (Figures 8.12B and 8.13). After the mastectomy scar is excised, the inferior flap is found to be very tight (Figure 8.12C). The latissimus flap is tunneled through from the back. A relaxing incision is made in the inferior skin flap, and an area of radiation-damaged skin from the superior lateral part of the wound is excised (Figures 8.12D and 8.14). The

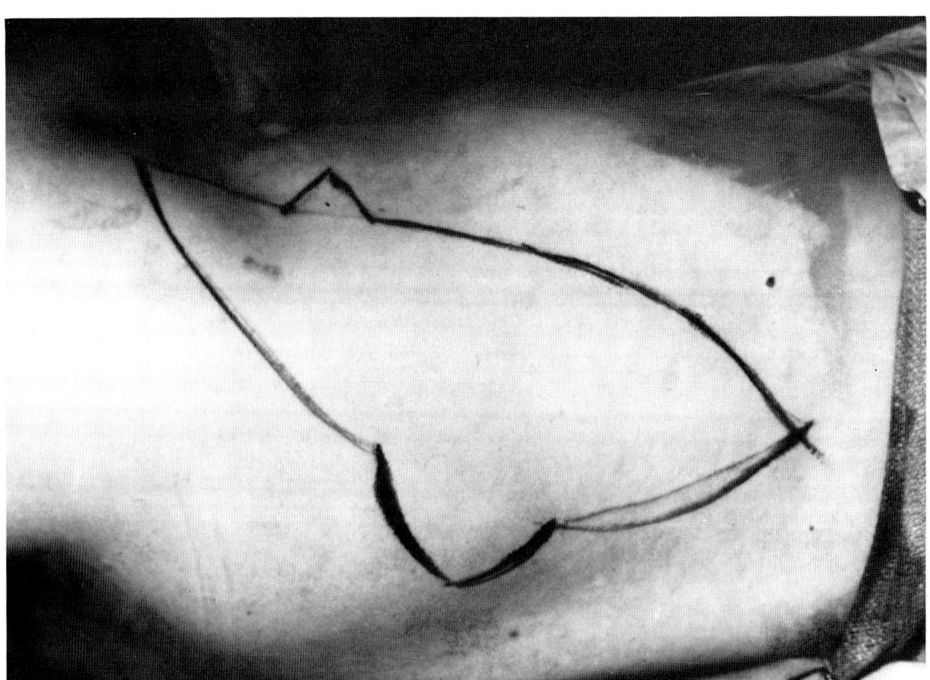

Figure 8.13. Skin paddle with superior and inferior darts. The superior dart (*top right of flap*) is designed so that it allows an area of radiation skin damage to be excised in the anterior axillary region. The inferior dart (*middle left of flap*) permits a relaxing incision to be made in the inferior flap and helps the inframammary fold to develop.

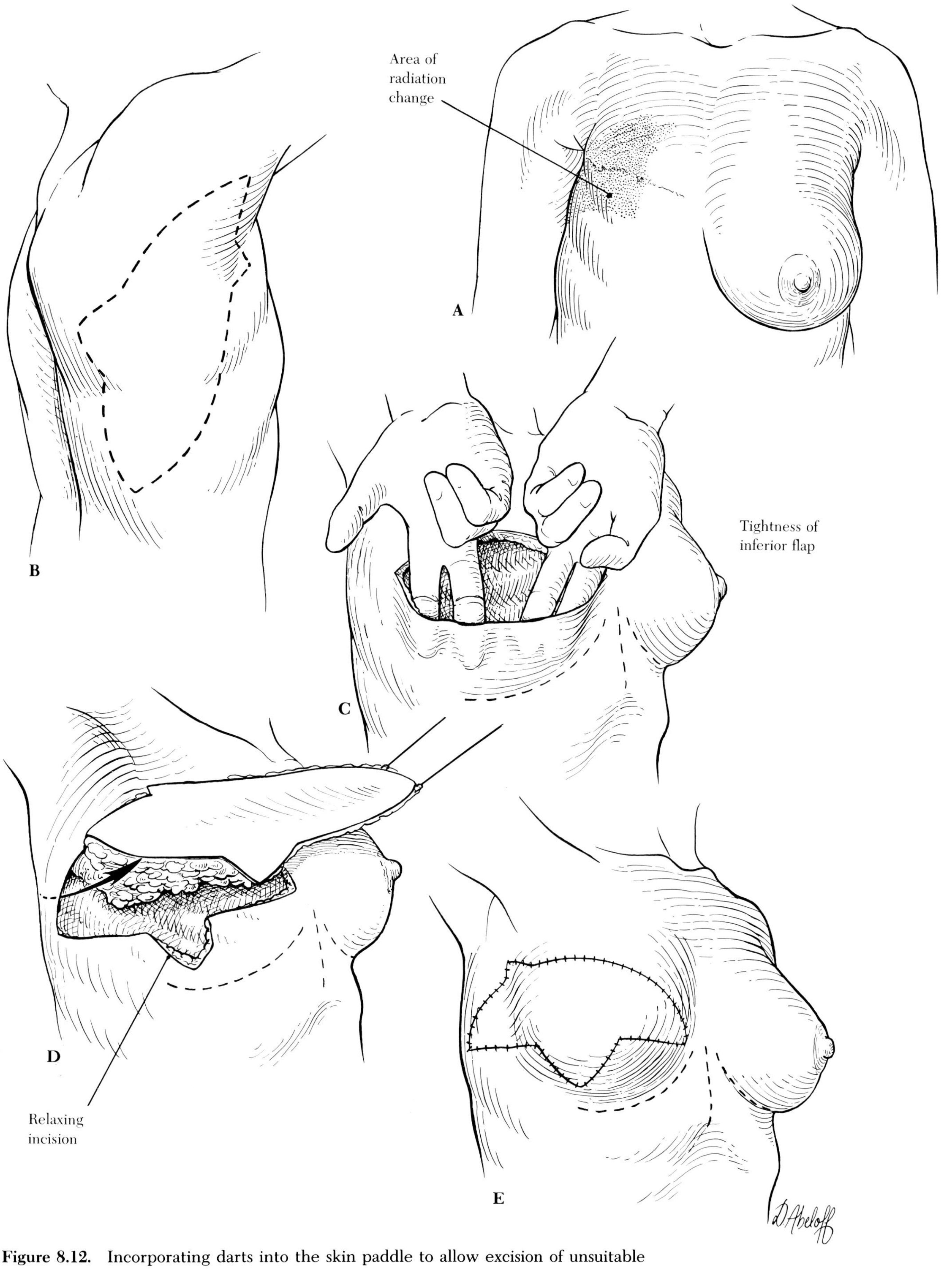

Figure 8.12. Incorporating darts into the skin paddle to allow excision of unsuitable skin and relaxation of the area of tight skin adherence. **A:** Area of radiation skin change. **B:** Outline of the latissimus paddle with darts incorporated. **C:** Tightness of the inferior flap. **D:** Latissimus flap tunneled through and then relaxing incisions made to incorporate the darts. **E:** Satisfactory breast mound produced with a silicone implant.

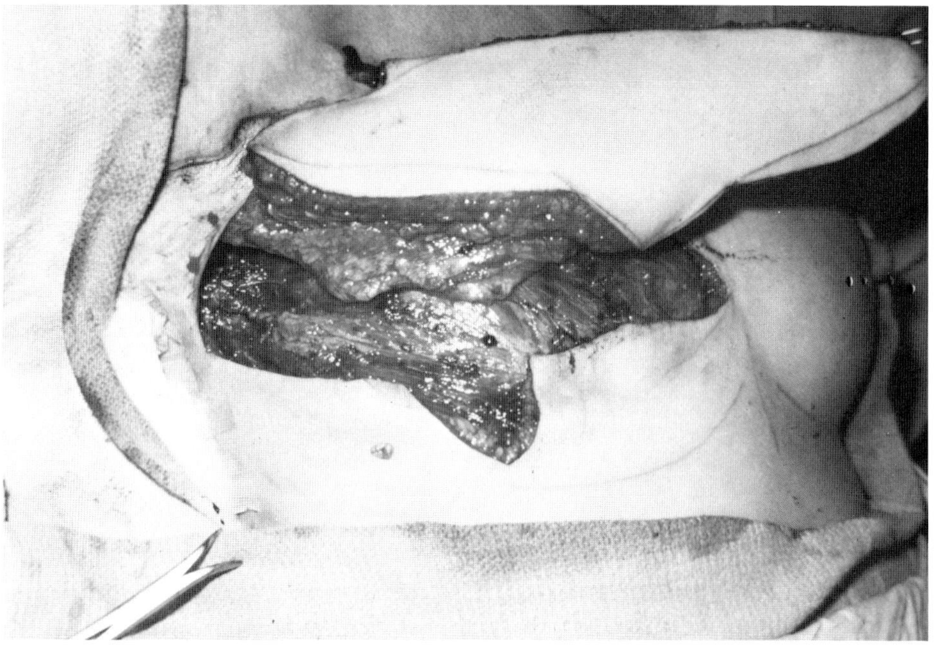

Figure 8.14. A latissimus flap with darts on the skin paddle is tunneled through to the anterior chest. The relaxing incision is then made in the inferior chest wall flap to coincide with the inferior dart. The superior dart is seen, but the area of excised radiation damage is hidden by the flap.

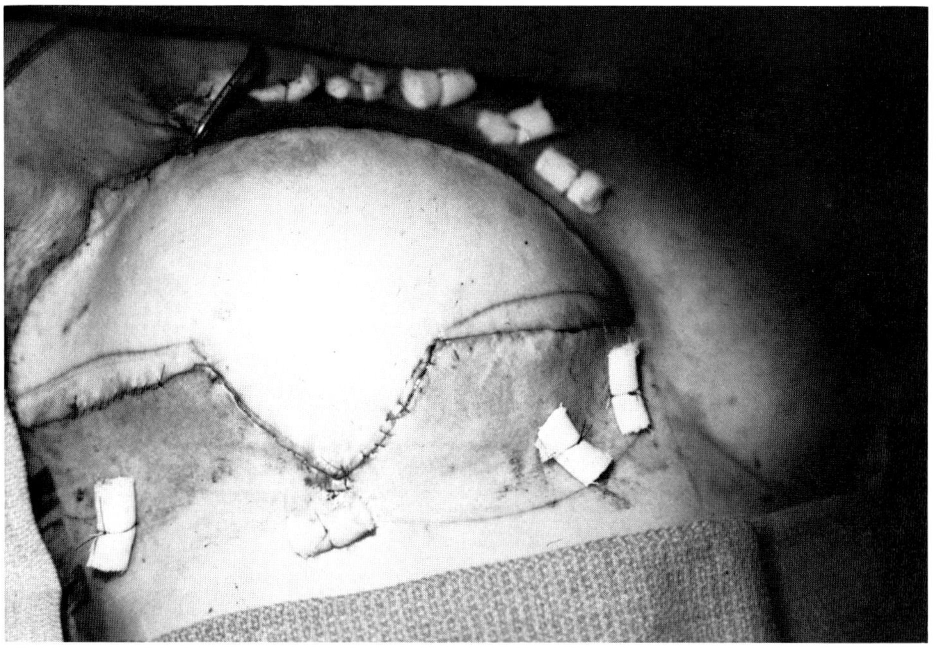

Figure 8.15. Flap inset with a silicone implant producing the breast mound (bolsters shown are rarely used now).

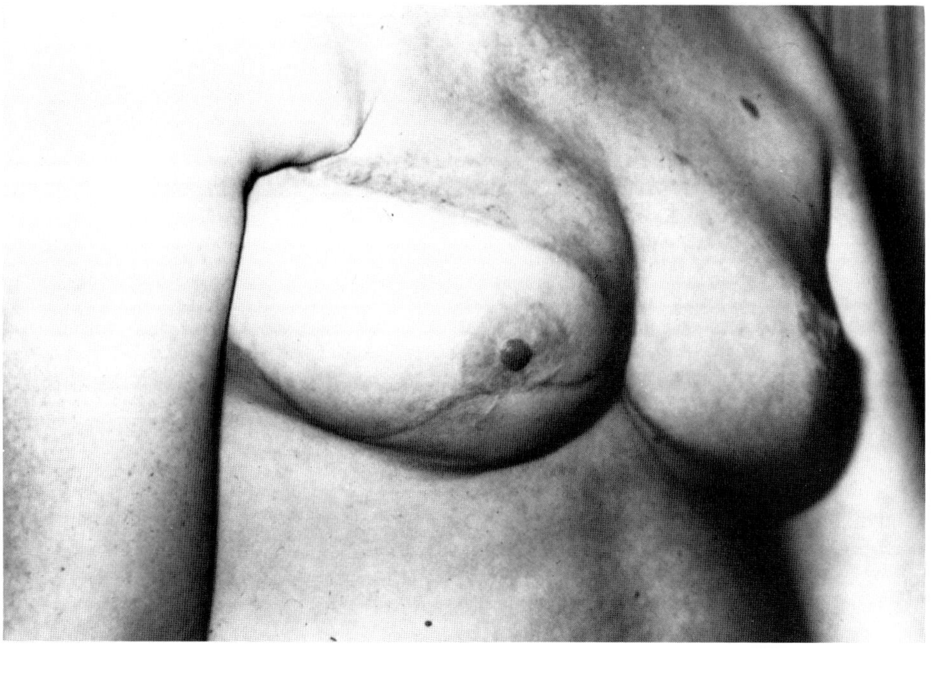

Figure 8.16. Final postoperative result of the patient in Figure 8.11–8.15.

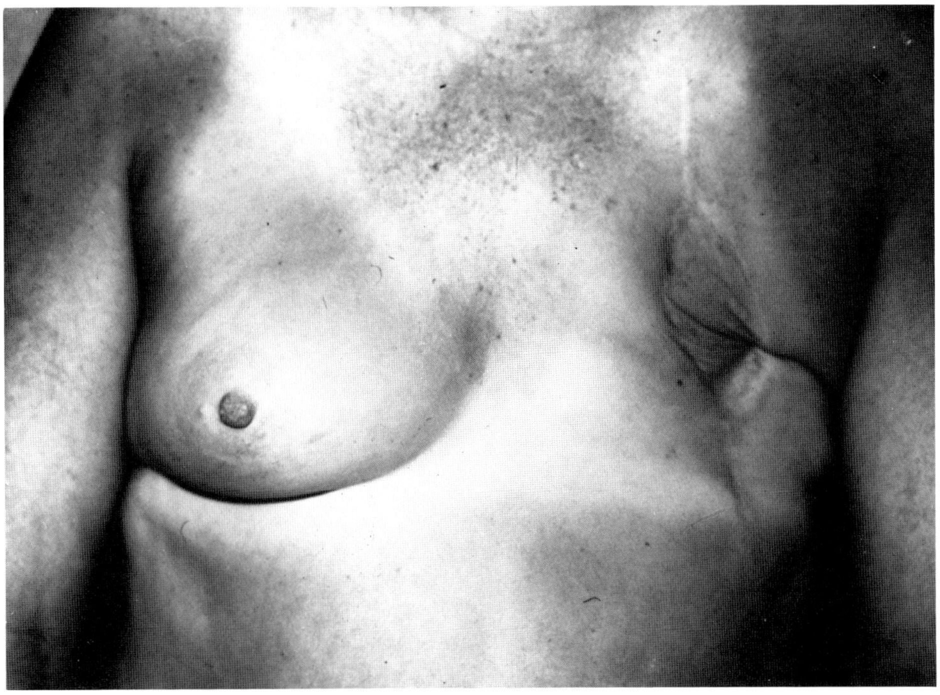

Figure 8.17. Depressed and adherent skin graft complicates the left modified radical defect.

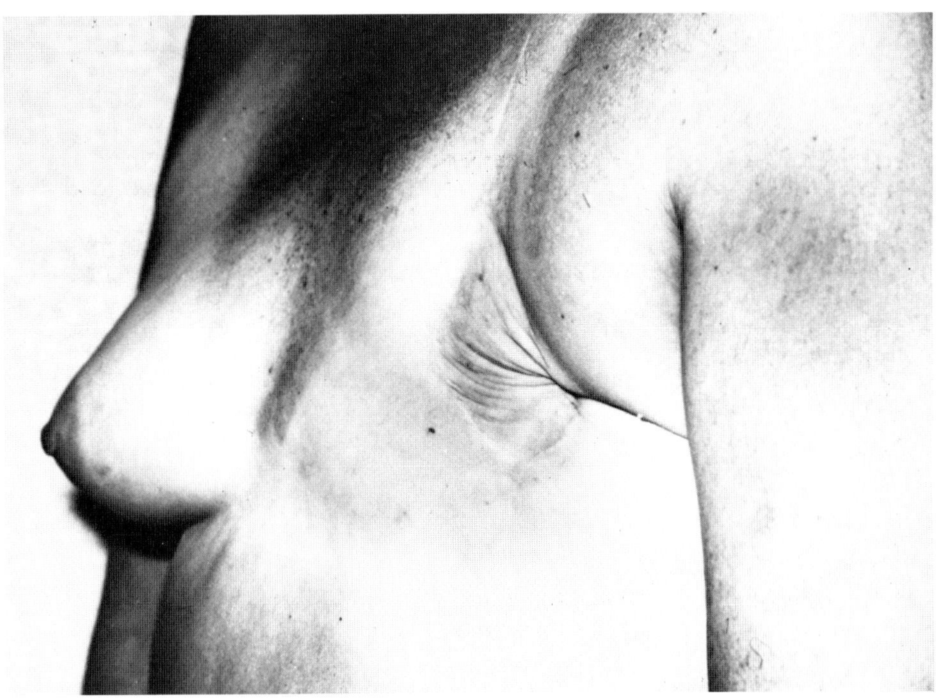

Figure 8.18. Oblique view of the patient in Figure 8.17.

modified latissimus skin muscle flap is inset, and a satisfactory breast mound is formed with a prosthesis (Figures 8.12E, 8.15, and 8.16).

2. An unsightly depressed and adherent skin graft complicates a satisfactory reconstruction (Figures 8.17 and 8.18). Here it is decided to excise the skin graft and incise along the inframammary crease (Figure 8.19A). A trefoil-shaped flap is planned (Figures 8.19B and 8.20). The flap is inset, providing enough skin relaxation to allow a breast mound shape to be developed with a prosthesis (Figure 8.19C). The final postoperative result is seen in Figures 8.21 and 8.22. The donor site closes as a T-shape.

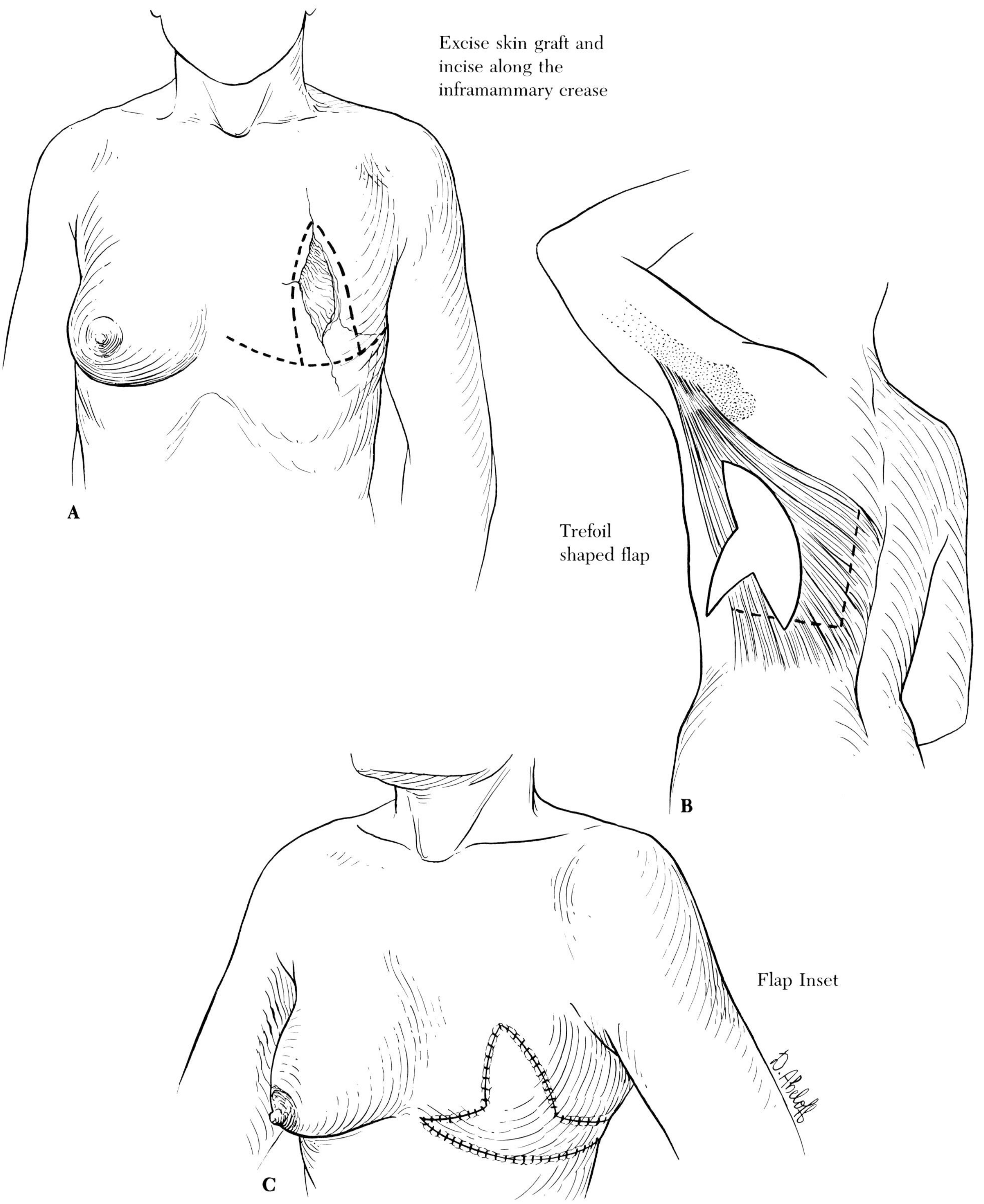

Figure 8.19. **A:** Outline of a skin graft excision and inframammary crease incision. **B:** Trefoil skin paddle planned. **C:** Flap inset with an underlying silicone implant to produce a breast mound.

3. A mastectomy scar has produced tightness both vertically and horizontally (Figures 8.23A and 8.24). A cruciate flap is designed (Figures 8.23B and 8.25). The scar is excised and then incised at right angles. A satisfactory full breast mound can be developed with an implant (Figures 8.23C, 8.26, 8.27, and 8.28). The donor site closes as a cross (Figures 8.23D and 8.29).
4. Occasionally the shape of the flap is dictated by the mastectomy scar (Figures 8.30A,B–8.32).

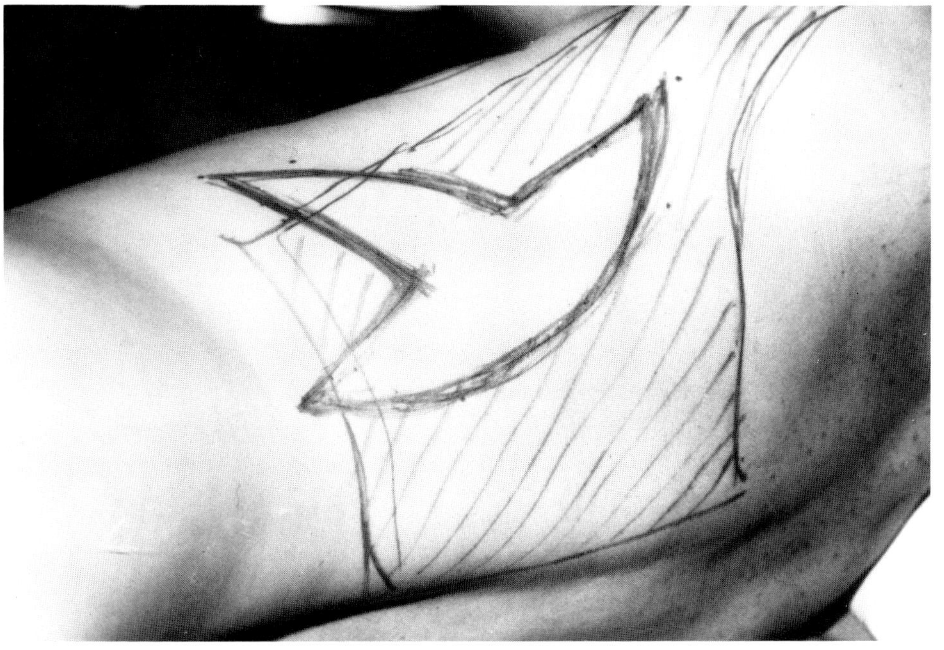

Figure 8.20. Trefoil skin paddle outlined.

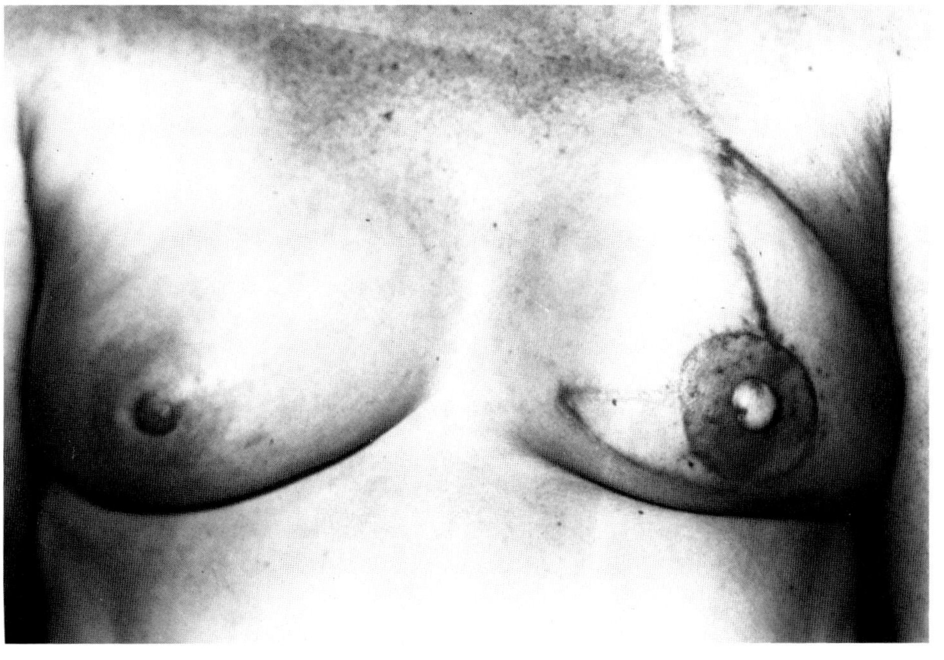

Figure 8.21. Anteroposterior (AP) view of the postoperative result after nipple-areola reconstruction. The trefoil flap gives the appearance of a crab claw.

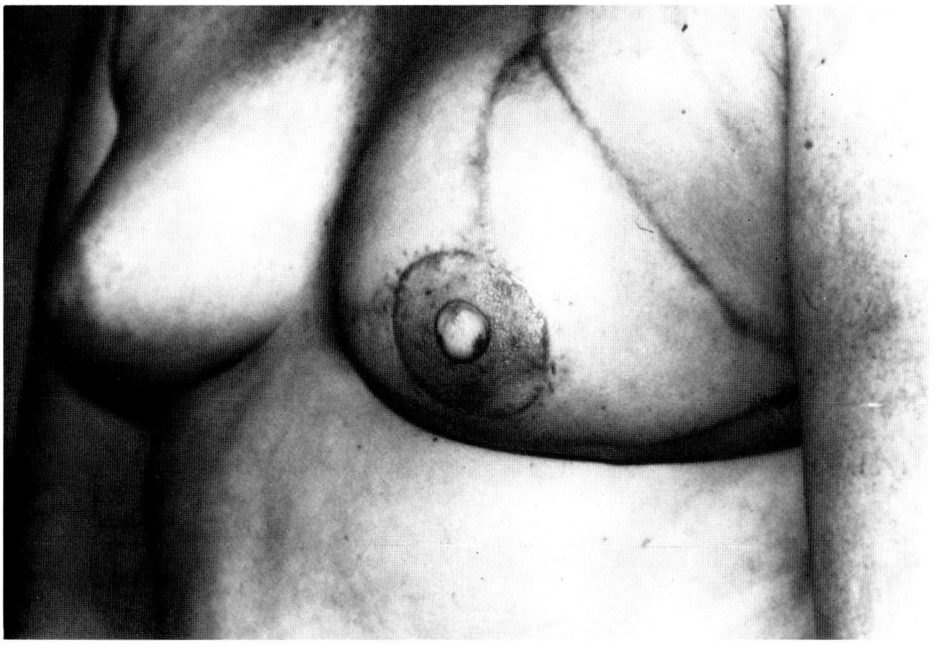

Figure 8.22. Oblique view of the postoperative result of the patient in Figures 8.17–8.21.

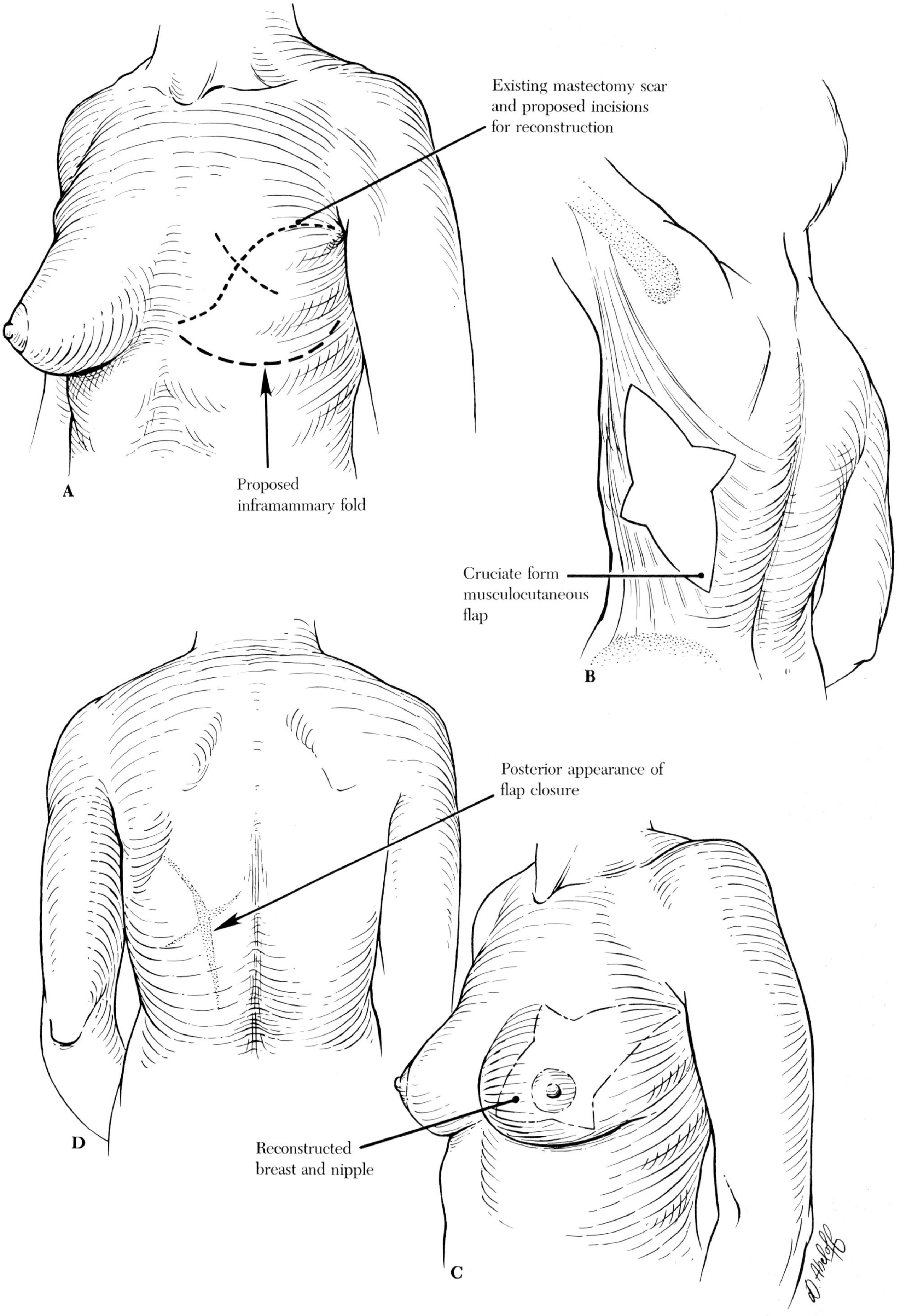

Figure 8.23. **A:** Left mastectomy scar and proposed lines of incision to allow chest wall relaxation. **B:** Cruciate flap design. **C:** Cruciate flap inset with underlying silicone implant producing slight ptosis to reconstructed breast. **D:** Donor site.

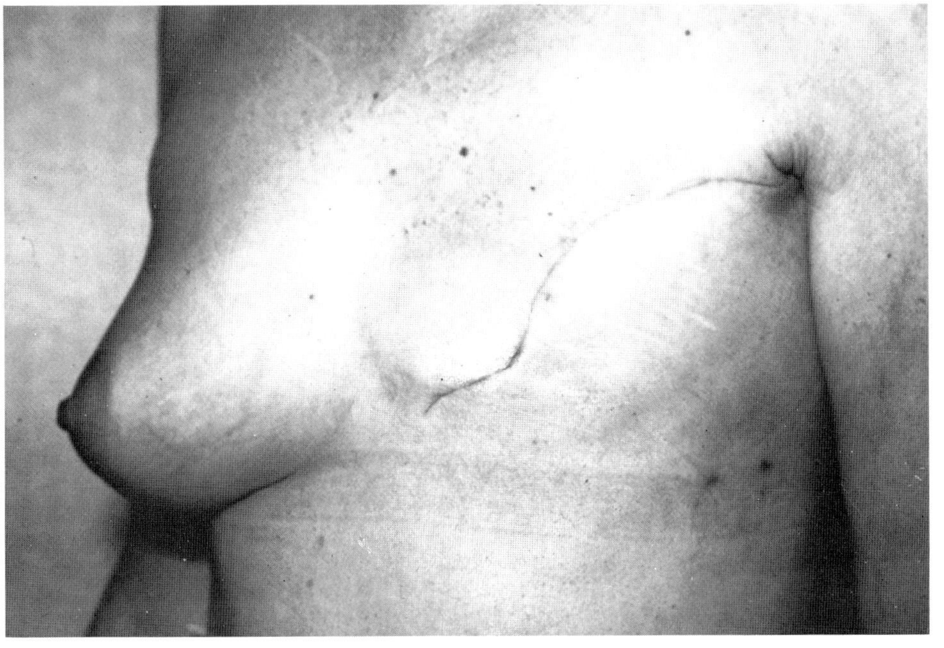

Figure 8.24. Tight left mastectomy scar with mildly ptotic right breast.

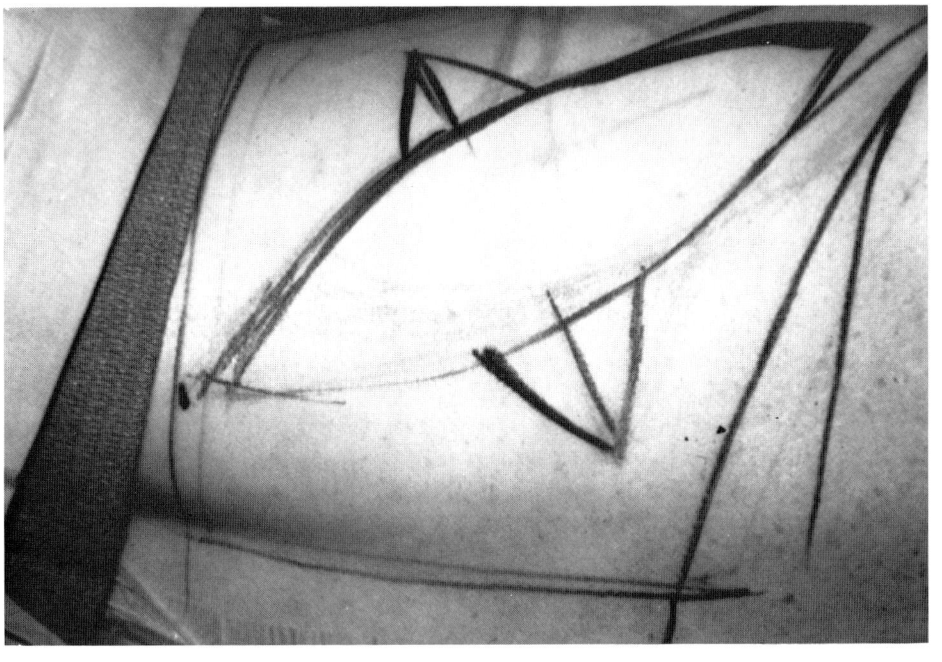

Figure 8.25. Outline of cruciate flap on left latissimus area.

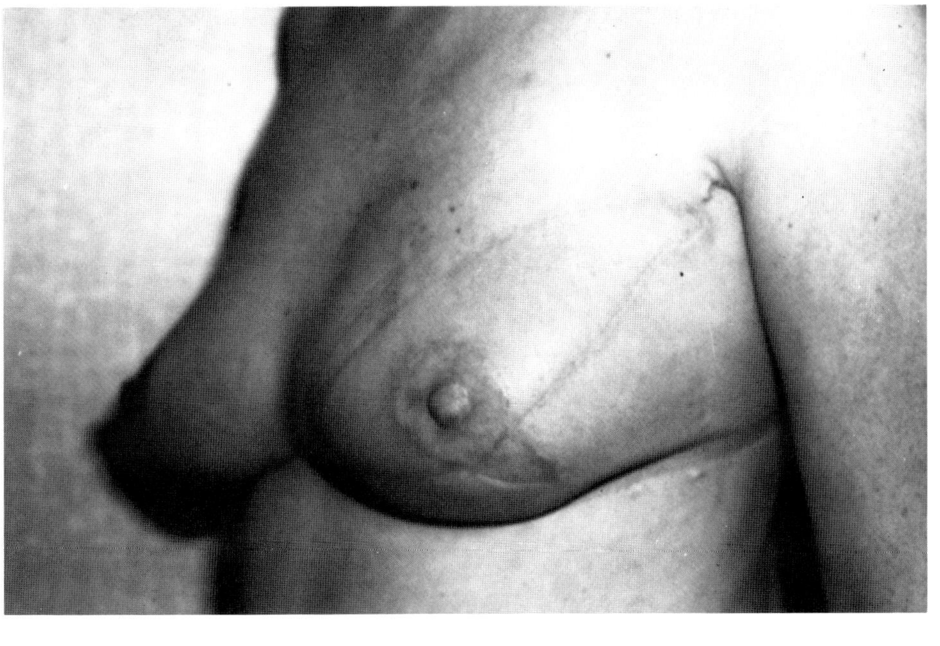

Figure 8.26. Left oblique postoperative view, cruciate flap inset with silicone implant produces slight ptosis to reconstructed breast. Nipple reconstructed with quadrapod flaps and areola formed from full thickness skin graft from inner thigh.

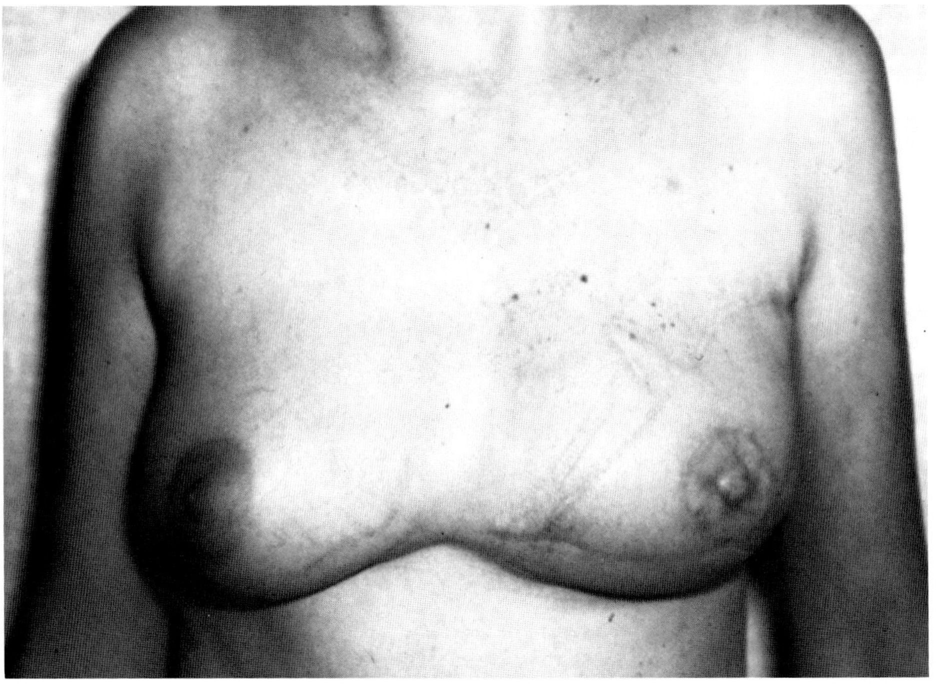

Figure 8.27. AP postoperative view.

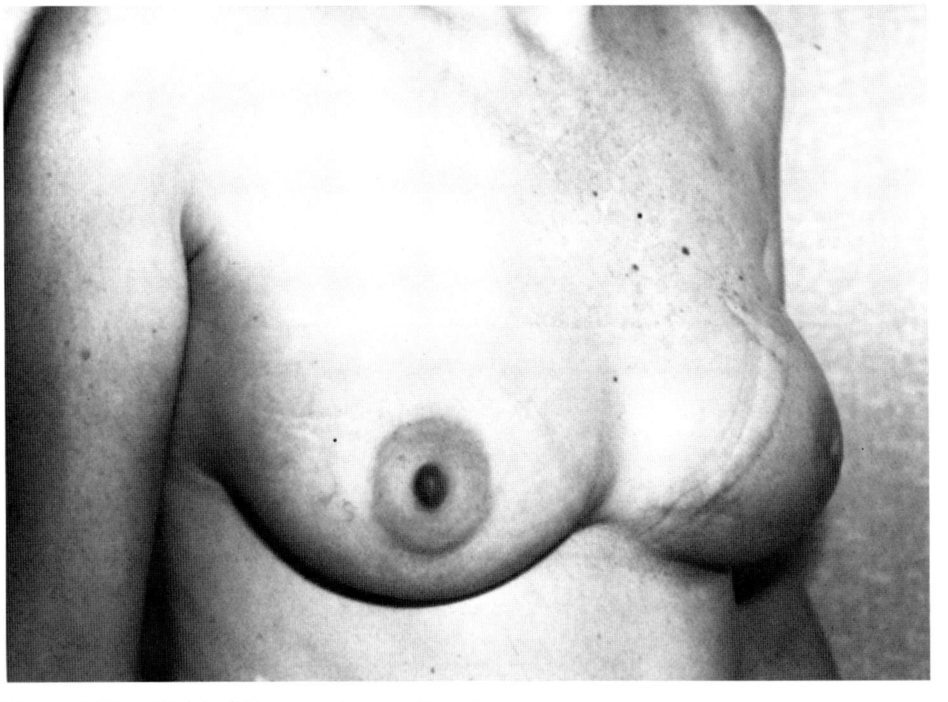

Figure 8.28. Right oblique postoperative view.

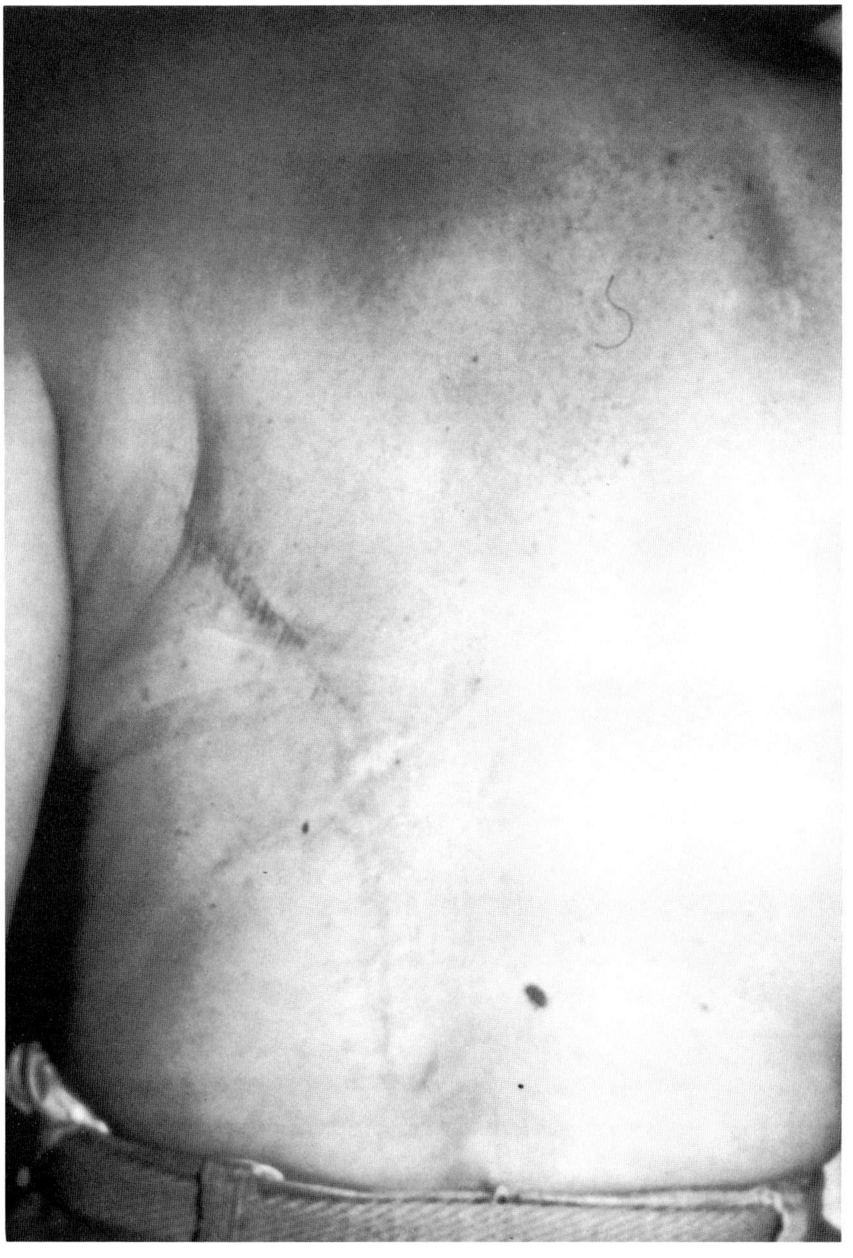

Figure 8.29. Left back scar showing primary closure.

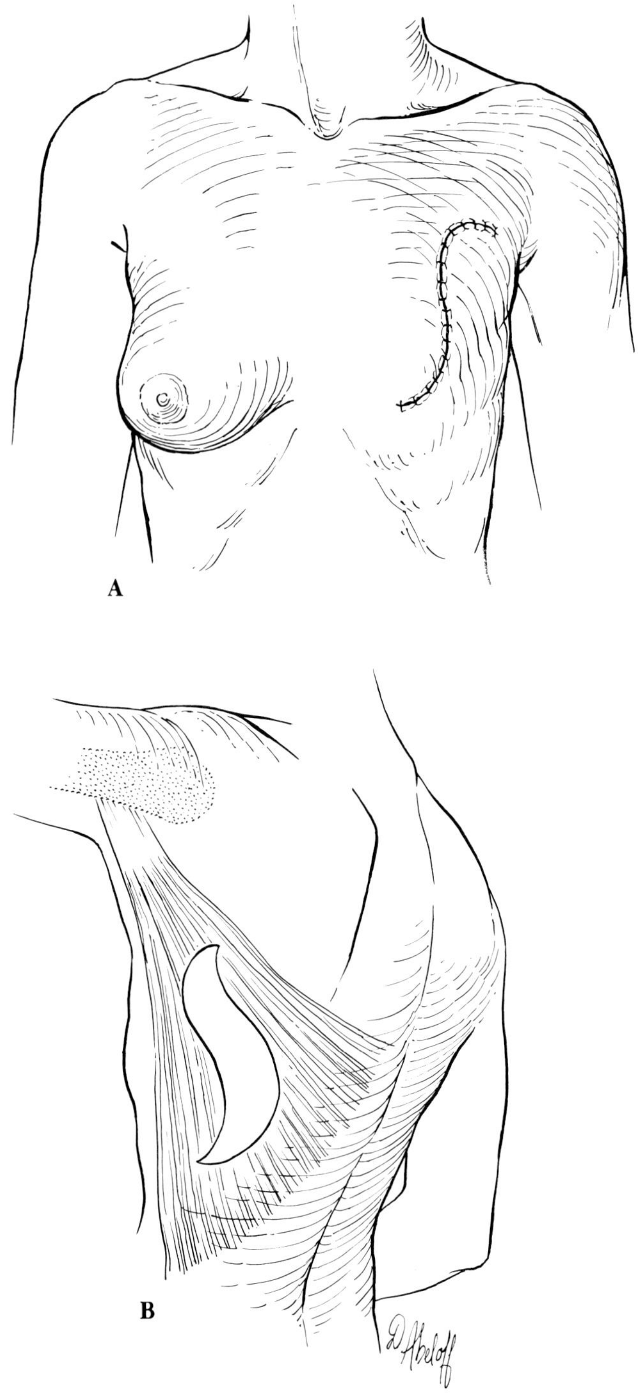

Figure 8.30. **A:** S-shaped mastectomy scar. **B:** S-shaped skin paddle design.

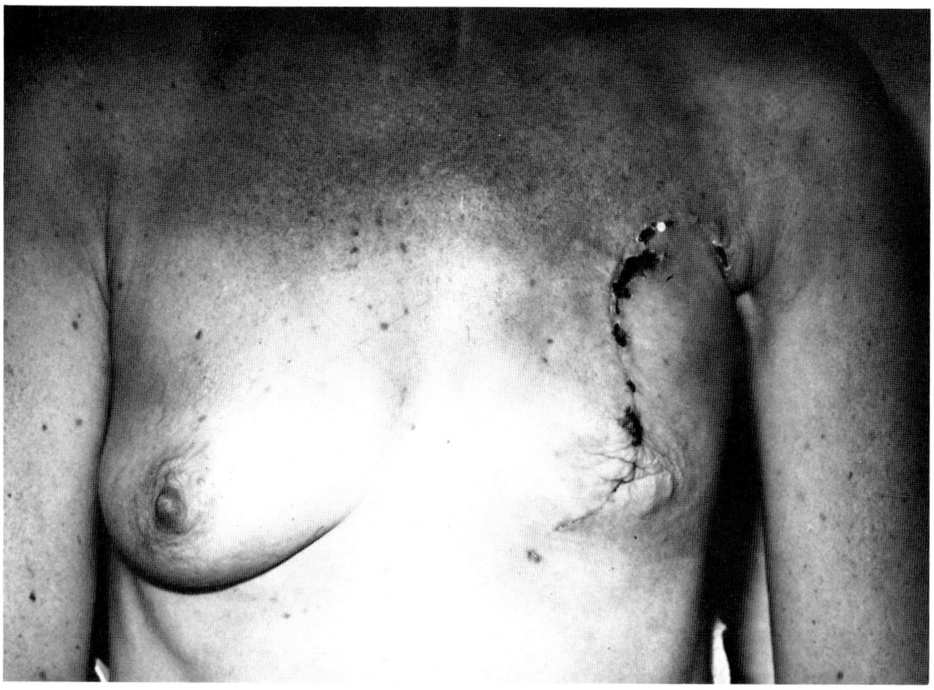

Figure 8.31. Preoperative AP view of a left modified mastectomy defect with an S-shaped scar.

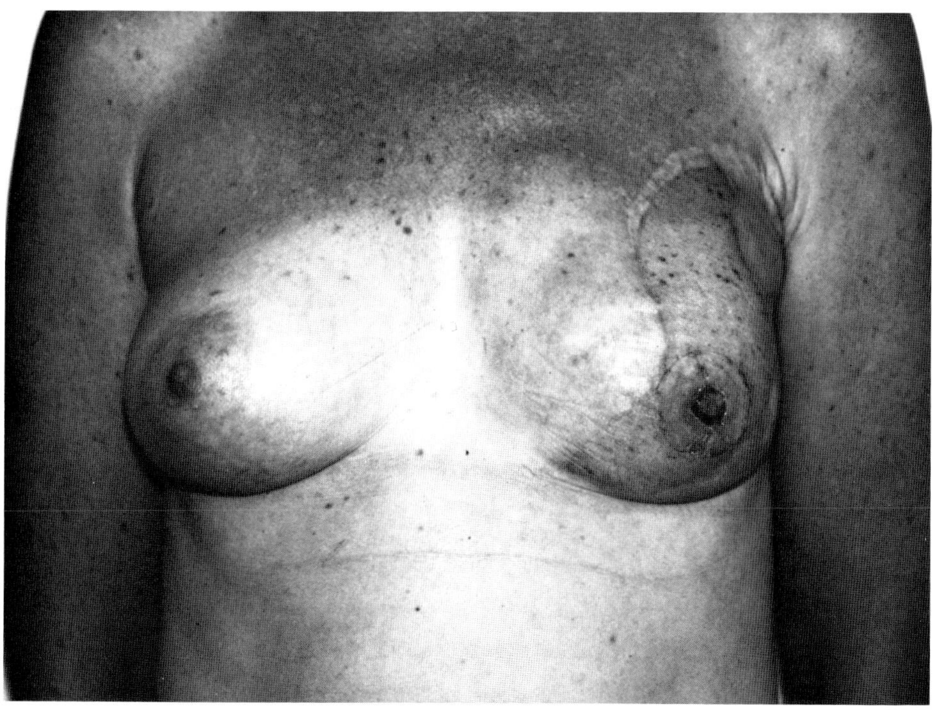

Figure 8.32. AP view of the postoperative result. The right breast was augmented for symmetry.

In the operation room the patient is placed in a midlateral position with the mastectomy site superior (Figures 8.33 and 8.34). A pillow is placed between the knees, and a roll is positioned below the dependent shoulder to prevent brachial plexus injury. A strip of wide adhesive tape secured to the operating table holds the hips in the correct position. The arm on the mastectomy side is extended in front of the patient and rests on a second Mayo stand which has been well padded to avoid pressure to the ulnar nerve (Figure 8.35A).

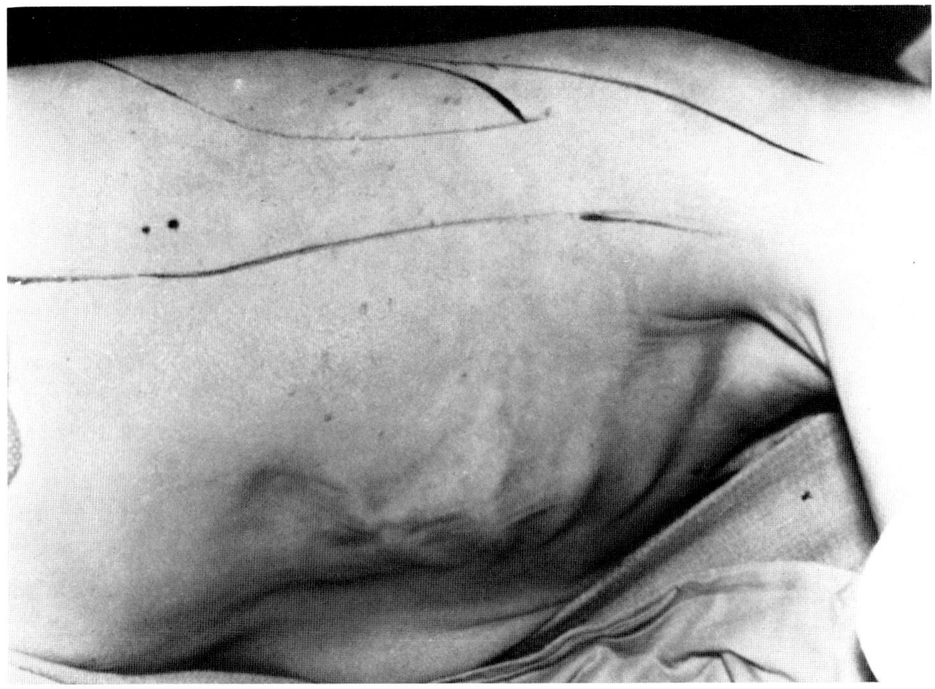

Figure 8.33. Patient positioned in the midlateral position on the operating table with the right mastectomy site visible.

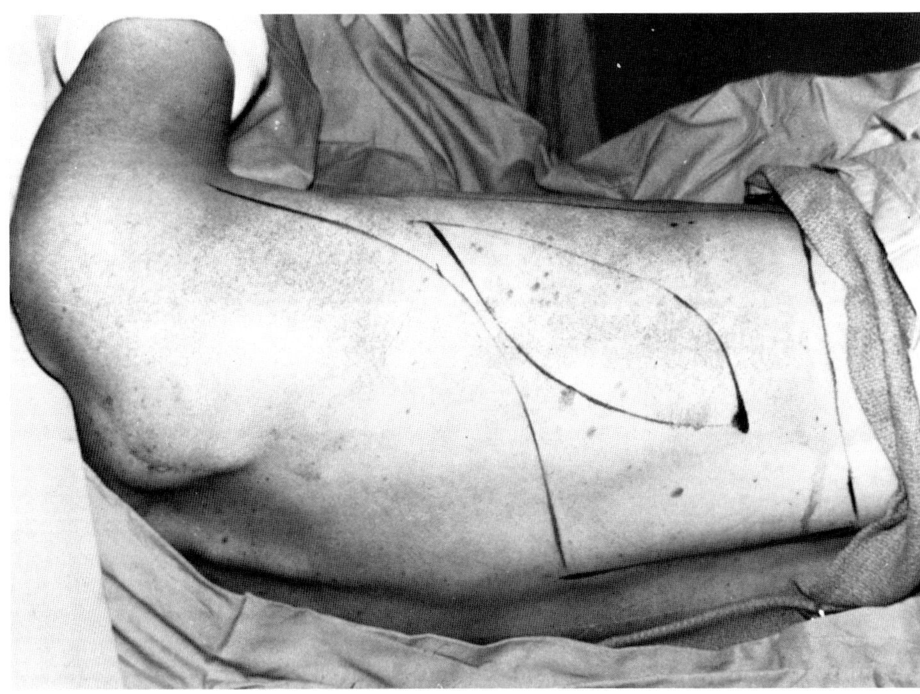

Figure 8.34. Patient in the midlateral position with the right latissimus flap and skin paddle outlined. The right arm is extended in front of the patient and supported on a sterile padded Mayo stand.

With the patient in this position, the skin of the upper arm and the anterior and posterior chest to beyond the midline is prepared. Sterile drapes are then applied. The upper arm is draped separately so that it can be moved freely during the operation.

The skin incision is made according to the outline of the paddle; the skin anteriorly is undermined until the anterior edge of the latissimus muscle is reached (Figure 8.35B). Scarring from the previous mastectomy operation may make this dissection difficult, and it may be hard to distinguish the latissimus muscle from the serratus anterior muscle (Figure 8.35C). (For this reason,

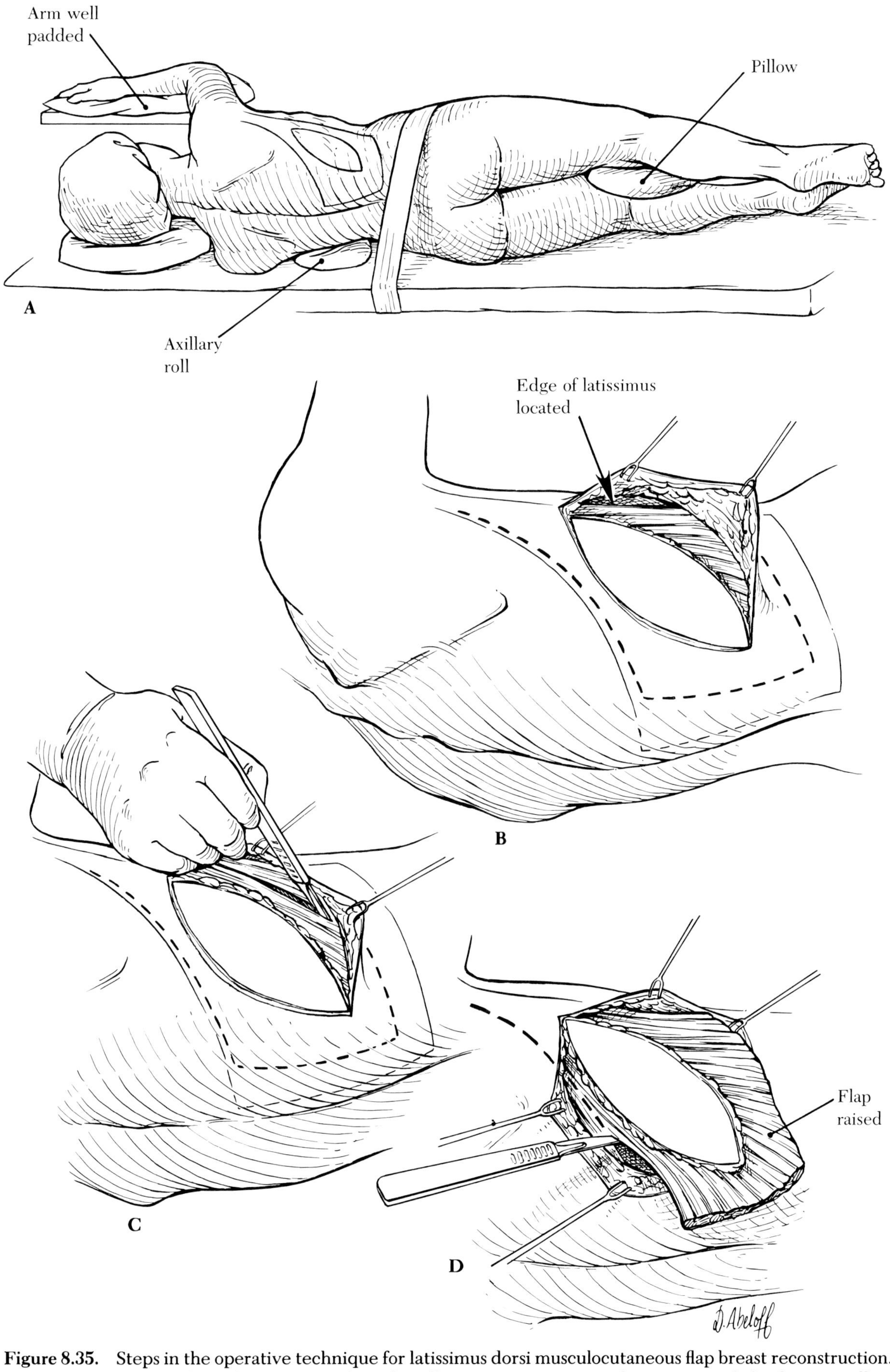

Figure 8.35. Steps in the operative technique for latissimus dorsi musculocutaneous flap breast reconstruction. **A:** Patient in the midlateral position with wide adhesive tape securing the position of the hips, a pillow between the knees, a roll under the chest, and arms on the mastectomy side extended and supported on a well-padded Mayo stand. **B:** Locating the anterior edge of the latissimus muscle. **C:** Sharp dissection may be necessary if scarring from the previous mastectomy makes the dissection difficult. **D:** Freeing of flap. **E:** Elevating the flap and noting the thoracodorsal artery and vein and branches to the serratus anterior msucle. **F:** Tunnel between back wound and anterior chest wound. **G:** Tunneling flap.

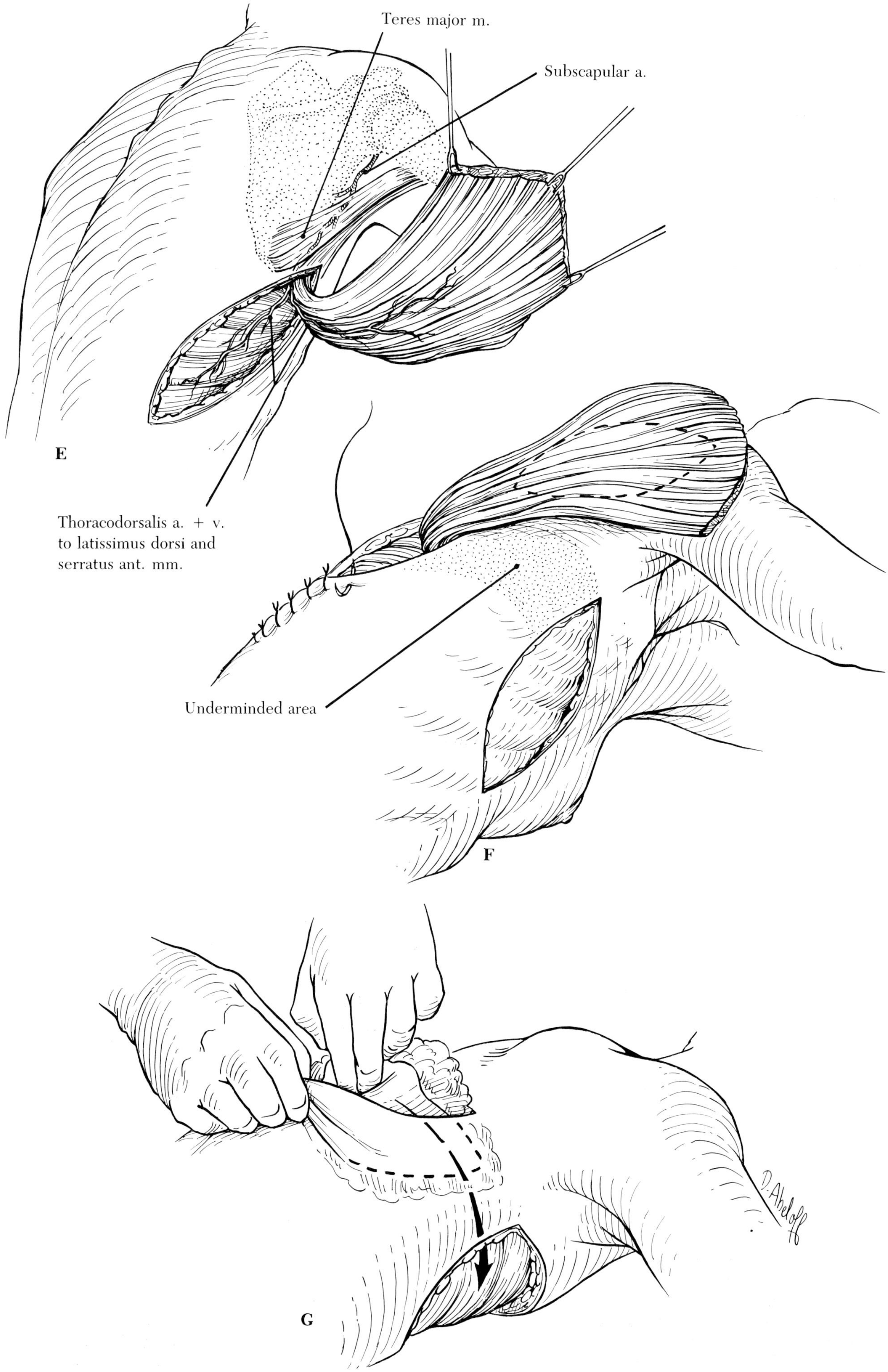
Teres major m.
Subscapular a.
E
Thoracodorsalis a. + v. to latissimus dorsi and serratus ant. mm.
Underminded area
F
G

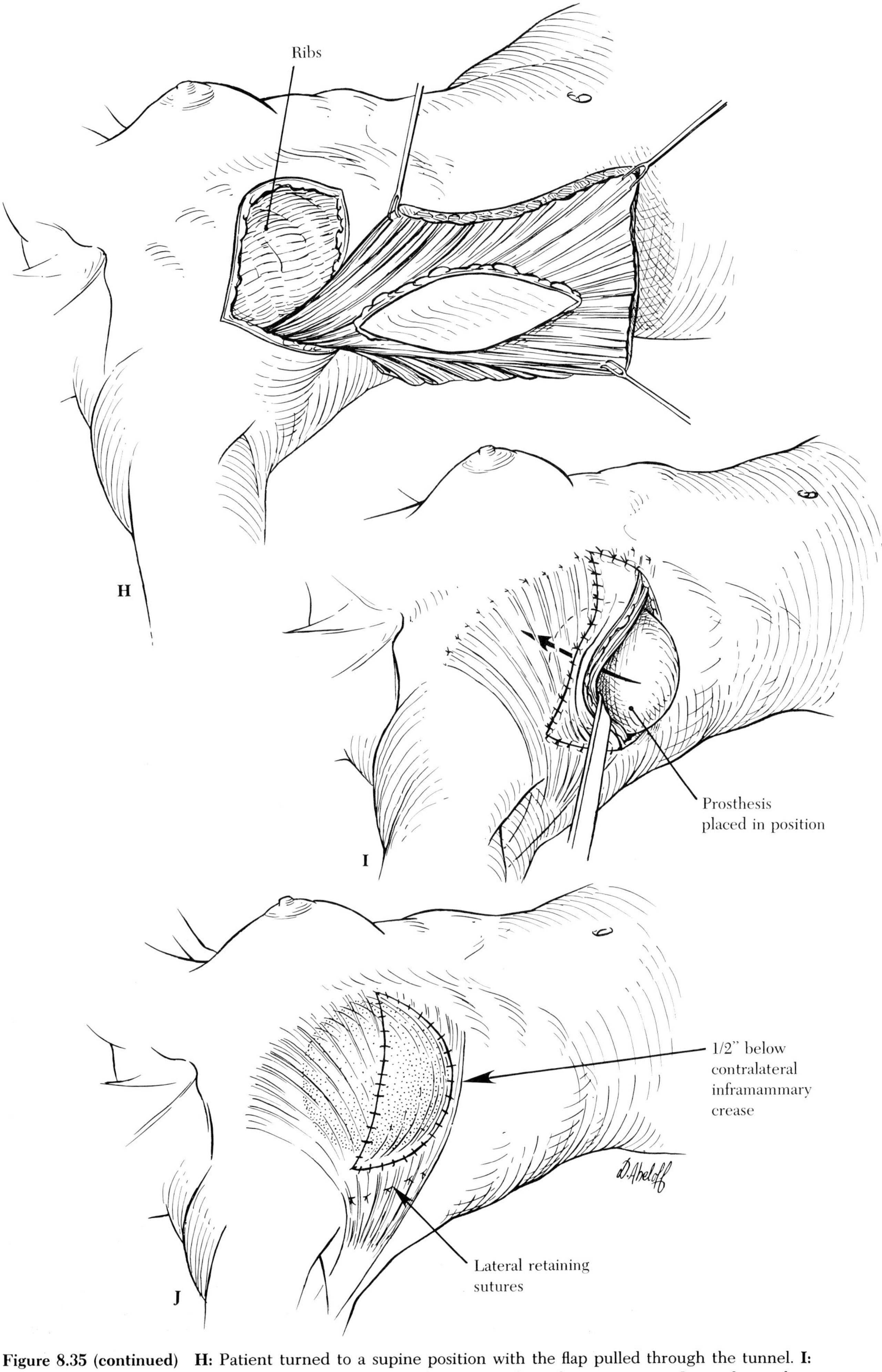

Figure 8.35 (continued) **H:** Patient turned to a supine position with the flap pulled through the tunnel. **I:** Flap partly inset and silicone implant being inserted. **J:** Flap inset with implant in position. Cavity for implant extends 0.5 inch below the contralateral inframammary crease. Sutures close off the cavity laterally.

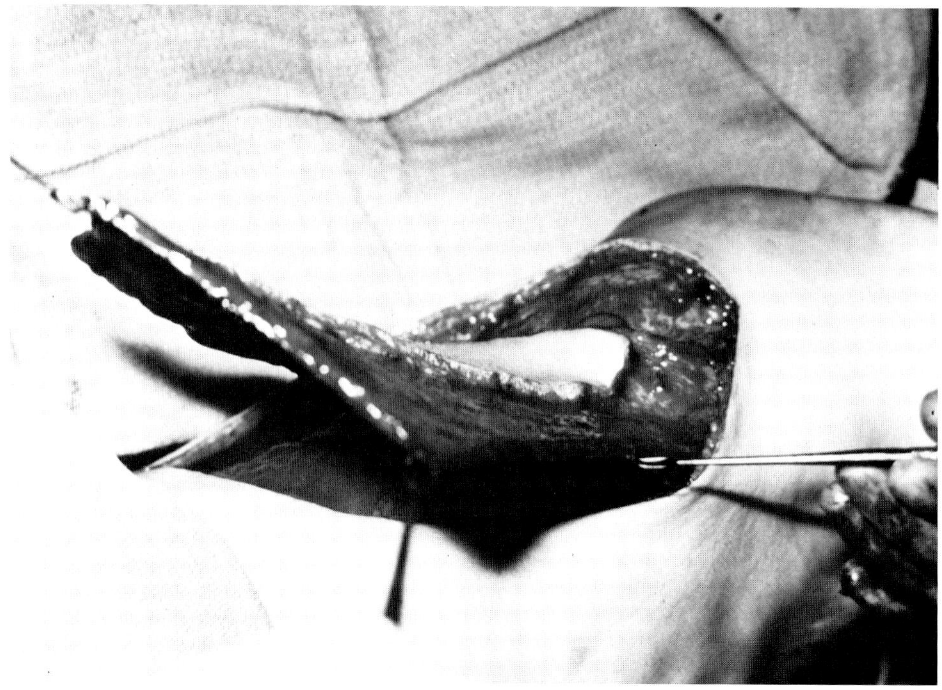

Figure 8.36. Thin atrophic latissimus muscle suggests damage to the nerve and possible obliteration of the thoracodorsal artery at the mastectomy operation.

some surgeons prefer to identify the muscle medially or posteriorly, at the initial part of the operation.) Once the anterior edge of the latissimus muscle has been identified, dissection proceeds inferiorly. Depending on how much muscle is required, it is divided transversely, beyond the extent of the skin paddle, across to the midline. Dissection then proceeds superiorly, freeing the latissimus from its spinous attachments. The freed inferior skin muscle flap is elevated (Figure 8.35D). Dissection is then performed on the undersurface of the flap toward the axilla. Perforating vessels are encountered, ligated, and divided. As the dissection extends superiorly, the muscle is freed from the trapezius and the spine of the scapula. At this point the latissimus lies inferior to the teres major muscle. As the muscle narrows toward its humeral attachment, dissection is performed with more care. If the latissimus muscle is very thin and atrophic, it is probable that the muscle has been denervated during the previous mastectomy operation (Figure 8.36). Because the nerve to the latissimus dorsi muscle and the thoracodorsal artery lie in close proximity in the axilla, it is possible that the artery was also obliterated. The thoracodorsal artery and vein can usually be identified on the undersurface of the flap, and the vascular branch from the thoracodorsal artery to the serratus anterior muscle can usually be located (Figure 8.35E). It is prudent to leave this branch to the serratus muscle intact until it is certain that the thoracodorsal artery is patent superiorly. Maxwell et al. showed that the latissimus dorsi musculocutaneous flap can be elevated in spite of ligation of the thoracodorsal artery so long as collateral circulation to the muscle is not interrupted (9). It is thus very important when elevating the flap toward the axilla to preserve any obvious collateral circulation, especially if the vessels seem to be larger than normal. It is possible, however, for the nerve to the latissimus dorsi to remain intact even if thoracodorsal vessels have been ligated. Therefore a normal-appearing muscle should not give one a false sense of security. If the thoracodorsal artery has been ligated superiorly near its origin, the serratus branch may be the main source of blood supply to the latissimus muscle by retrograde flow (Figures 8.37 and 8.38). When the thoracodorsal vessels are found intact, the surgeon may elect to skeletinize the pedicle, facilitating transposition of the flap. This also allows the flap to be made into a neurovascular island pedicle if desired by dividing the insertion to the humerus. It must be added that the flap can often be mobilized enough for tunneling anteriorly without visualizing the vessels (Figure 8.39).

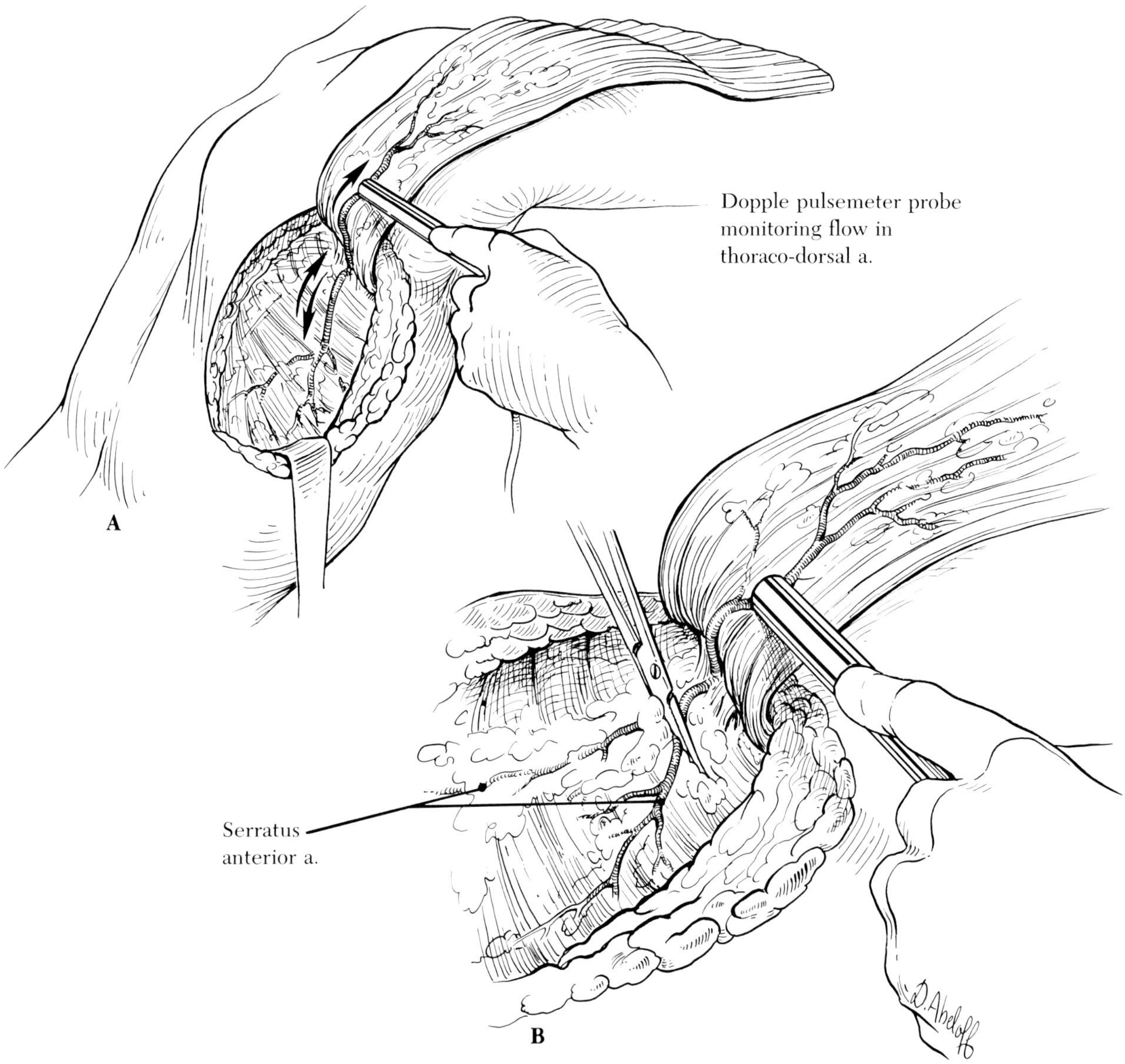

Figure 8.37. **A:** Monitoring the blood flow in the thoracodorsal artery. **B:** Pressure on the branch to the serratus anterior artery occludes the blood flow. If flow is still present in the thoracodorsal artery, it can be assumed that normal flow is present. If flow is halted in the thoracodorsal artery, however, it suggests that retrograde flow from the serratus branch is present and that the thoracodorsal artery may have been obliterated proximally at the previous mastectomy operation.

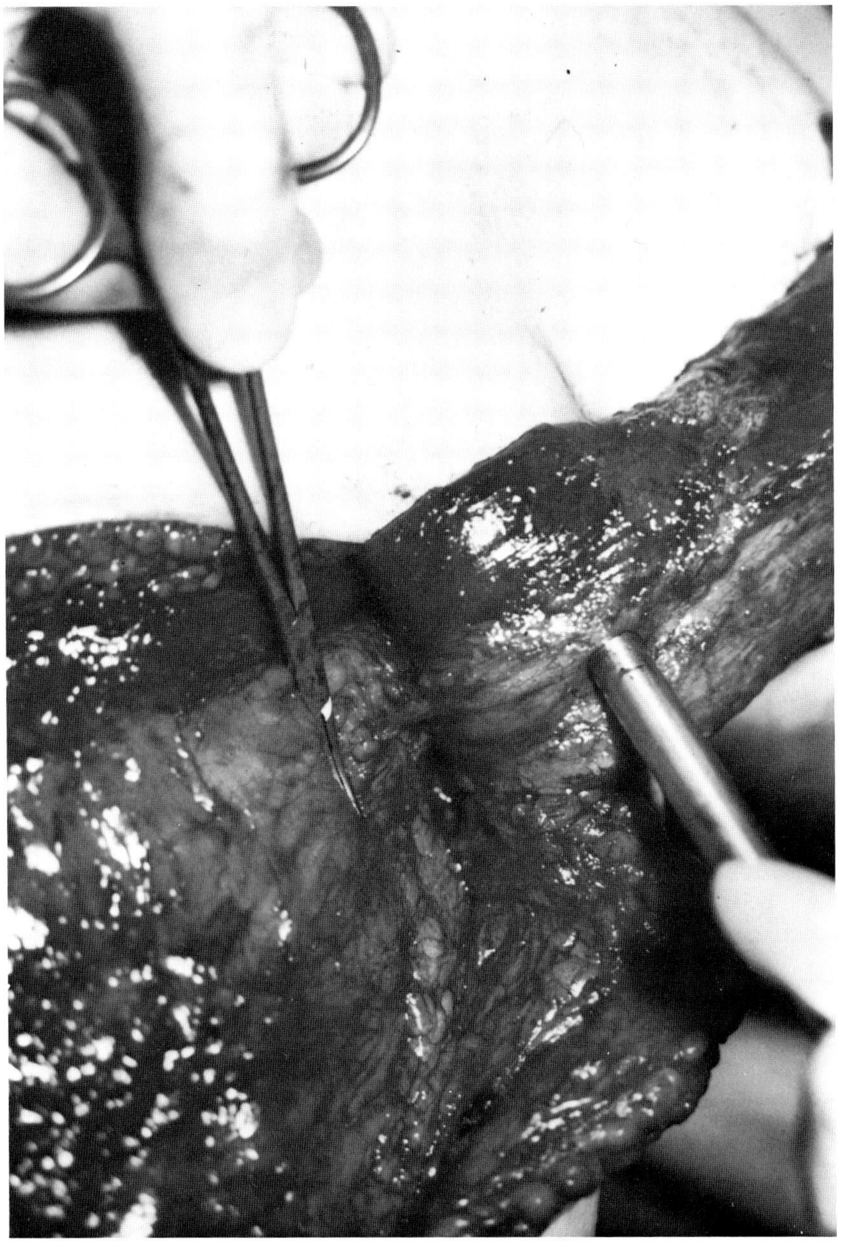

Figure 8.38. As in Figure 8.37.

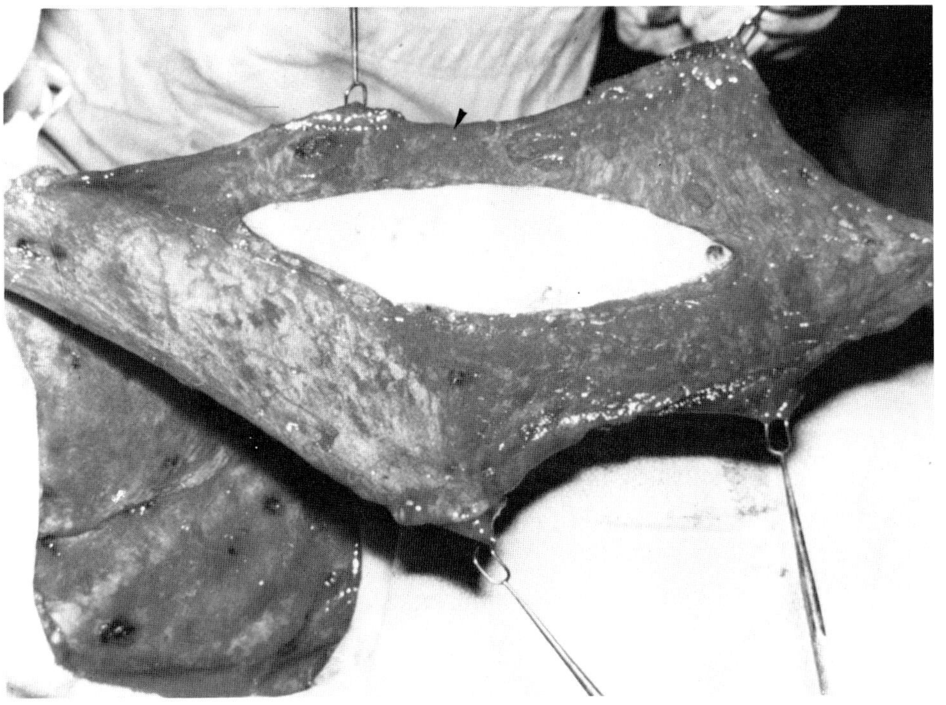

Figure 8.39. Latissimus dorsi musculocutaneous flap freed except from the humeral attachment.

At this point, an incision is made on the anterior chest (Figure 8.35F). This may include the mastectomy scar, or it can be placed independent of the scar if the latter is located too high. The skin is undermined between the chest incision and the posterior incision until a tunnel is developed (Figure 8.33F). The musculocutaneous latissimus dorsi flap can then be passed in a posterior to anterior direction. (Figures 8.35G,H, 8.40, and 8.41). It is important to make the tunnel high in the axilla to prevent the formation of an unsightly lateral bulge. A drain is placed in the posterior wound and brought out through a dependent position; the back wound is then closed.

The muscle skin flap, having passed through the tunnel, can be tacked with temporary sutures to the anterior chest wound while the patient is turned to a supine position. As an alternative, the flap may be placed in a sterile glove while the patient is repositioned and reprepping and redraping of the anterior chest is done. The flap is then inset (Figure 8.42).

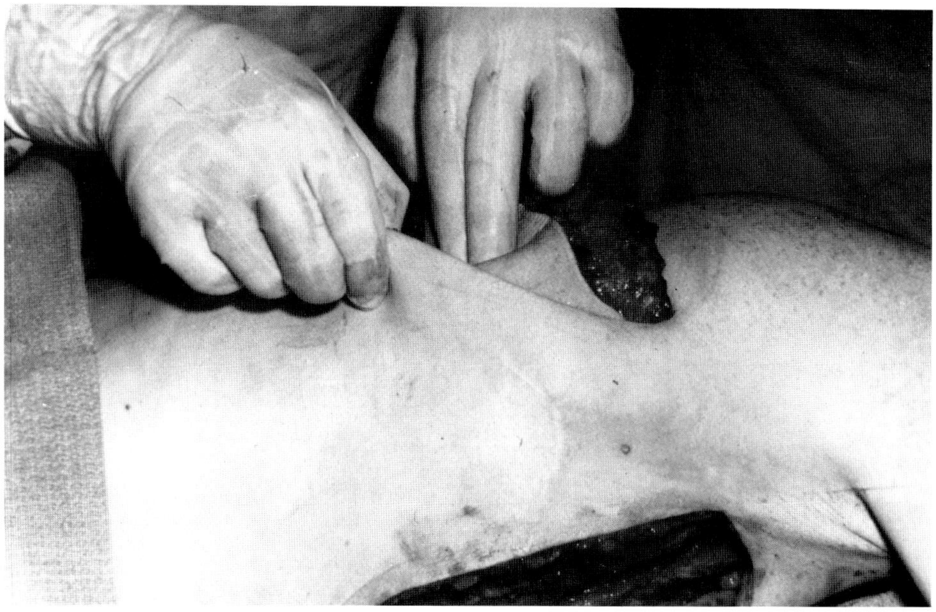

Figure 8.40. Passing the flap front to back through the tunnel into the anterior chest wound.

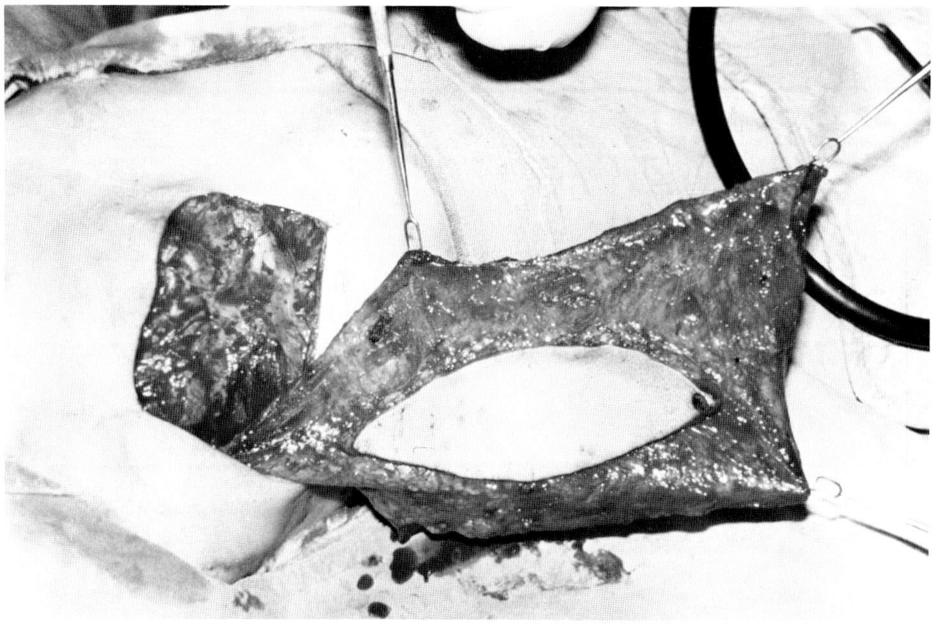

Figure 8.41. Latissimus dorsi musculocutaneous flap after being tunneled through the axilla is demonstrated on the right anterior chest. The excised mastectomy scar has opened up because of tension of the tight chest wall.

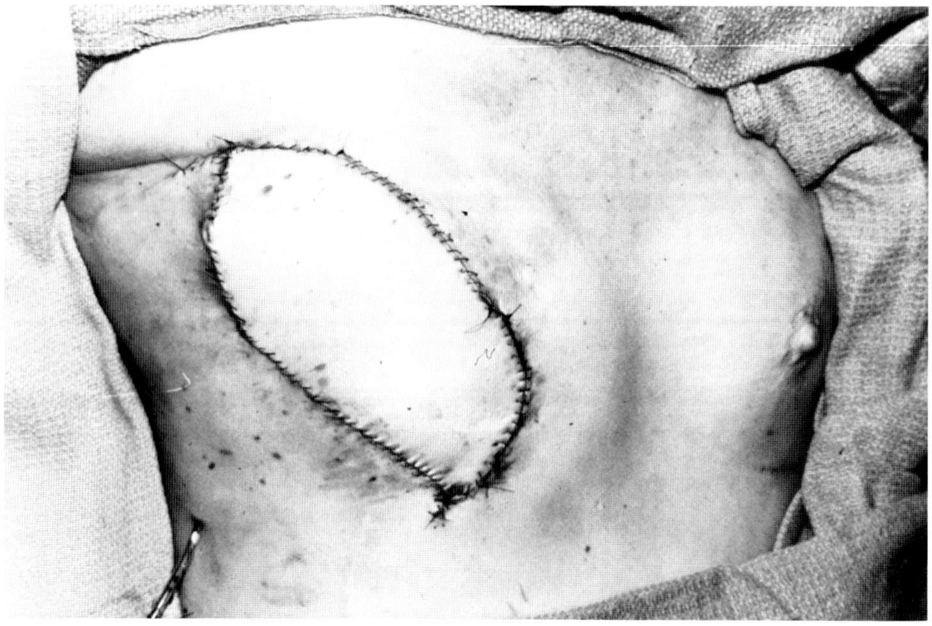

Figure 8.42. Flap inset, with a small silicone implant to match the small contralateral breast.

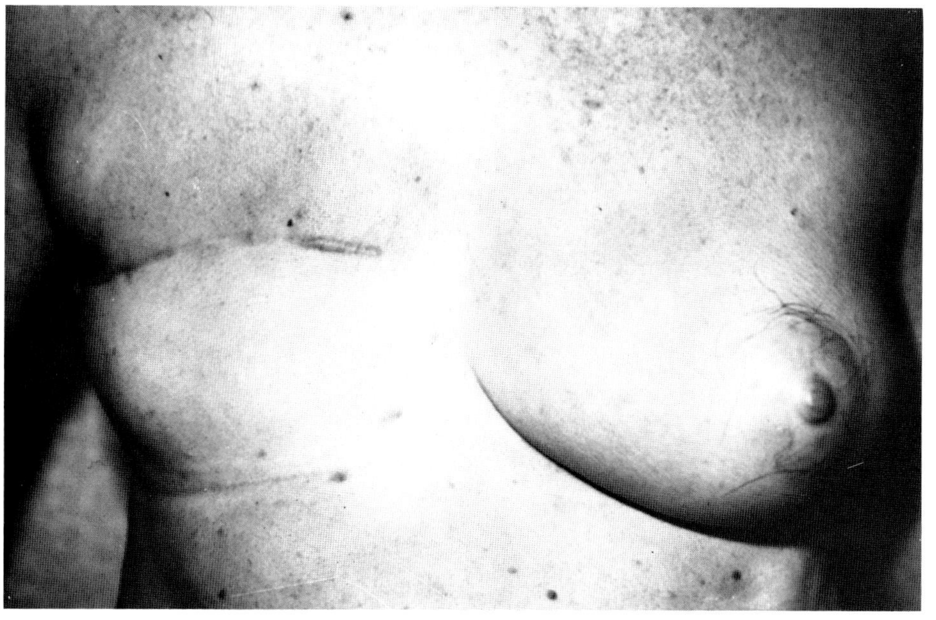

Figure 8.43. Right transverse mastectomy scar.

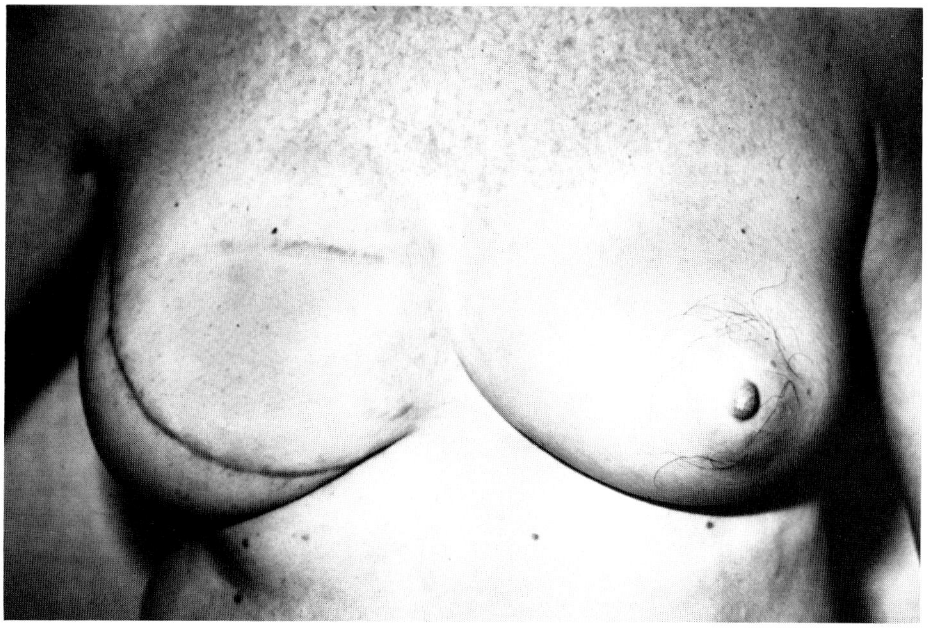

Figure 8.44. Ignoring the transverse mastectomy scar, the skin paddle is inset obliquely downward and medially across the greatest diameter of the breast to produce a hammock effect for the implant.

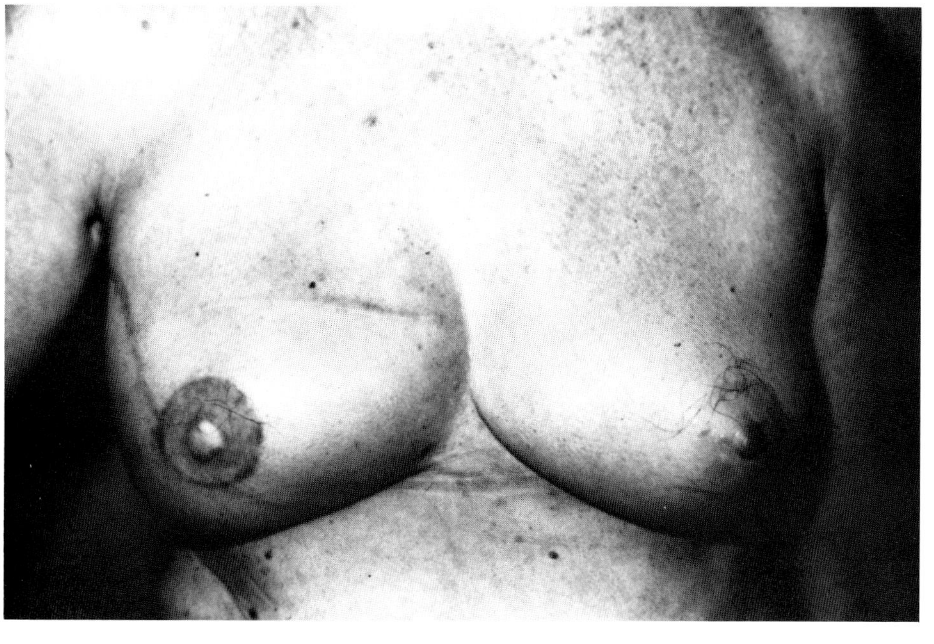

Figure 8.45. The hammock effect, several weeks later, after nipple areola reconstruction, is more evident than in Fig. 8.44.

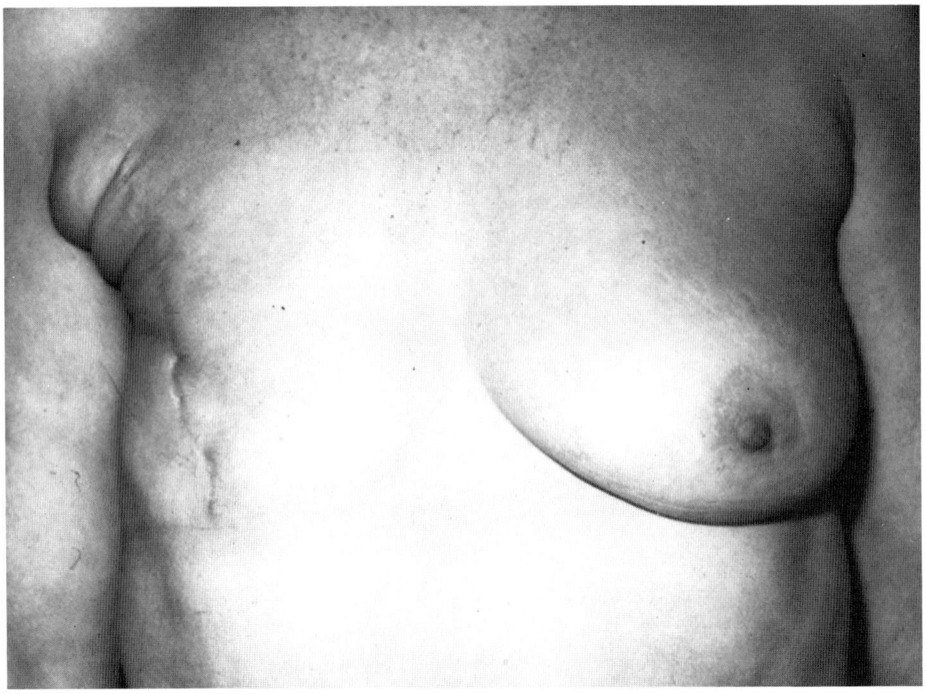

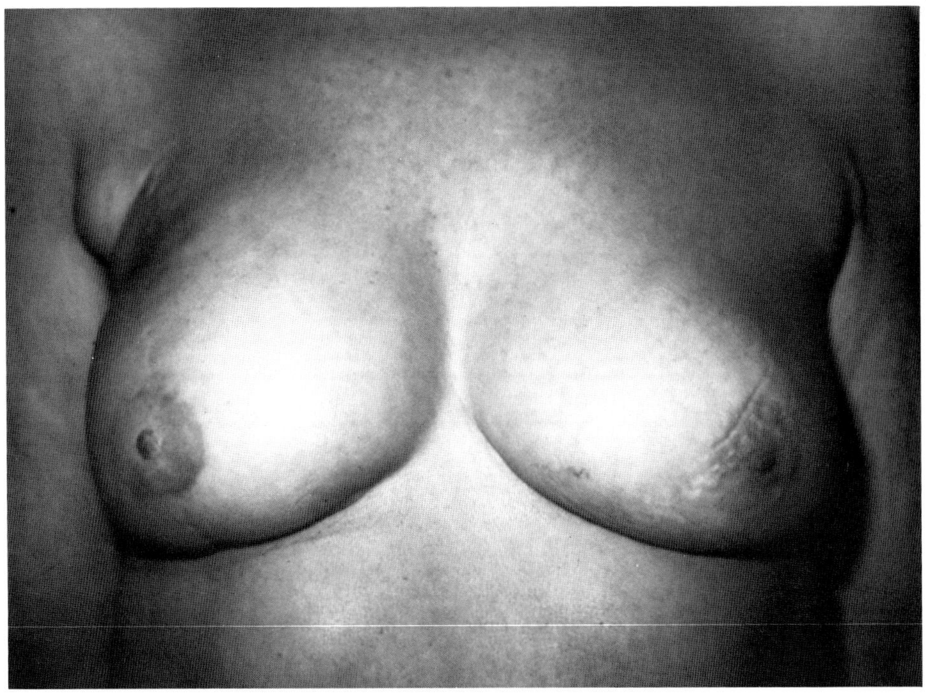

Figure 8.46. **Top:** Right oblique mastectomy scar. **Bottom:** Final reconstruction showing flap inset in the line of the mastectomy scar.

Placement of a Paddle on the Anterior Chest Wall

To achieve the most natural looking breast reconstruction, the skin paddle should be inset obliquely downward and medially across the greatest diameter of the breast, producing a hammock effect. This often means ignoring the mastectomy scar (Figures 8.43–8.45). If the mastectomy scar is oblique, it makes the reconstruction easier (Figures 8.46 and 8.47).

If the anterior chest scar is "bad," being either wide and hypertrophic or very tight and unyielding, a good breast mound shape cannot be obtained unless the "check rein" effect of the scar is removed. In this situation the flap may be inset obliquely by dividing the scar and producing a "Z-plasty effect" (Figures 8.48 and 8.49). Occasionally, high placement of the flap is indicated, e.g., when there is a skin graft with an obvious depression and an unaesthetic appearance high on the chest wall (Figures 8.50 and 8.51).

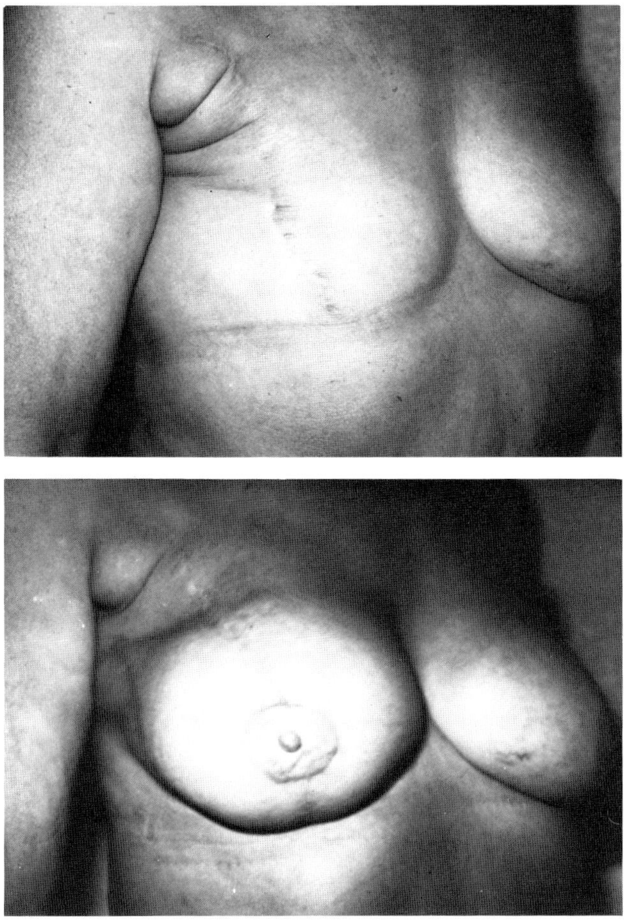

Figure 8.47. Oblique views of the same patient as in Figure 8.46.

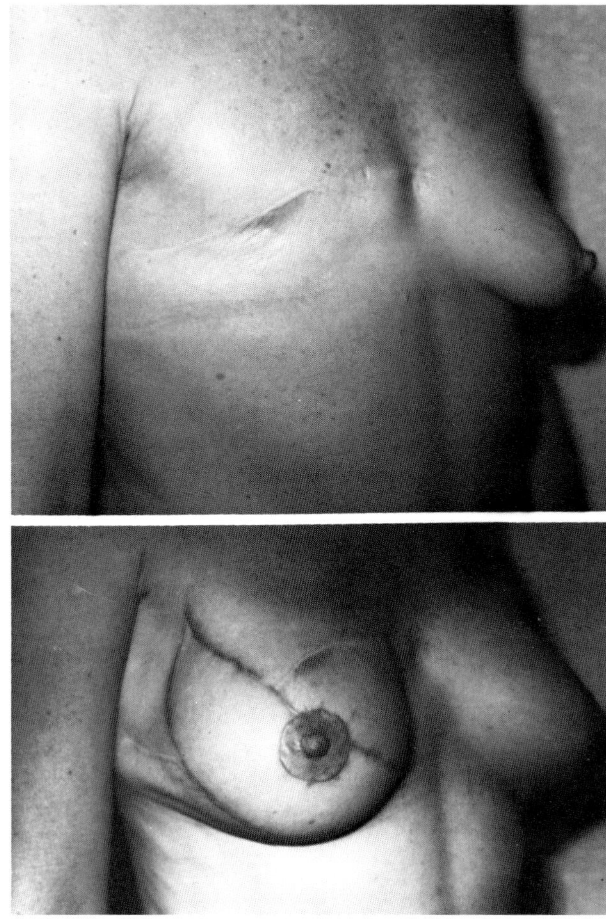

Figure 8.48. **Top:** Tight unyielding right transverse mastectomy scar. **Bottom:** Flap inset obliquely through the scar releases the "check rein" effect. The left breast has been augmented for symmetry.

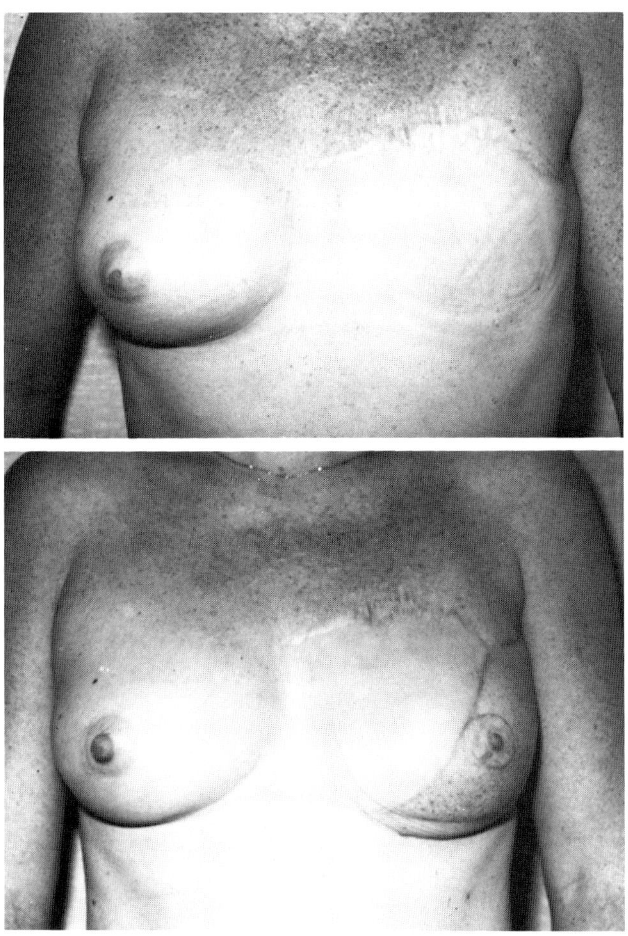

Figure 8.49. **Top:** Wide tight left transverse mastectomy scar. **Bottom:** Flap inset obliquely through the scar releases tightness. The freckled appearance of the flap is less noticeable in this position than if placed in the transverse mastectomy scar.

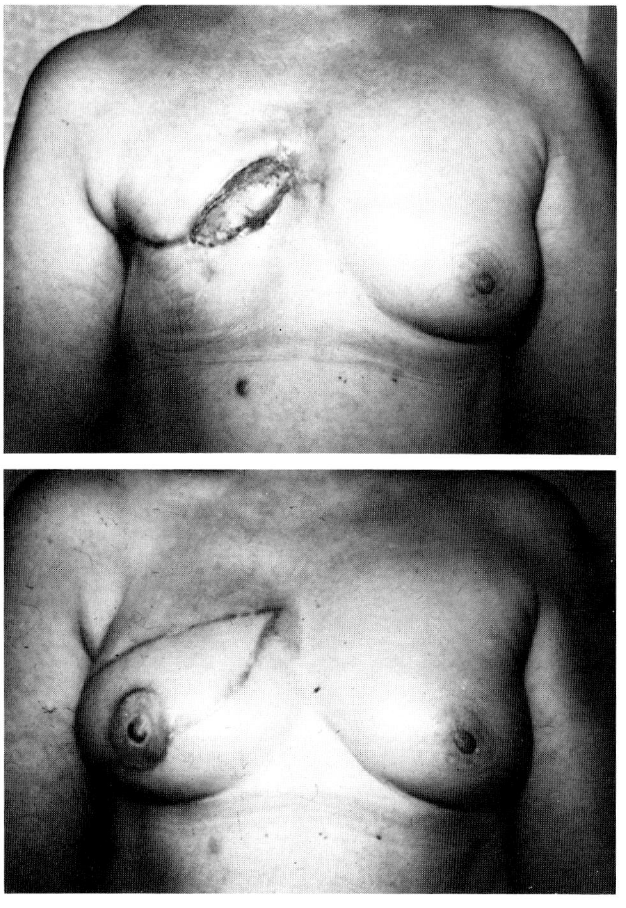

Figure 8.50. **Top:** Right mastectomy deformity with unaesthetic depressed skin graft high on the chest wall. **Bottom:** It is necessary to excise the skin graft and inset the flap in the high position in order to get a satisfactory result.

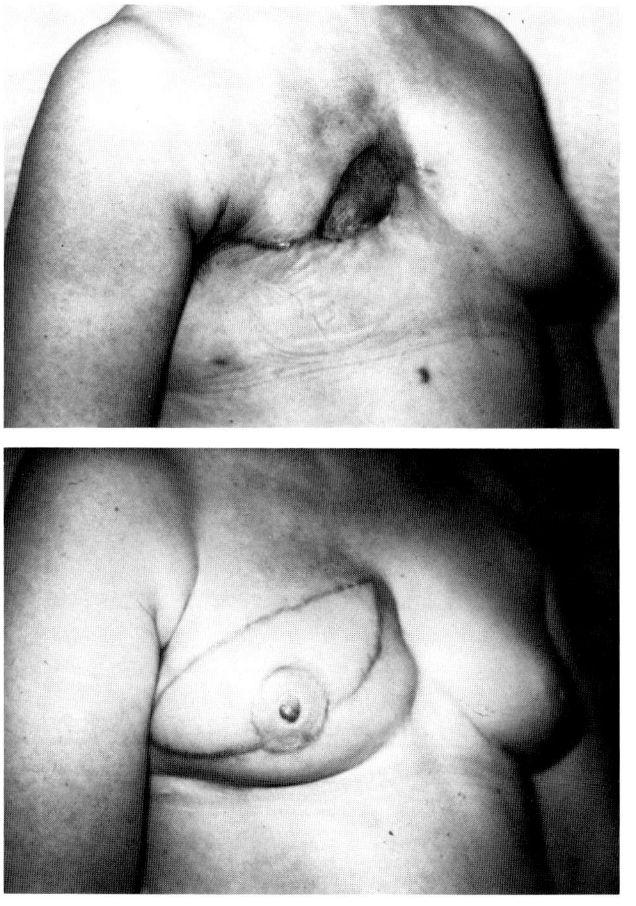

Figure 8.51. Oblique view of the patient in Figure 8.50.

Recreating the Anterior Axillary Fold

In the classic radical mastectomy, the most obvious postoperative deformity is the marked anterior axillary fold extending to the chest wall and the associated deep depression underneath the clavicle (Figure 8.52A). This can be corrected to a greater or lesser degree with the use of the muscular pedicle of the latissimus dorsi flap. The flap can be made into a neurovascular island by detaching the humeral head. The detached head can then be brought anteriorly and sewn to the fascia around the pectoralis major muscle stump or the coracoid process (Figure 8.52C). However, a simpler and probably more effective way is to double the pedicle on itself (Figures 8.52B and 8.54).

With a radical mastectomy, the anterior chest skin is undermined medially to the sternum, superiorly to the clavicle, and inferiorly to 0.5 inch below the proposed inframammary crease. The latissimus dorsi muscle is then sutured to the periosteum of the sternum and the clavicle (Figures 8.53 and 8.55).

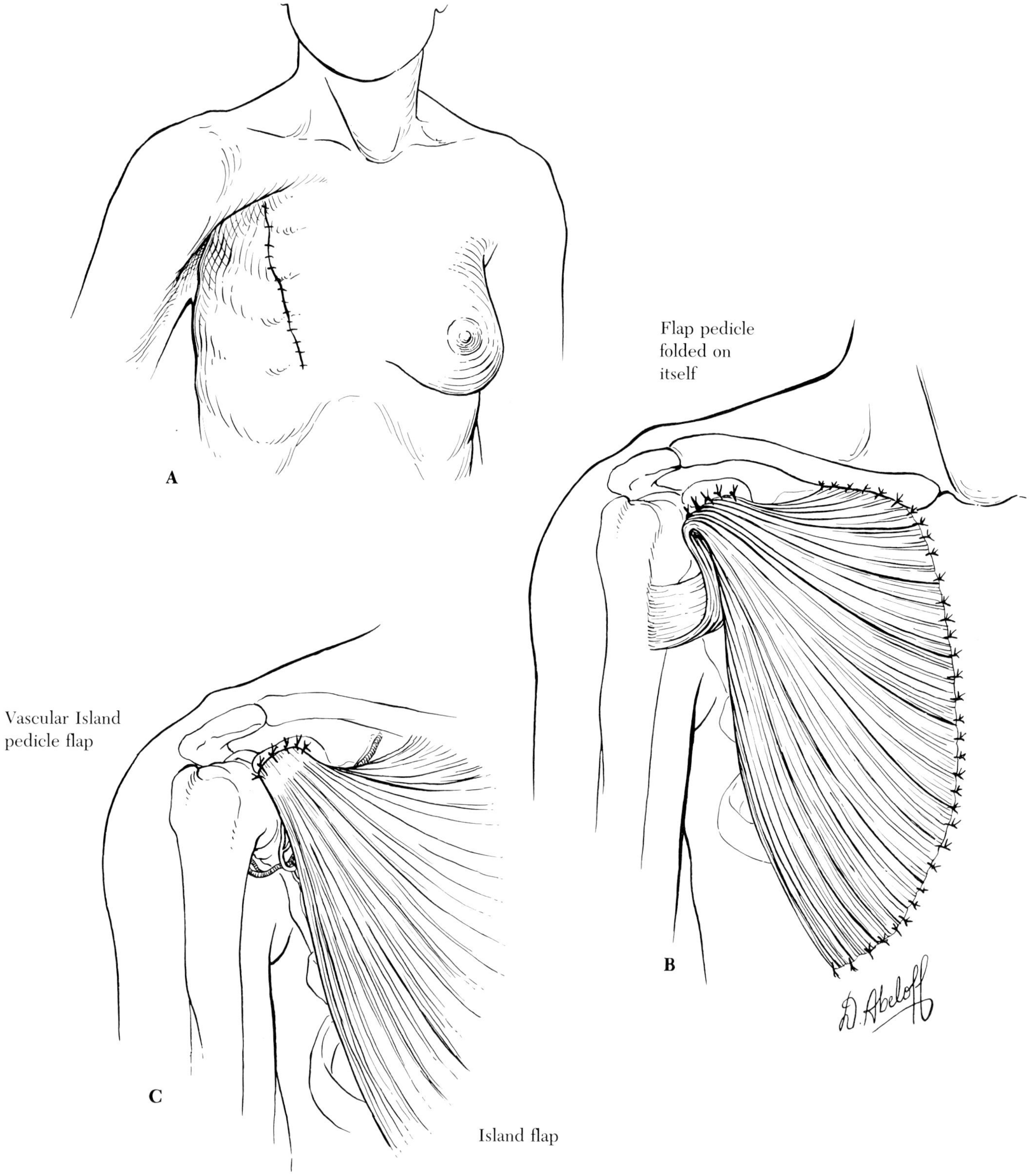

Figure 8.52. **A:** Typical deformity resulting from a classic radical mastectomy. **B:** Pedicle of the latissimus muscle doubled on itself and attached to the coracoid process. **C:** Detached humeral head of the latissimus muscle sutured to the coracoid process.

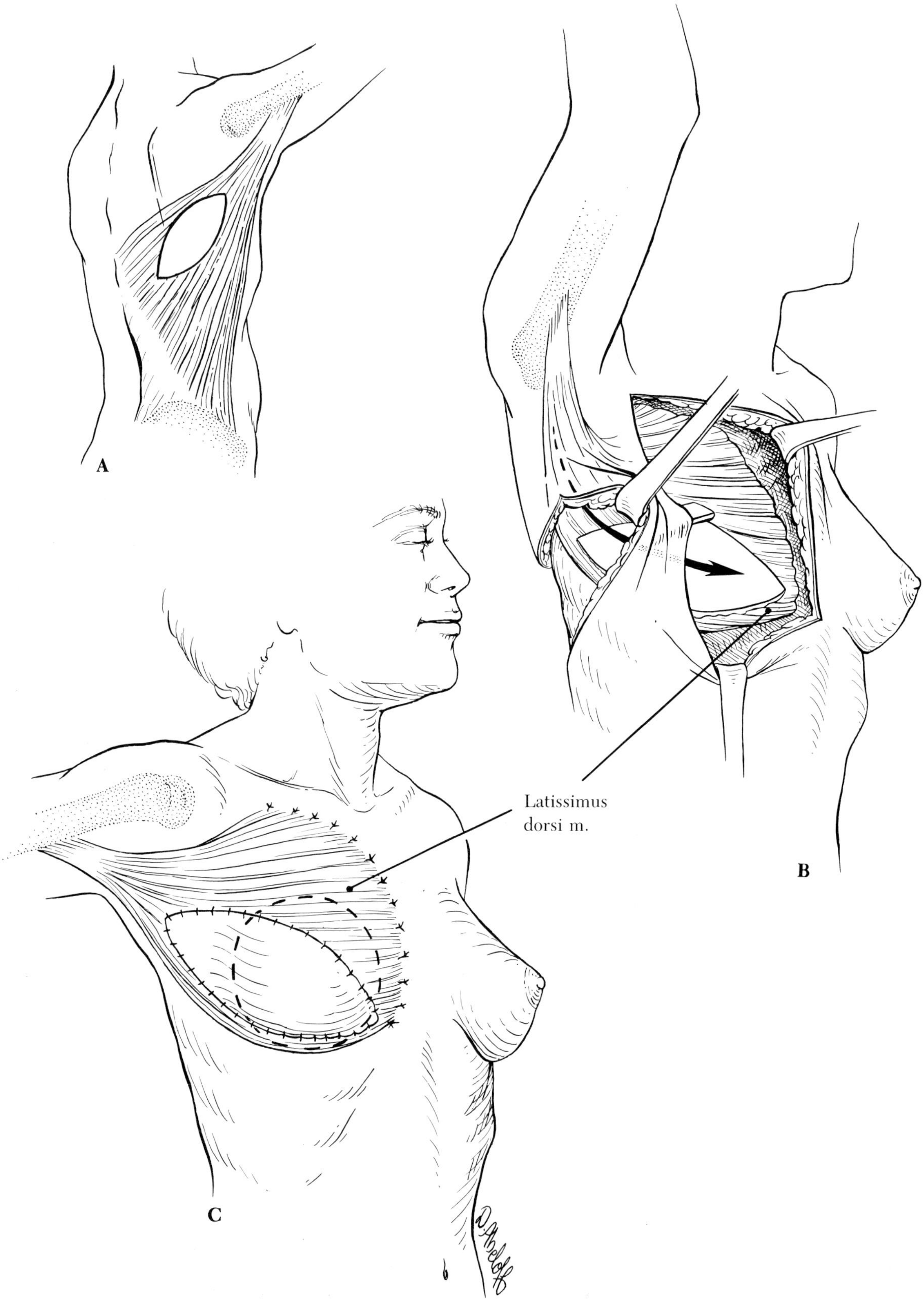

Figure 8.53. Reconstruction of a radical mastectomy defect using the latissimus dorsi musculocutaneous flap. **A:** Note the position of the skin paddle toward the posterior edge of the muscle, leaving a large amount of muscle anteriorly. **B:** Flap passed through a tunnel in the axilla. **C:** Muscle sutured to fascia over the medial half of the clavicle and the lateral edge of the sternum. A skin paddle is inset with the implant in place.

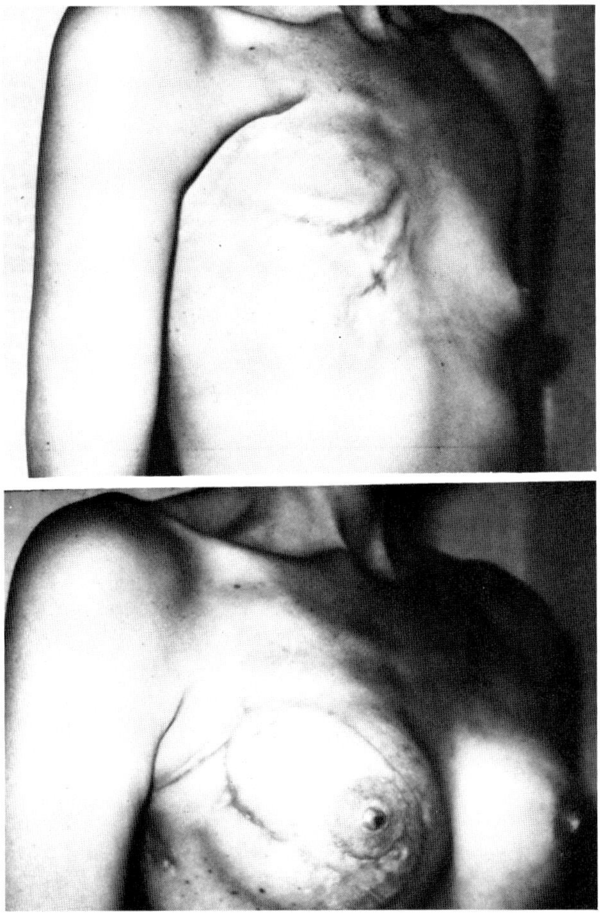

Figure 8.54. **Top:** Right radical mastectomy showing a fold from the axilla and the depression underneath. **Bottom:** Postoperative result with axillary deformity corrected by the latissimus muscle folded on itself and sutured to the coracoid process. The left breast is reconstructed following a subcutaneous mastectomy.

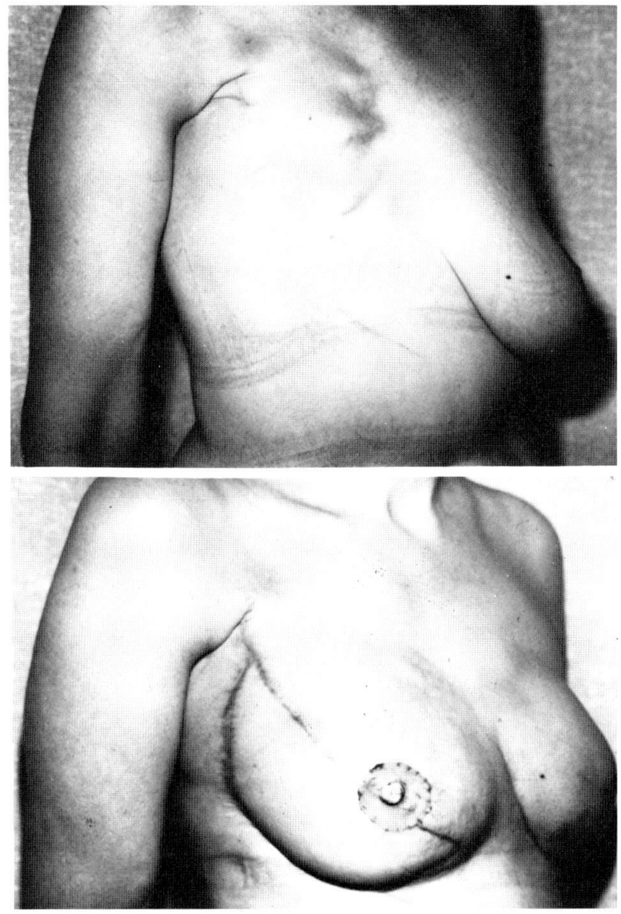

Figure 8.55. **Top:** Right radical mastectomy defect with a prominent rib cage. **Bottom:** Right breast reconstruction using a latissimus dorsi musculocutaneous flap with a large amount of muscle anteriorly to cover the rib cage and a silicone gel implant. The left breast is seen following subcutaneous mastectomy, a skin envelope reduction, and a subpectoral implant.

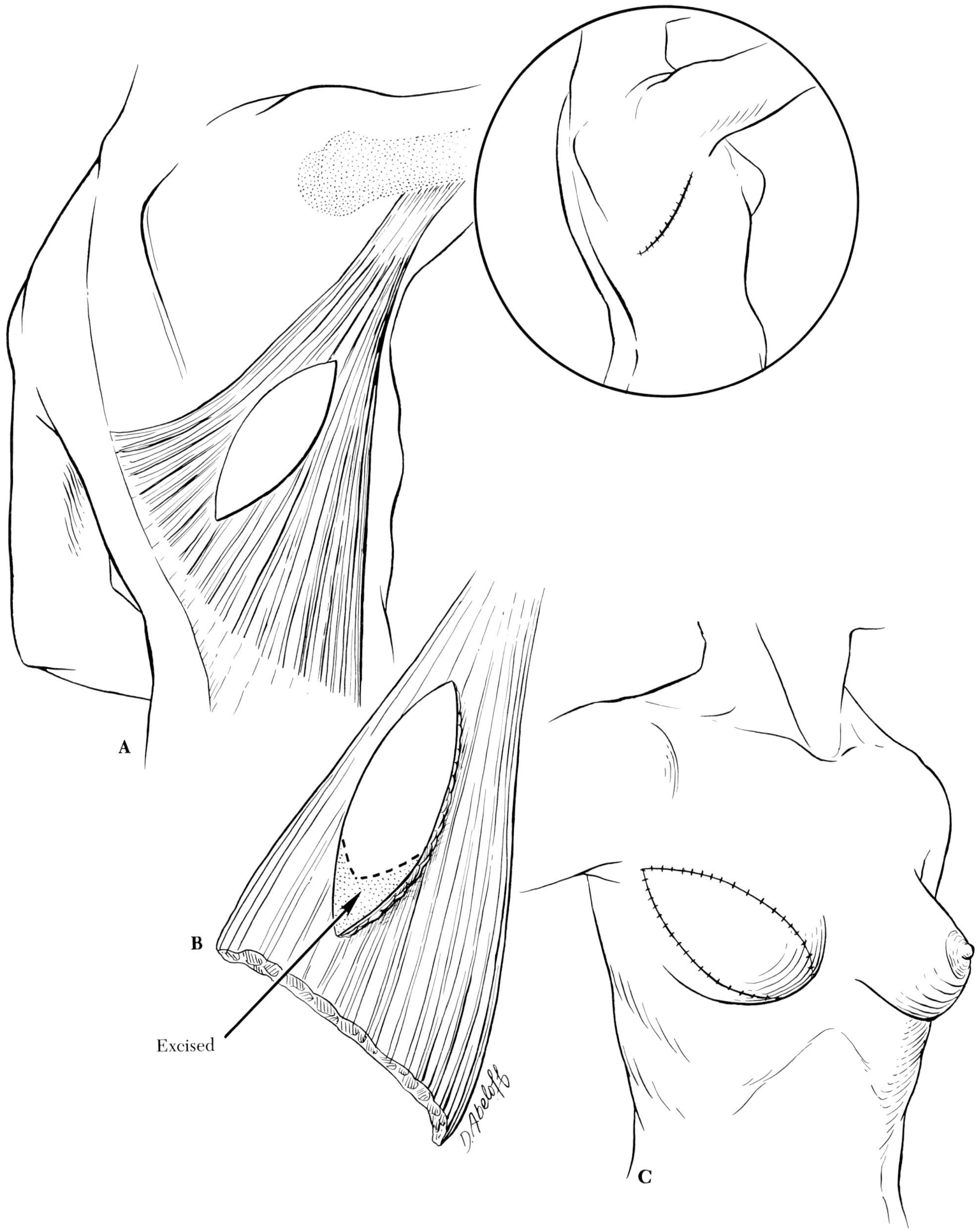

Figure 8.56. **A:** Elliptical shape of the paddle allows a straight line closure without a "dog ear" deformity. **B:** The inferior end of the paddle is truncated by excising the stippled area. **C:** When inset the blunt truncated inferior end produces a fullness in the skin envelope that allows a ptotic appearance to develop.

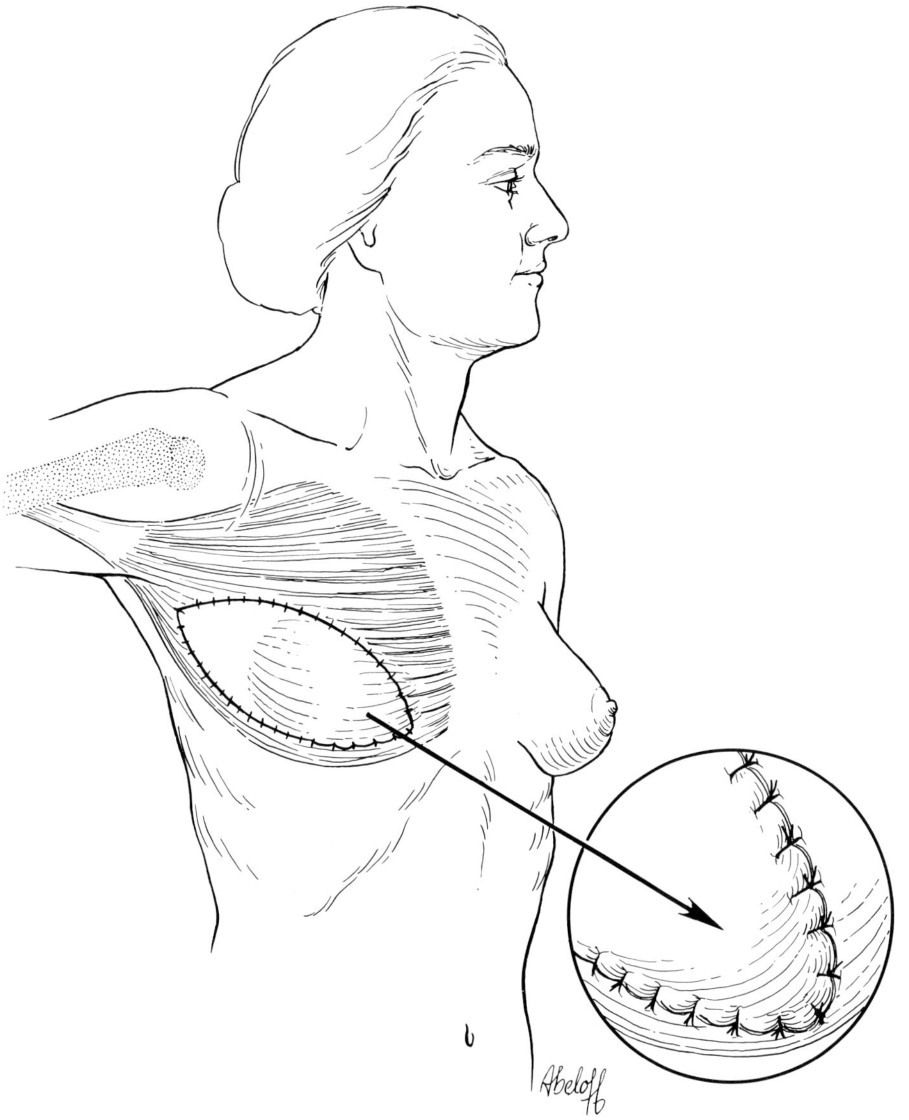

Figure 8.57. The length of the paddle is made somewhat longer than the chest wound. When the paddle is inset, the inferior end can be puckered to produce a fullness.

Obtaining Ptosis

A natural looking reconstructed breast usually has some degree of ptosis. Apart from placing a crescent-shaped flap in the inframammary crease, the following techniques also help to obtain the ptotic effect. 1) The paddle may be truncated (Figure 8.56) to allow greater fullness in the inferior part of the breast mound. 2) The paddle may be puckered by sutures to produce a fullness inferiorly (Figure 8.57). 3) A series of W-plasties may be created inferiorly on the skin paddle and a series of cuts made on the inferior chest wall flap (Figure 8.58A,B) to coincide with the W-plasties when the flap is inset (Figures 8.57C,D, 8.59, and 8.60).

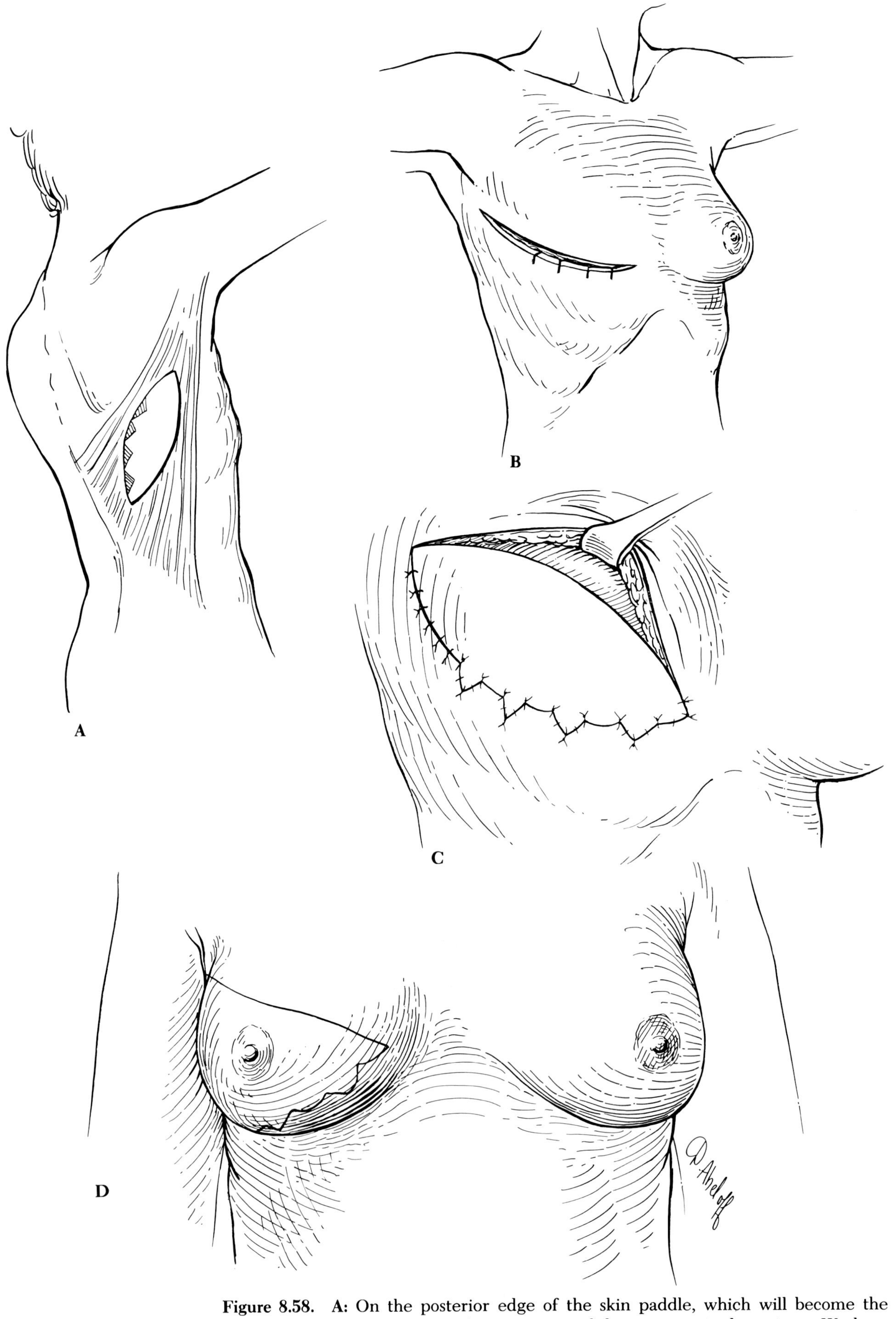

Figure 8.58. **A:** On the posterior edge of the skin paddle, which will become the inferior edge on the anterior chest, a series of darts are excised to give a W-plasty appearance. **B:** A number of small relaxing incisions are made on the inferior chest flap to coincide with the apices on the paddle. **C:** Insetting flap. **D:** Ptosis of the flap develops inferiorly.

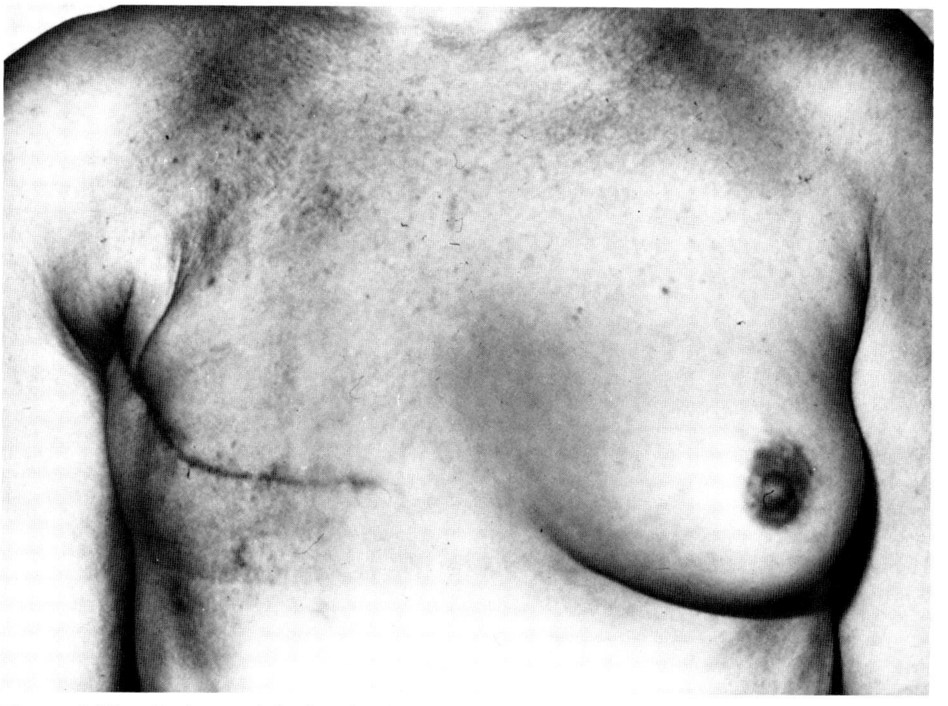

Figure 8.59. Right modified radical mastectomy with a tight mastectomy scar. Chest wall inferior to the scar did not relax after the mastectomy scar was excised.

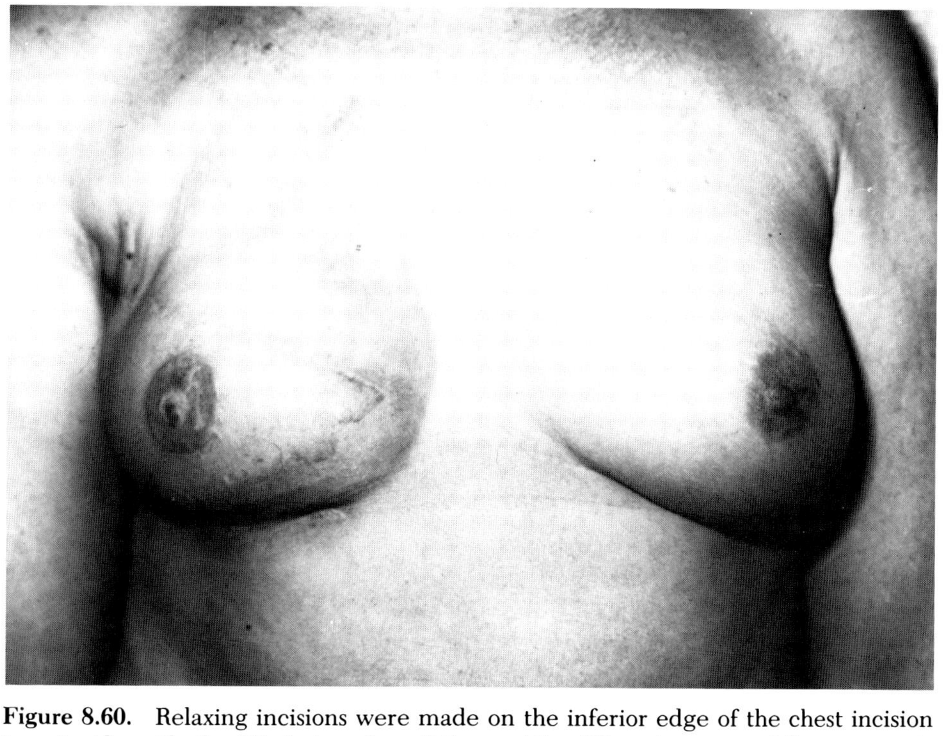

Figure 8.60. Relaxing incisions were made on the inferior edge of the chest incision to coincide with the W-plasty edge of the paddle. When inset a satisfactory ptotic breast shape developed.

Position of the Implant

Before the skin paddle is sutured into position laterally, a silicone prosthesis, commensurate with the size of the other breast or at least compatible with the patient's height and configuration, is inserted beneath the latissimus muscle (Figure 8.61). Because there is a tendency in the reconstructed breast for the implant to "ride up" during the process of healing, the pocket for the implant is dissected approximately 0.5 inch below the level of the contralateral inframammary crease. This should result in the final location of the implant at the correct level.

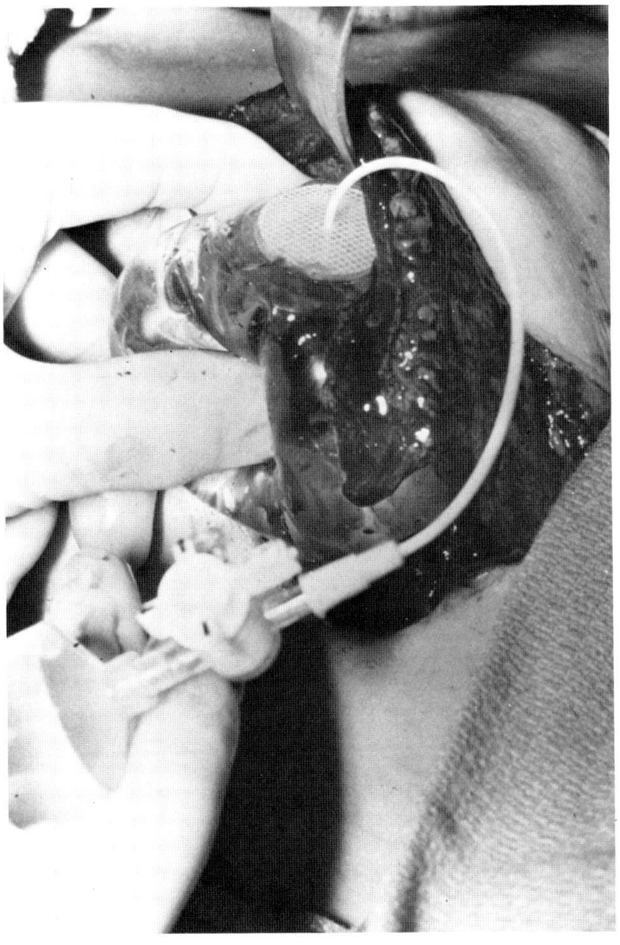

Figure 8.61. A bilumen style implant, with a catheter in place through the self-sealing valve, is placed under the flap for a trial of size. Isotonic sterile saline can be added or subtracted to match the size of the contralateral breast. The implant is then removed, the catheter withdrawn, and the implant reinserted with the valve facing posteriorly.

The lateral edge of the latissimus muscle is then sutured to the lateral chest wall, usually to the serratus muscle, to prevent the prosthesis from falling laterally. The inferior edge of the muscle is attached to the chest wall at the lower level of dissection. Final closure of the skin flap is then performed. As in the back, wound drains are inserted.

With the modified radical mastectomy, the superior edge of the transferred latissimus muscle flap is sewn to the inferior edge of the pectoralis muscle (Figure 8.62B). A subpectoral pocket is then developed, and the prosthesis is inserted behind the combined muscle flap. The inferior edge of the transposed latissimus muscle can sometimes be turned up to form a hammock in which the prosthesis lies. Final skin closure is performed to reconstruct the breast mound.

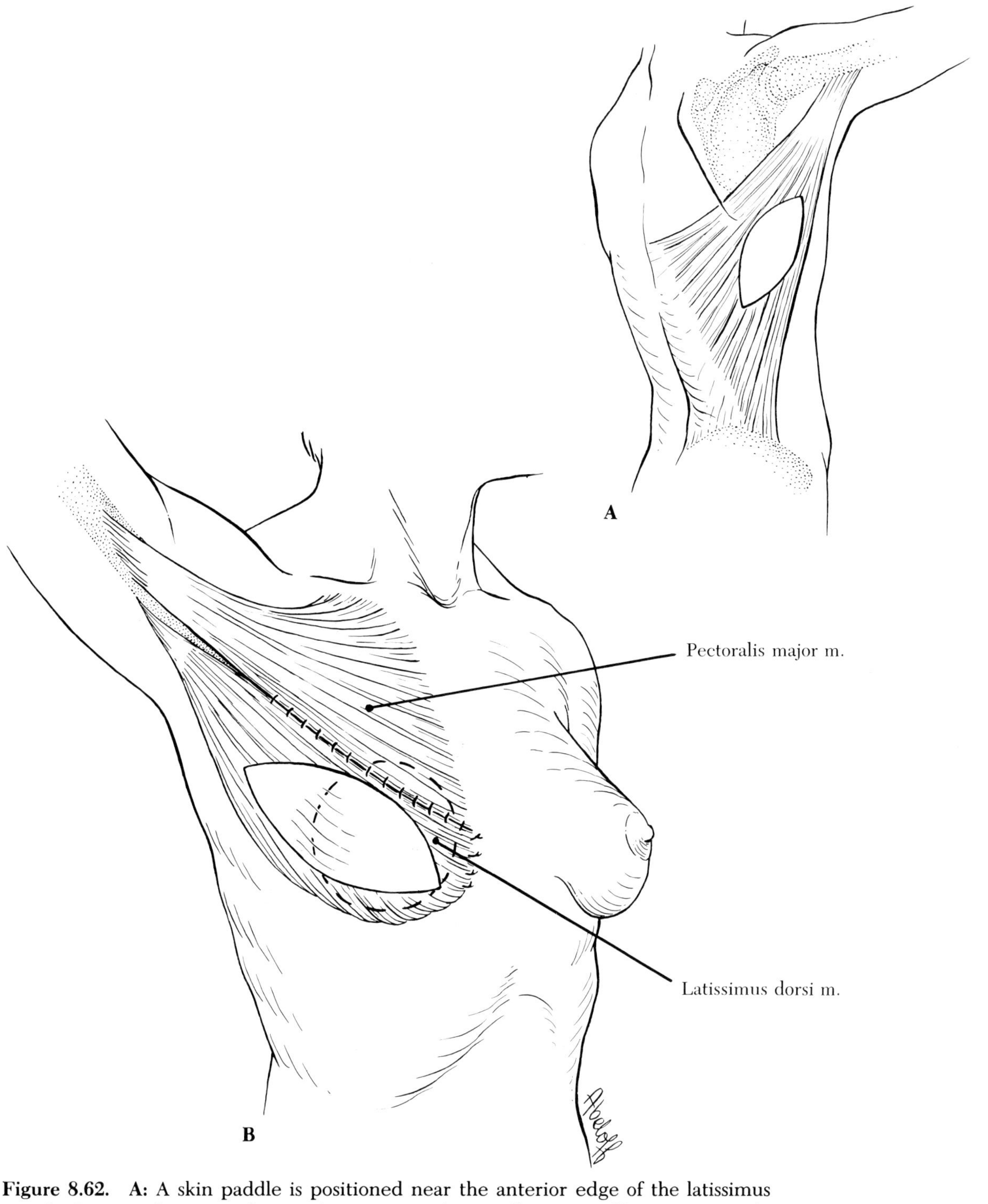

Figure 8.62. A: A skin paddle is positioned near the anterior edge of the latissimus muscle. Because the pectoralis muscle is intact, only a small amount of latissimus muscle is required. **B:** The superior edge of the latissimus flap is sutured to the inferior edge of the pectoralis muscle. A subpectoral pocket is developed, and the implant is inserted behind the combined muscle flap.

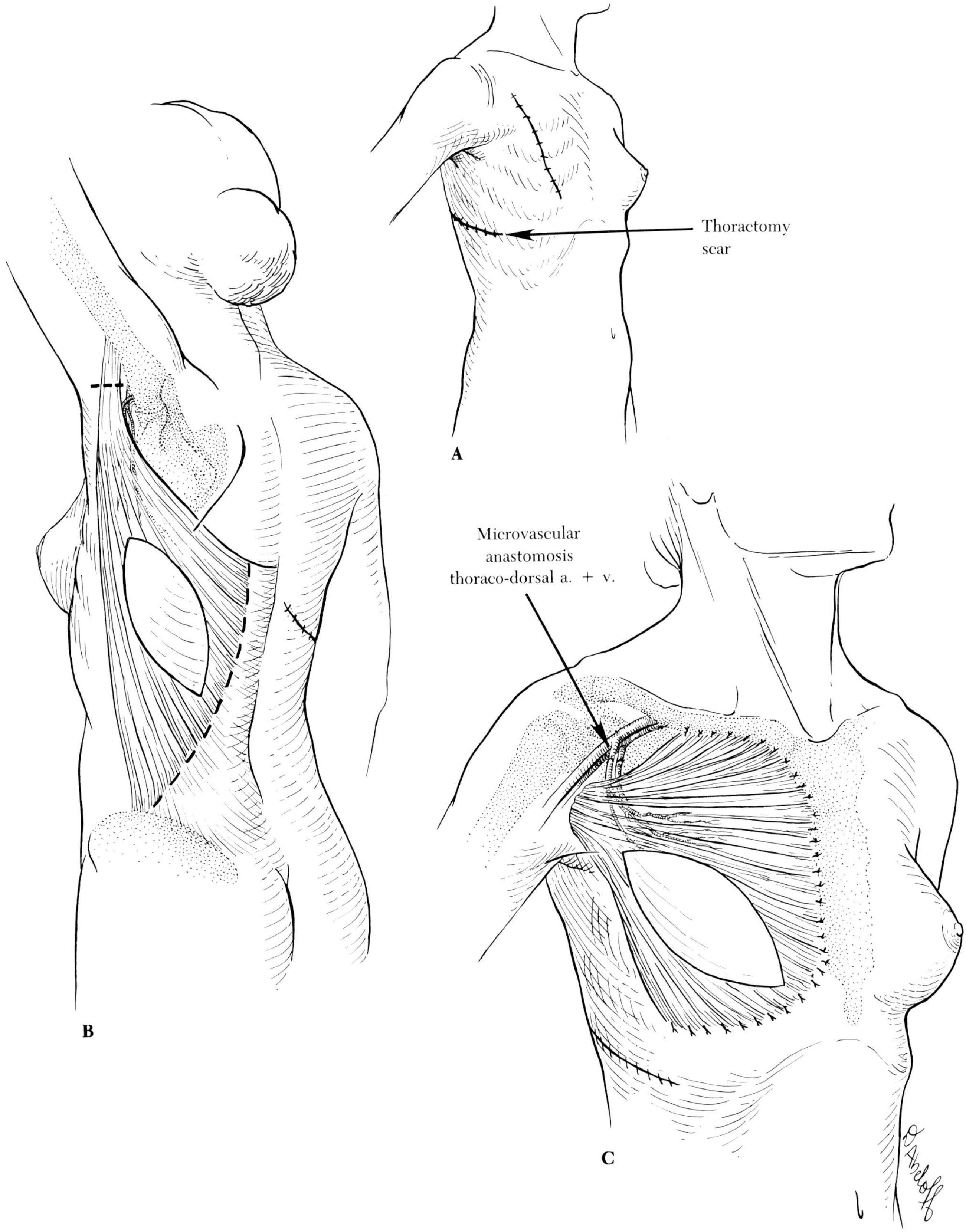

Figure 8.63. **A:** Right radical mastectomy with ipsilateral thoracotomy scar. **B:** Proposed free flap from the left side. **C:** A left latissimus dorsi musculocutaneous flap is inset to correct the right radical mastectomy defect after microvascular anastomosis of the thoracodorsal arteries and veins.

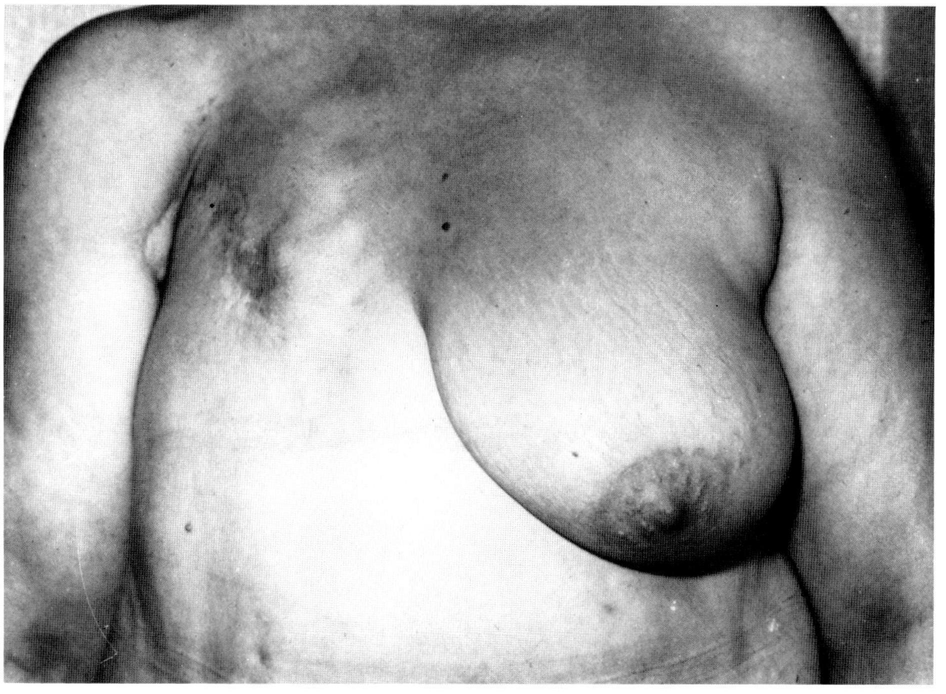

Figure 8.64. AP view of a right radical mastectomy defect.

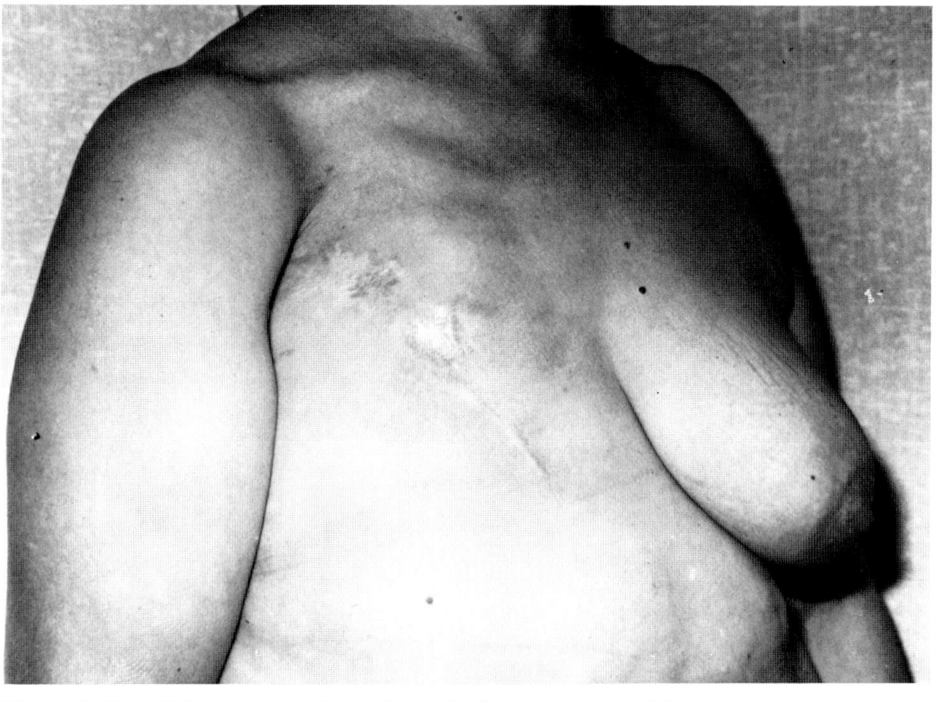

Figure 8.65. Oblique view of a right radical mastectomy defect.

Free Flaps

Occasionally, patients seek reconstruction who have undergone a radical mastectomy as well as an associated ipsilateral thoracotomy which has transected the latissimus dorsi muscle (Figures 8.63A, 8.64–8.66). This prohibits use of the latissimus dorsi muscle from the same side because of the scar.

One solution is to use a contralateral latissimus dorsi musculocutaneous flap, as a free flap (3,5,6,13,14) (Figure 8.63B,C). The thoracodorsal artery on the left latissimus dorsi musculocutaneous free flap was anastomosed by microvascular technique to the thoracodorsal artery on the mastectomy side on the right; the veins were similarly anastomosed. The muscle was sutured to the clavicular and sternal periosteum (Figures 8.67–8.69). Another latissimus dorsi free flap, for the same indication, is shown in Figures 8.70–8.72 .

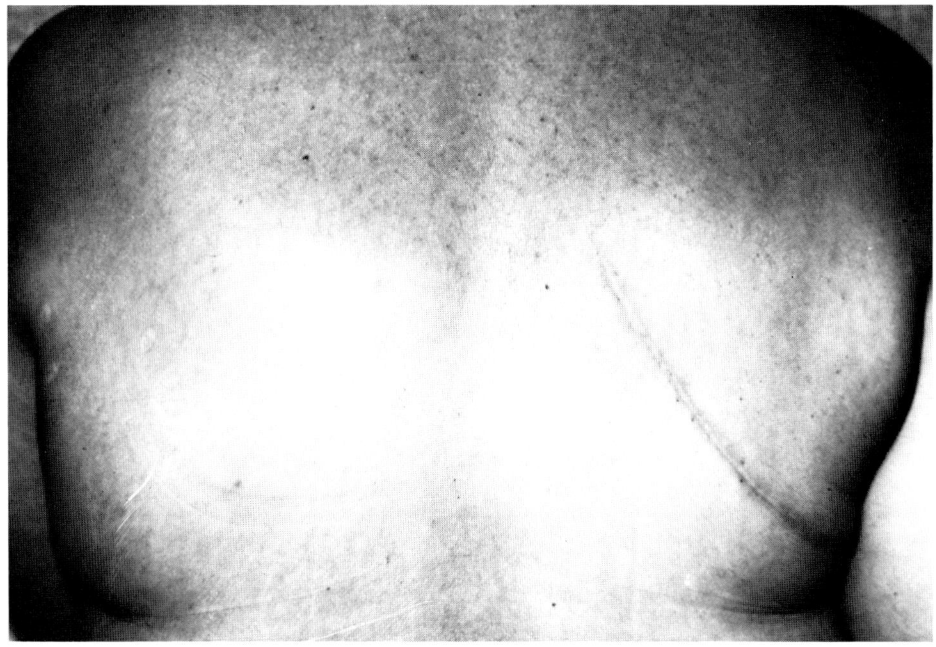

Figure 8.66. Right posterior thoracotomy scar on the same patient as in Figures 8.62 and 8.63.

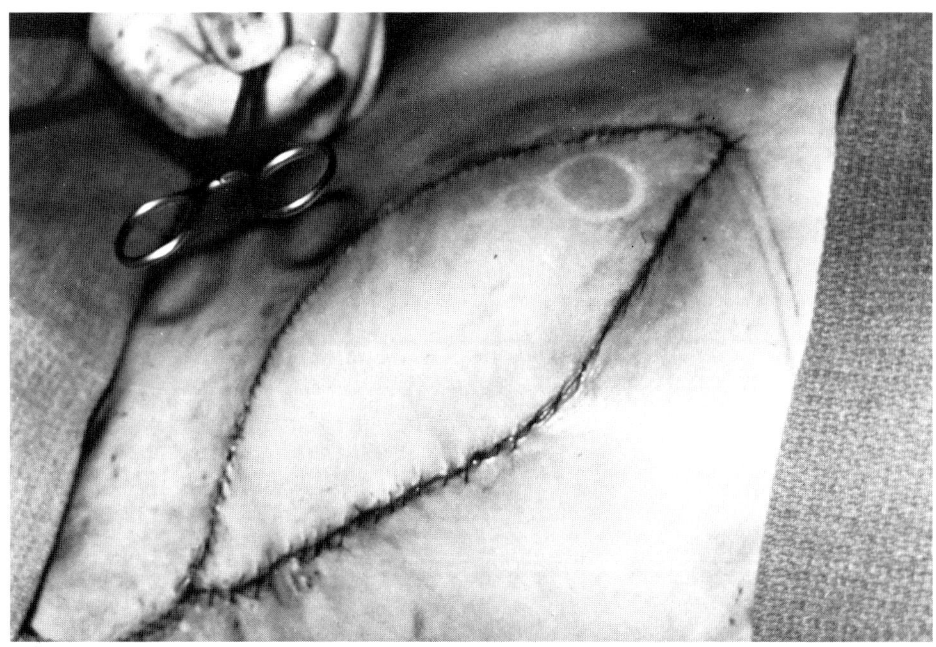

Figure 8.67. Blanch test performed on the free flap.

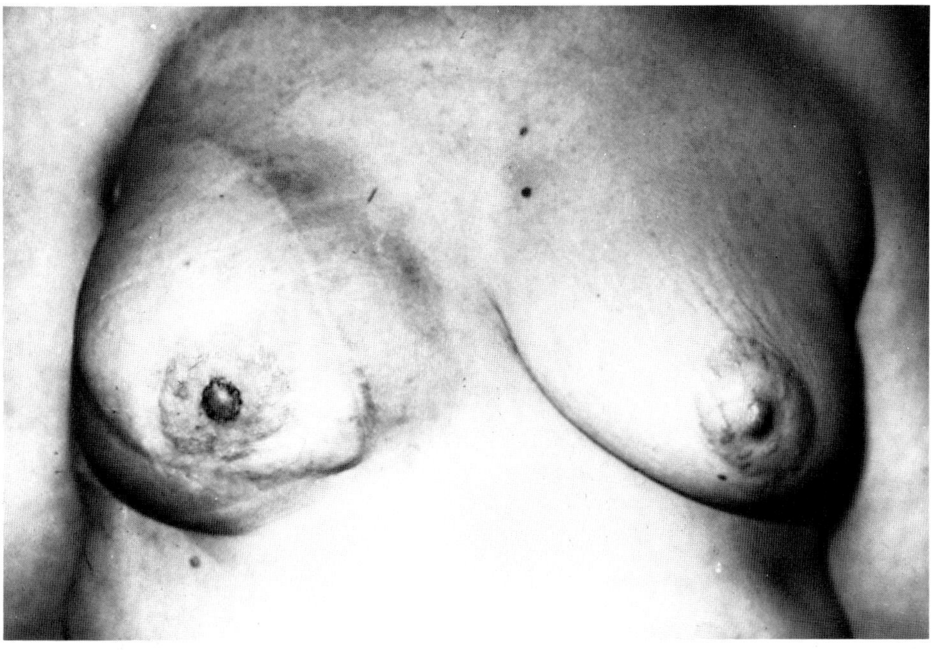

Figure 8.68. AP view of the postoperative result, latissimus dorsi musculocutaneous free flap.

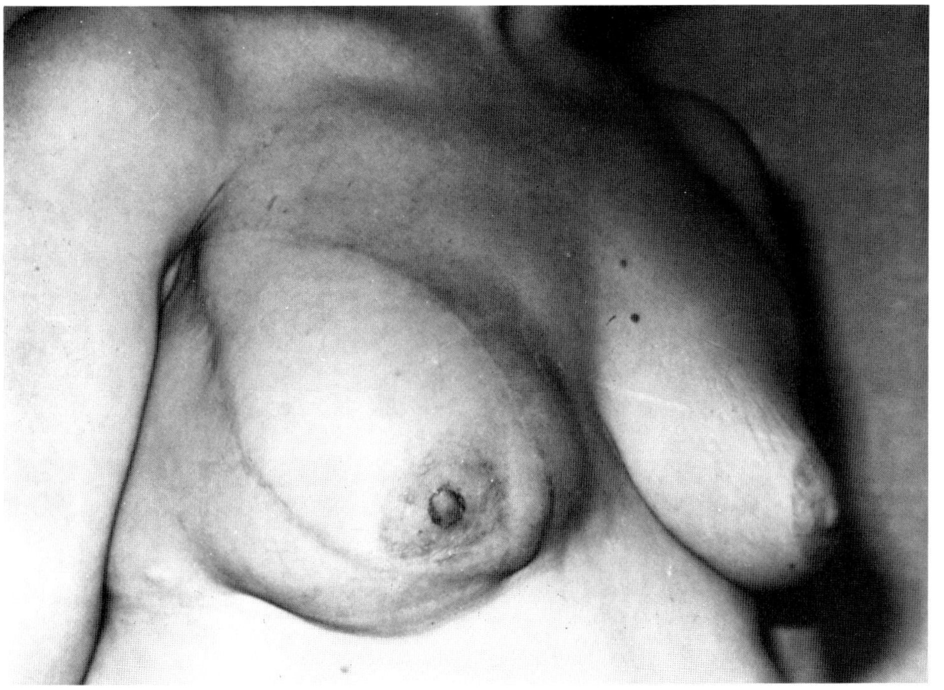

Figure 8.69. Oblique view of the postoperative result in the patient in Figure 8.66.

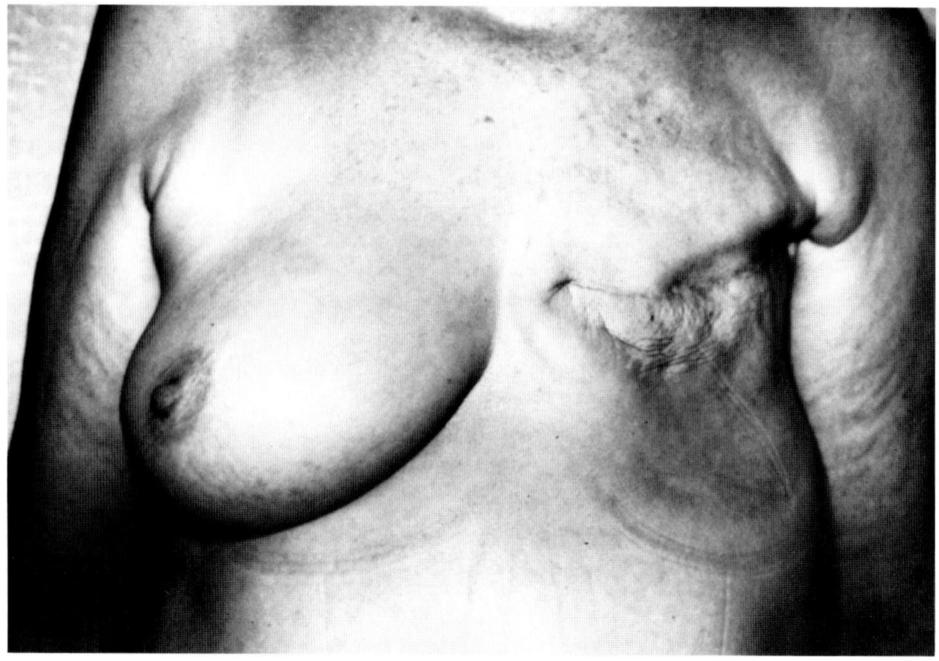

Figure 8.70. AP view of a left mastectomy defect.

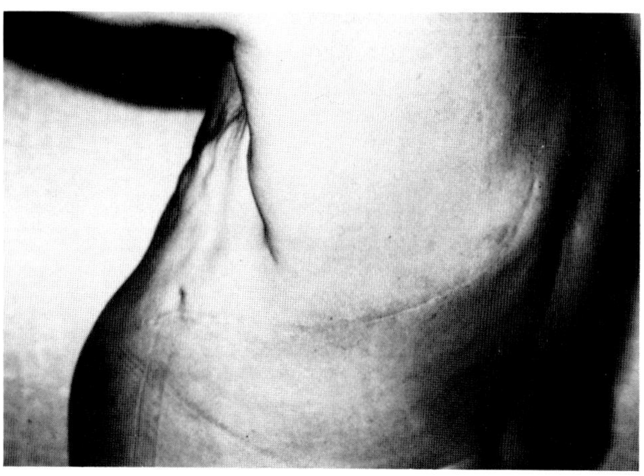

Figure 8.71. Left posterior thoracotomy scar.

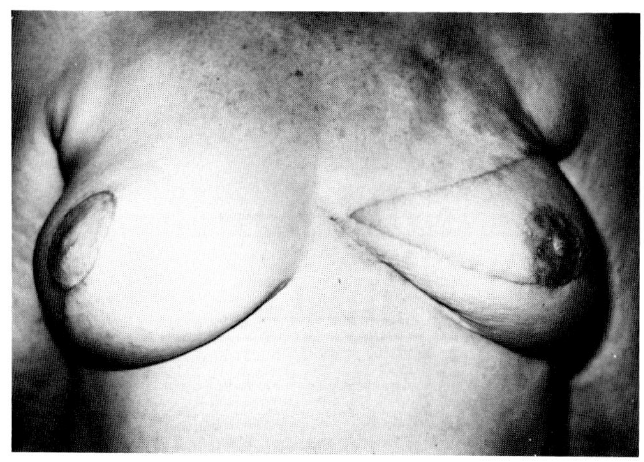

Figure 8.72. AP postoperative view of a latissimus dorsi musculocutaneous free flap.

Today the transverse abdominal island flap or the vertical rectus abdominus musculocutaneous flap seems to offer a more suitable solution to this particular problem (4).

Modification of the Latissimus Dorsi Musculocutaneous Flap

James J. Ryan

The Ryan modification of the foregoing procedures locates the skin pedicle in the midlateral chest area and transposes the skin muscle flap as a pedicle instead of an island. In a modified radical mastectomy a small amount of muscle is taken, whereas in the more radical procedure the whole of the muscle is taken with the flap. When reconstructing a radical mastectomy by this technique, the trailing muscle is folded on itself under the skin flap and can be brought superior to it (Figures 8.73–8.75).

Three problems are avoided with this modification. First, there is usually marked disparity in thickness and pigmentation between back skin and breast skin, whereas the thickness and color of the lateral chest skin very closely matches that of the ventral body skin. Second, a back donor site is an extensor and working surface of the trunk and has a limited amount of skin that can be removed and closed primarily. A neutral midlateral site facilitates primary closure and is camouflaged easily by almost all clothing as well as by the arm in its resting position. Third, intraoperative positional change for the patient, particularly if bilateral breast surgery is to be carried out in a modified mastectomy patient in the same operative stage, can be avoided by a midlateral rather than a back donor site.

Postoperative Complications of Latissimus Dorsi Musculocutaneous Flap

Incorrect Sizing and Positioning of the Implant

It is not unusual to discover a few weeks postoperatively that the size and/or position of the prosthesis is incorrect. A secondary procedure is indicated if the error is markedly noticeable and disturbing to the patient. An adjustment can often be made at the second stage when the nipple-areola complex is reconstructed.

It is not difficult to correct the size of the implant, and lowering a "too high" implant is also relatively easy. The inferior healed incision is opened and the implant removed. The inferior level of the breast cavity is lowered by sharp dissection. Slight overcorrection is usually advised as there is a tendency for the implant to "rise" again.

Raising an implant is more difficult (Figure 8.76). To make the correction, a line is drawn on the inside of the breast cavity, on the chest wall, to correspond to the level of the desired inframammary crease. The pseudolining of the breast cavity below this line is then folded on itself. Interrupted sutures are used to secure the fold to the line (Figure 8.76D). Similarly, if the implant falls too far laterally when the patient lies supine, the lateral excess cavity can be reduced by the "infolding" technique.

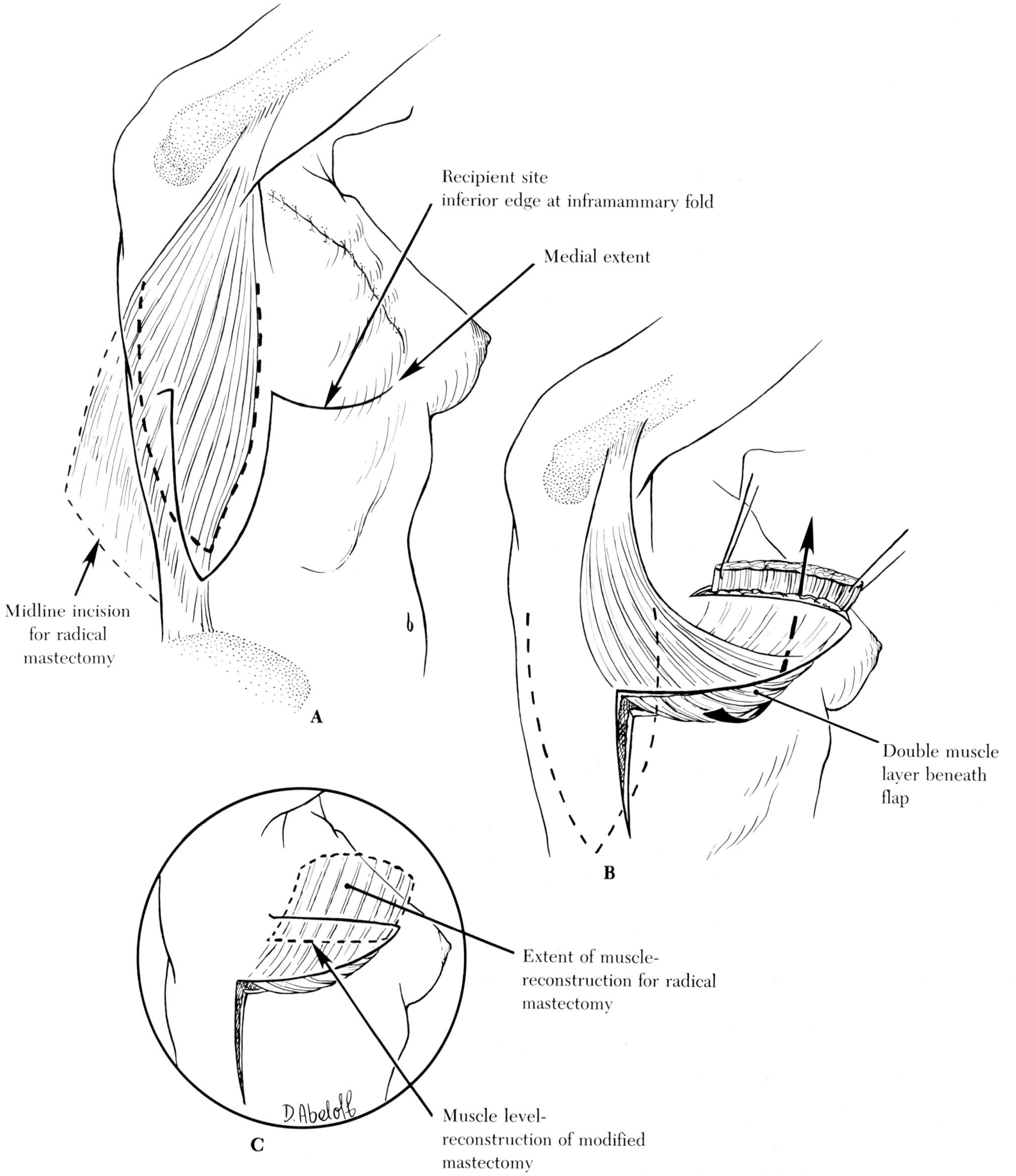

Figure 8.73. Latissimus dorsi musculocutaneous pedicle flap (Ryan modification).

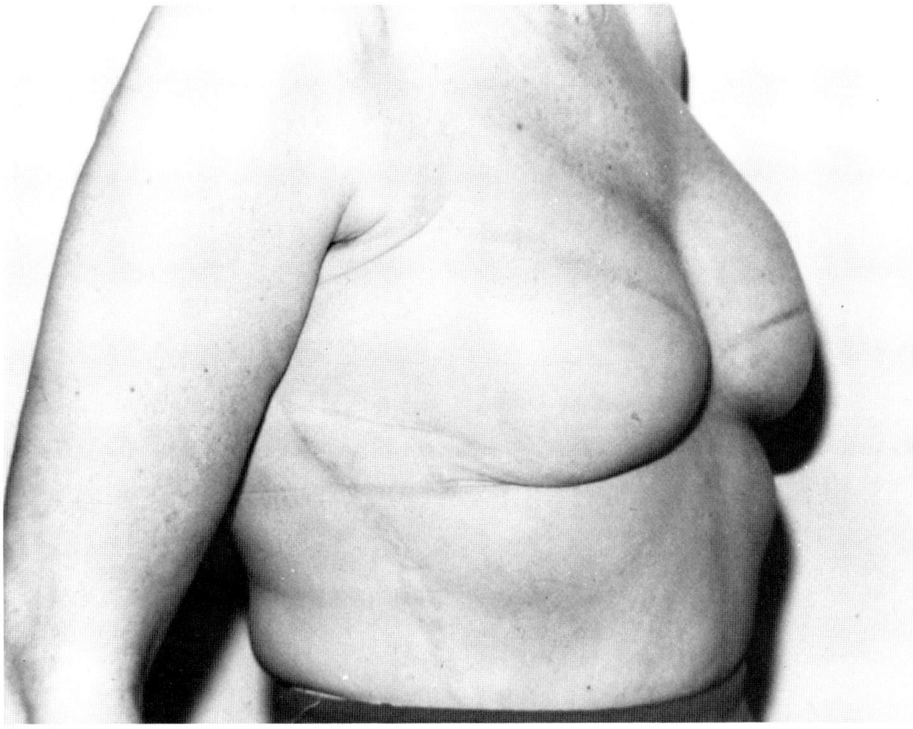

Figure 8.74. Oblique postoperative view of a staged bilateral reconstruction following staged modified radical mastectomies for bilateral carcinoma. Invasive adenocarcinoma in the left breast developed 1 year after the mastectomy had been performed on the right side for carcinoma. Note the donor scar on the right midlateral site and transposition of the modified latissimus dorsi musculocutaneous pedicle flap.

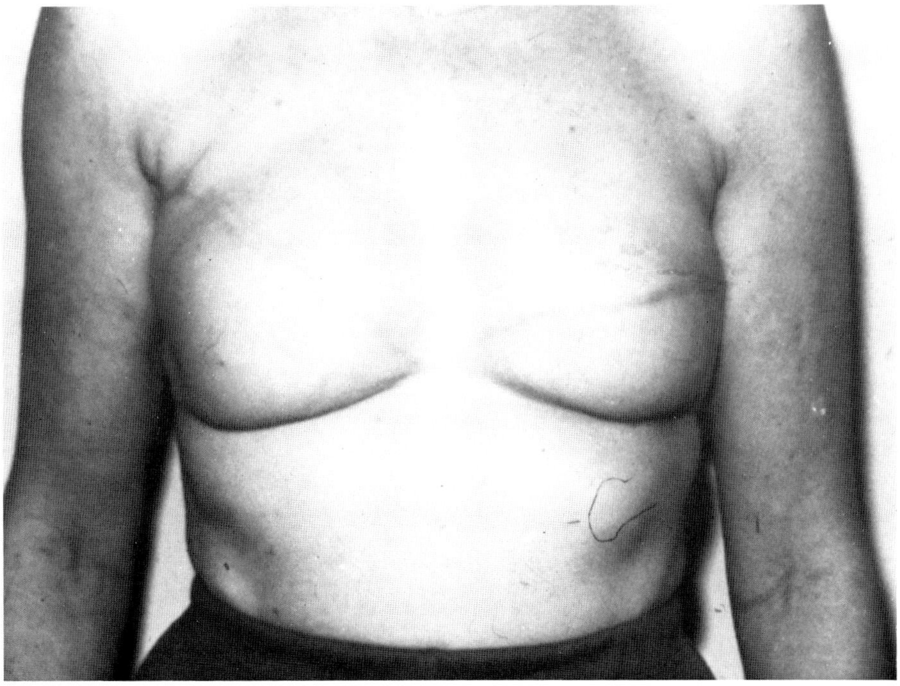

Figure 8.75. AP postoperative view of the result in the patient in Figure 8.72.

Insufficient Muscle Coverage of the Implant

When the pectoralis major has atrophied inferiorly and insufficient latissimus muscle has been transposed anteriorly, the outline of the silicone implant may become too obvious. Kinking of the outer shell of a bilumen implant may occur when there is insufficient fill and the skin flap is too thin (Figures 8.77–8.79). This may require replacement of the implant or an extra volume of saline to the outer shell.

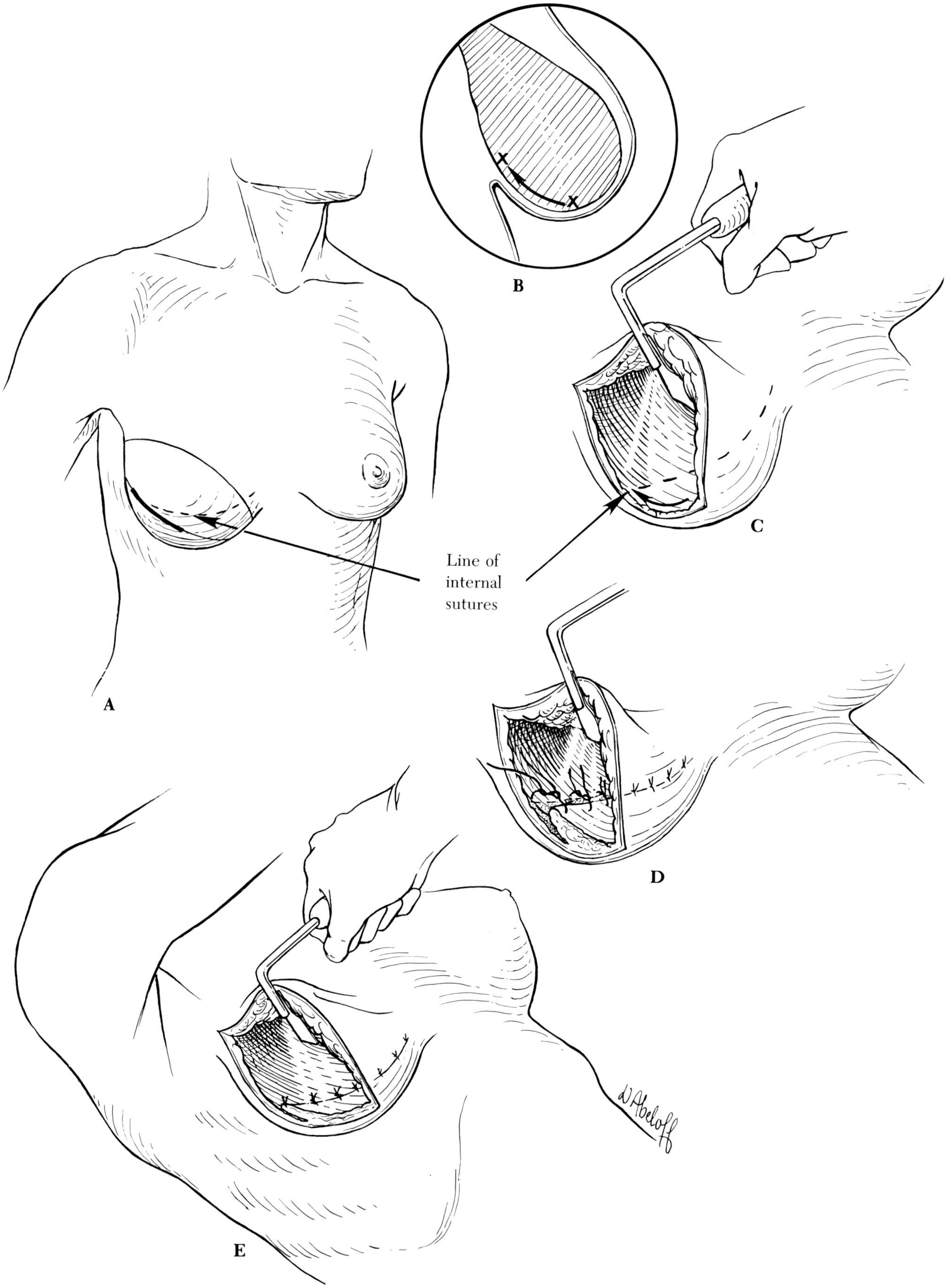

Figure 8.76. **A:** A lower incision is opened, the implant is removed, and a line is drawn inside the cavity on the chest wall to correspond to the level of the desired inframammary crease. **B:** The extent of raising the cavity is shown. **C:** Inside the breast cavity, with the implant removed, showing the line of sutures. **D:** Lining of the breast cavity folded on itself and sutured into position. **E:** Lower extent of breast cavity raised.

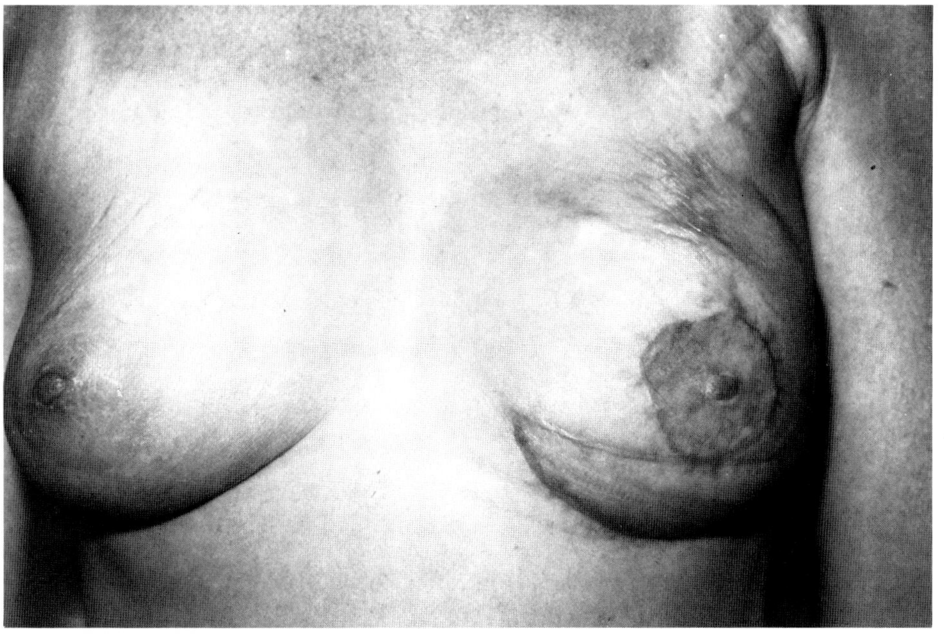

Figure 8.77. Knuckle of kinked outer shell of an implant showing through a thin skin flap.

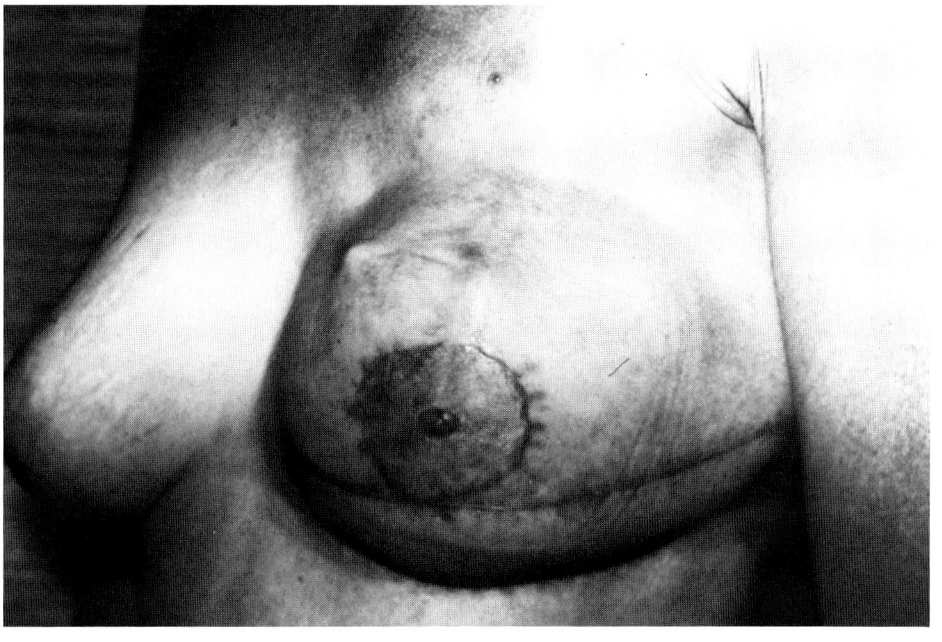

Figure 8.78. Outline of an implant and kinking of the outer shell was obvious through atrophy of the pectoralis muscle inferiorly and insufficient latissimus muscle transferred.

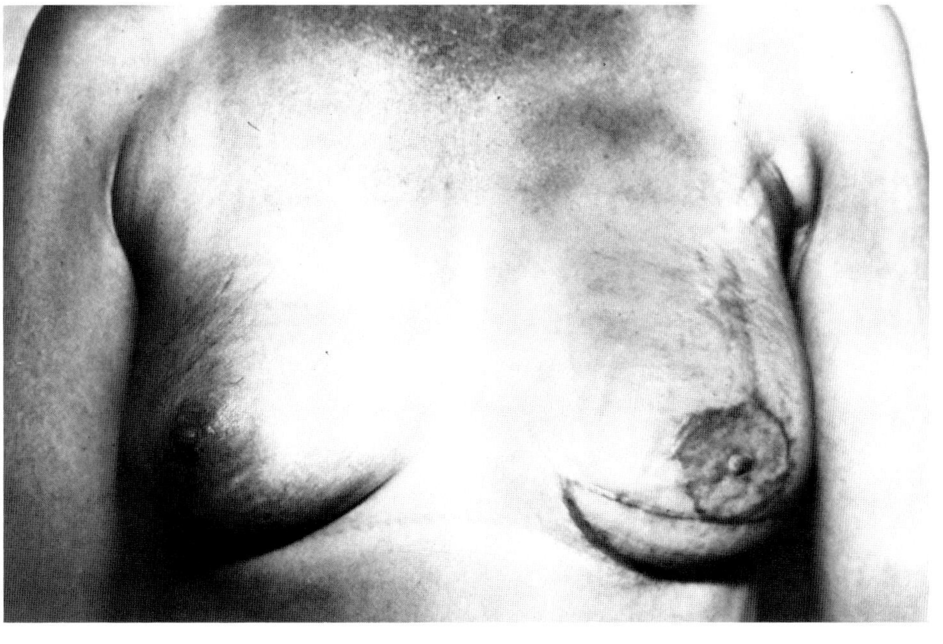

Figure 8.79. The appearance improved (from that in Figures 8.77 and 8.78) by replacing the round implant with a Birnbaum style.

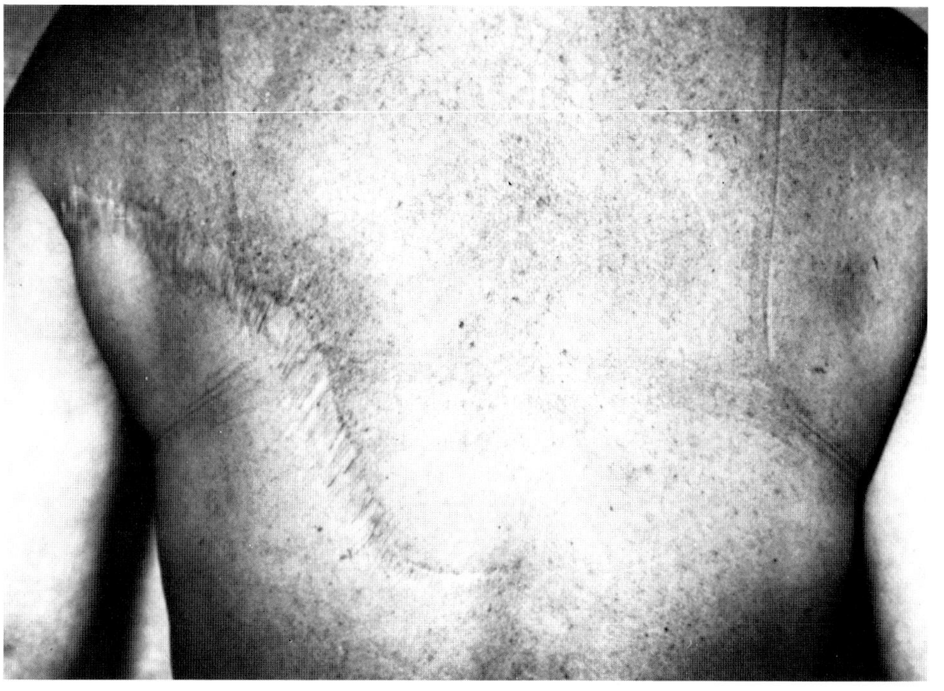

Figure 8.80. Widening of the back scar sometimes makes it very obvious.

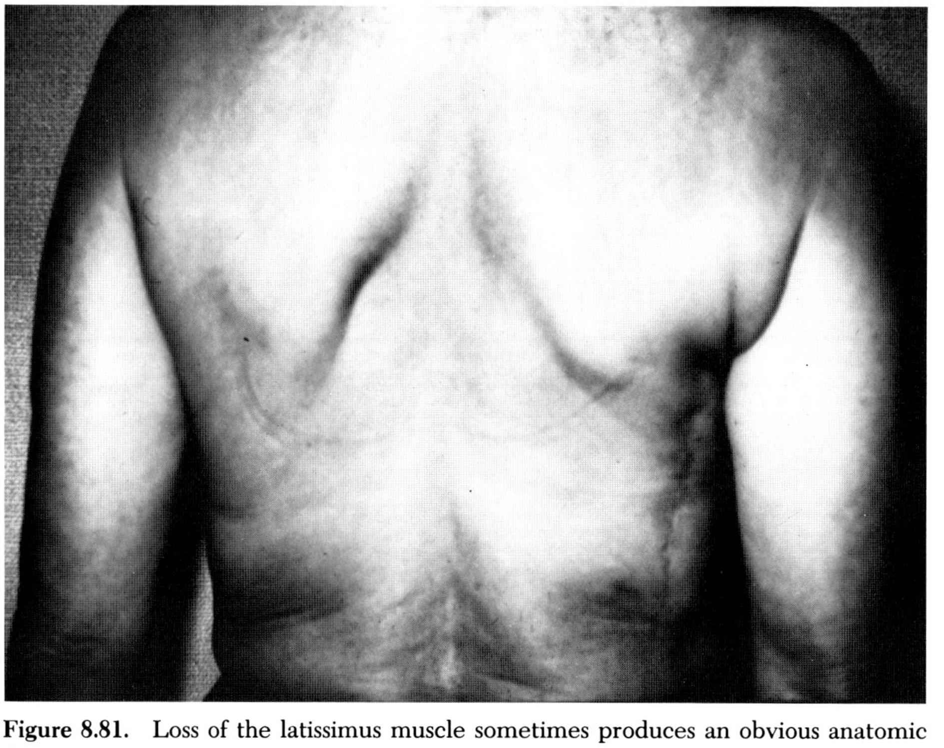

Figure 8.81. Loss of the latissimus muscle sometimes produces an obvious anatomic depression.

Back Defect

One disadvantage of the latissimus dorsi flap is the associated scar and defect of the back. In some individuals this can be quite obvious (Figures 8.80 and 8.81), whereas in others it is less so (Figure 8.82).

Partial or Complete Loss of the Flap

Occasionally, the distal tip of the skin paddle undergoes a superficial slough. Very rarely, complete loss of the paddle occurs (Figure 8.83). This happens when the thoracodorsal artery has been obliterated during the radical mastectomy but it is not recognized preoperatively that this has occurred and during elevation of the flap the collateral circulation is destroyed. In other cases where

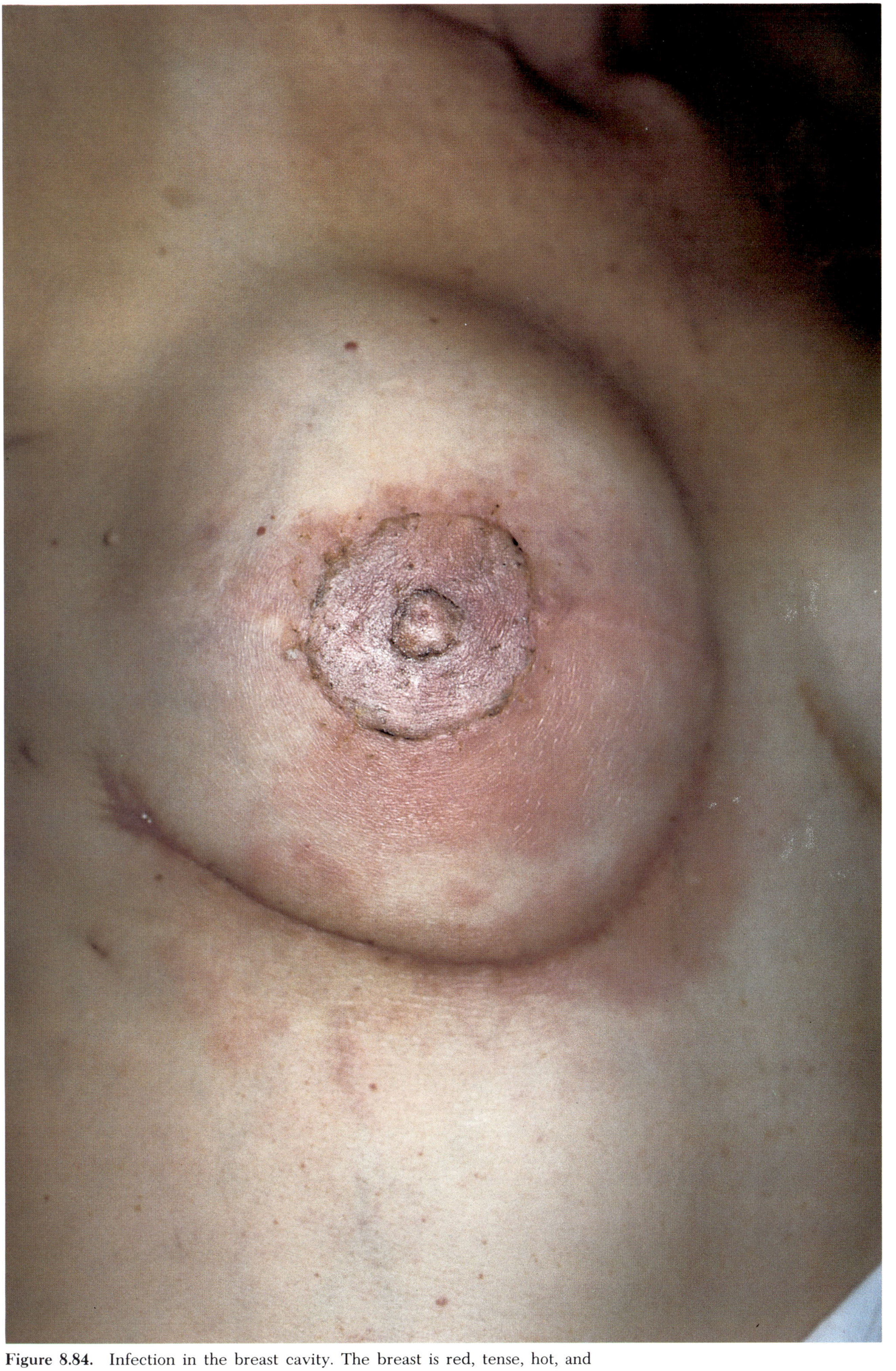

Figure 8.84. Infection in the breast cavity. The breast is red, tense, hot, and tender. The implant was removed and the breast cavity drained.

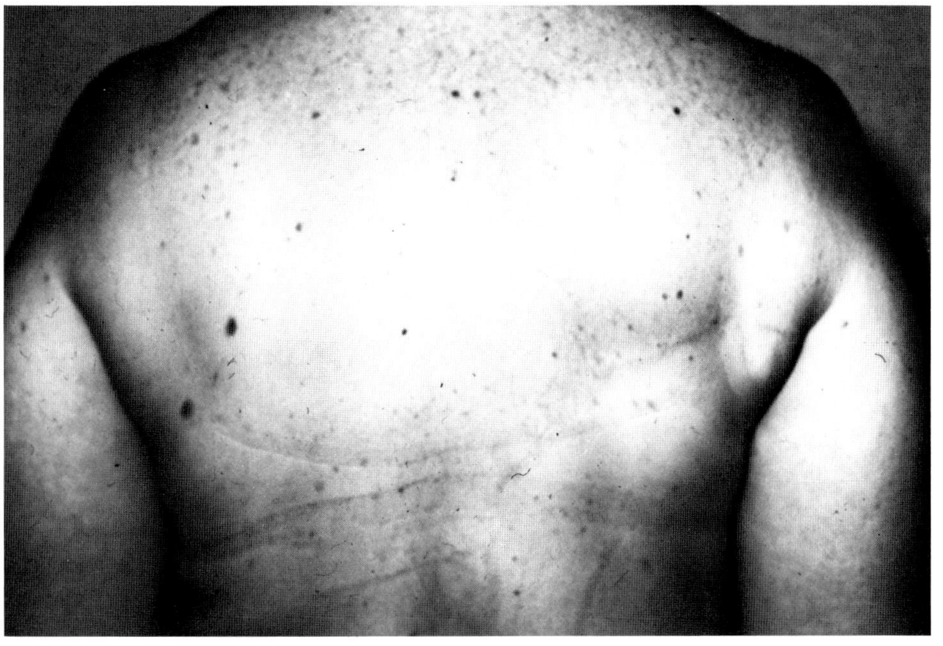

Figure 8.82. Other scars are less obvious.

the thoracodorsal artery has been previously obliterated, flaps have been raised and transposed successfully (9). In these cases the humeral pedicle has been dissected only enough to allow transposition of the flap, and the collateral circulation has been carefully preserved.

Infection of the Breast Cavity

Infection of the breast cavity following reconstructive surgery is rare. Patients complain of discomfort and tightness in the reconstructed breast 2–3 weeks after the operation and are found on examination to be pyrexial and toxic, with redness, induration, and tenderness of the affected area. The implant must be removed and the breast cavity drained. The implant can then be reinserted several months later when the infection has healed (Figure 8.84).

Seroma

The reported incidence of seroma developing in the back wound is approximately 10%. Needle aspiration is effective in treating these cases.

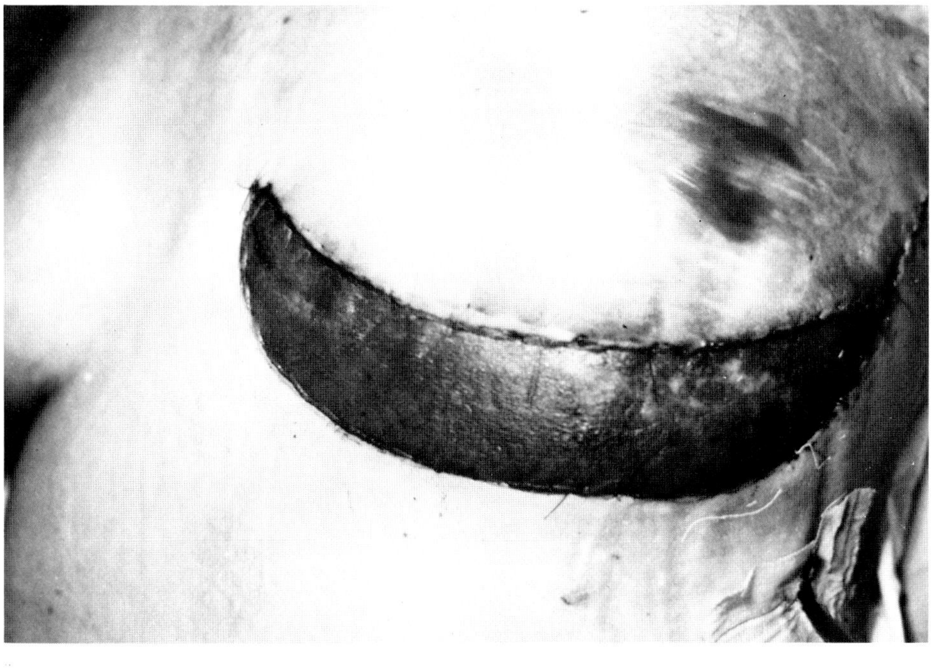

Figure 8.83. Total necrosis of the skin paddle occurred in this case. The thoracodorsal artery had been obliterated during the mastectomy, a fact that was not appreciated until after the collateral circulation had been divided.

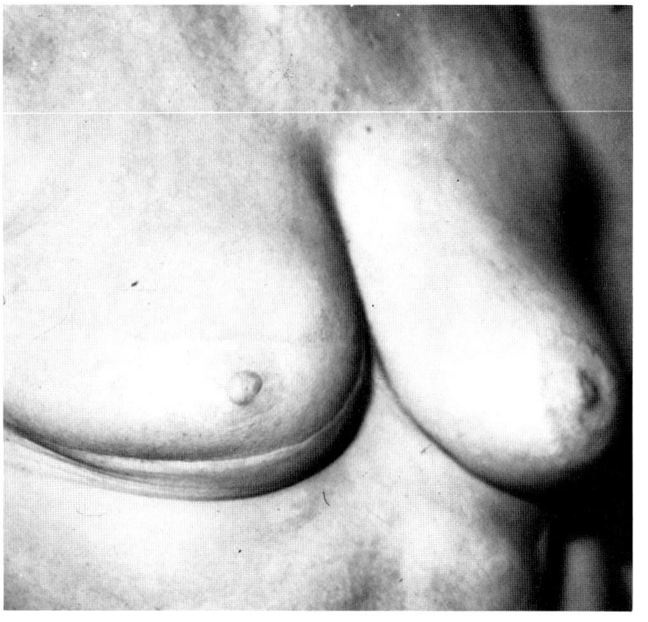

Figure 8.85. If a transverse flap is used, a "double bubble" appearance may result.

Double Bubble Appearance

If a transverse flap is used, a "double bubble" appearance may result (Figure 8.85). This may be avoided by inserting the flap downward and medially in an oblique direction.

References

1. Bostwick J, Nahai F, Wallace JG, et al, 1979: Sixty latissimus dorsi flaps. Plast Reconstr Surg 63:21.
2. Bostwick J, Vasconez LO, Jurkiewicz MJ, 1978: Breast reconstruction following radical mastectomy. Plast Reconstr Surg 61:682–693.
3. Daniel RK, Williams HB, 1973: The free transfer of skin flaps by microvascular anastomoses. Plast Reconstr Surg 52:16–31.
4. Drever JM, 1981: Total breast reconstruction. Ann Plast Surg 7:54–61.
5. Fujino T, Harashina T, Enomato J, 1976: Primary breast reconstruction after a standard radical mastectomy by a free flap transfer. Plast Reconstr Surg 58:371–374.
6. Gant TD, Serafin D, Buncke H Jr, 1981: Free flap reconstruction of the breast. In: Post-Mastectomy Reconstruction, edited by TD Gant, LO Vasconex, pp 161–173. Williams & Wilkins, Baltimore.
7. Gant TD, Vasconez LO, 1981: Latissimus dorsi musculocutaneous flap breast reconstruction. In: Post-Mastectomy Reconstruction, edited by TD Gant, LO Vasconez, pp 69–89. Williams & Wilkins, Baltimore.
8. Mathes SJ, Hanai F, 1979: Clinical Atlas of Muscle and Musculocutaneous Flaps. Mosby, St. Louis.
9. Maxwell GP, McGibbon BM, Hoopes JG, 1979: Vascular consideration in the use of the latissimus dorsi myocutaneous flap following mastectomy with axillary dissection. Plast Reconstr Surg 64:771–780.
10. McCraw, JB, Dibbell DG, 1977: Experimental definition of independent myocutaneous vascular territories. Plast Reconstr Surg 60:212–220.
11. McCraw JB, Dibbell DG, Carraway JH, 1977: Clinical definition of independent myocutaneous vascular territories. Plast Reconstr Surg 60:341–352.
12. Millard DR Jr, 1982: Breast aesthetics when reconstructing with the latissimus dorsi musculocutaneous flap. Plast Reconstr Surg 70:161–171.
13. O'Brien B, et al, 1974: Free flap transfer with microvascular anastomosis. Br J Plast Surg 27:220.
14. Serafin D, Georgiade NG, Given KS, 1978: Transfer of free flaps to provide well-vascularized thick cover for breast reconstruction after radical mastectomy. Plast Reconstr Surg 62:527–536.

9

Rectus Abdominus Musculocutaneous Flaps

Introduction

Bernard M. McGibbon

Over the past 50 years a number of flap operations have evolved. Based on an ever-increasing knowledge of the field, they have been stepping stones to the present use of abdominal flaps for breast reconstruction.

In 1937 Webster used the superficial inferior epigastric artery and the superior thoracic and long thoracic arteries to design a multistaged tubed bipedicled flap (24). Shaw and Payne in 1946 developed a one-stage arterialized single-pedicle flap based on the inferior epigastric and circumflex iliac arteries (20). The impressive studies by Fujino in 1967 resulted in the contribution of perforator vasculature to circulation in flaps (12). Tai and Hasegwa (22), Bohmert (1,2), Cronin et al. (4), and Brown et al. (3) during the 1970s all used the information regarding axial blood supply and perforator vasculature to raise transverse abdominal flaps based on the superior epigastric artery. More recently, the concept of the musculocutaneous flap has resulted in the evolution of three flaps based on the rectus abdominis muscle and supplied by the superior epigastric vessels (15). The use of these three flaps in reconstructing the breast is discussed in this chapter (5,7).

The vertical rectus abdominus flap, described here by Drever, is a musculocutaneous flap. The perforating vessels from the superior epigastric artery augment the blood supply to the skin from the underlying muscle. Drever is so confident about this blood supply that he elevates the superior part of the skin flap from the muscle and converts that part into a random flap (9,10,17).

The contralateral rectus abdominus submammary flap uses a small segment of rectus muscle as a carrier for the perforating cutaneous branches of the superior epigastric artery (14). The part of the flap over the muscle is musculocutaneous; the rest of the flap is axial. Vasconez discusses its use and the meticulous technique required (23). The results can be spectacular, and the donor site is well hidden.

The transverse abdominal island flap is much larger than the preceding two but is designed on sound surgical and anatomic principles. It allows a significant amount of skin, subcutaneous fat, and rectus muscle to be transferred to the breast area. Similar to the contralateral submammary flap, it is partly musculocutaneous and partly axial. It is technically challenging but safe if kinking of the vascular pedicle is prevented by not folding the rectus in an accordion fashion. This operation (11,13,18,19) is discussed by both Hartrampf and McGibbon.

Points of Surgical Anatomy

The central abdominal skin and fat are nourished by large vessels perforating the anterior rectus sheath (Figure 9.1) (15). These perforators form a rich plexus around Scarpa's fascia and in the subdermal plane of the abdominal wall. They probably communicate laterally with the thoracolumbar vascular complex and even cross the midline, communicating with the opposite rectus perforators. These rectus perforators have their origin from the superior and inferior epigastric vascular systems. The superior and inferior epigastric vessels

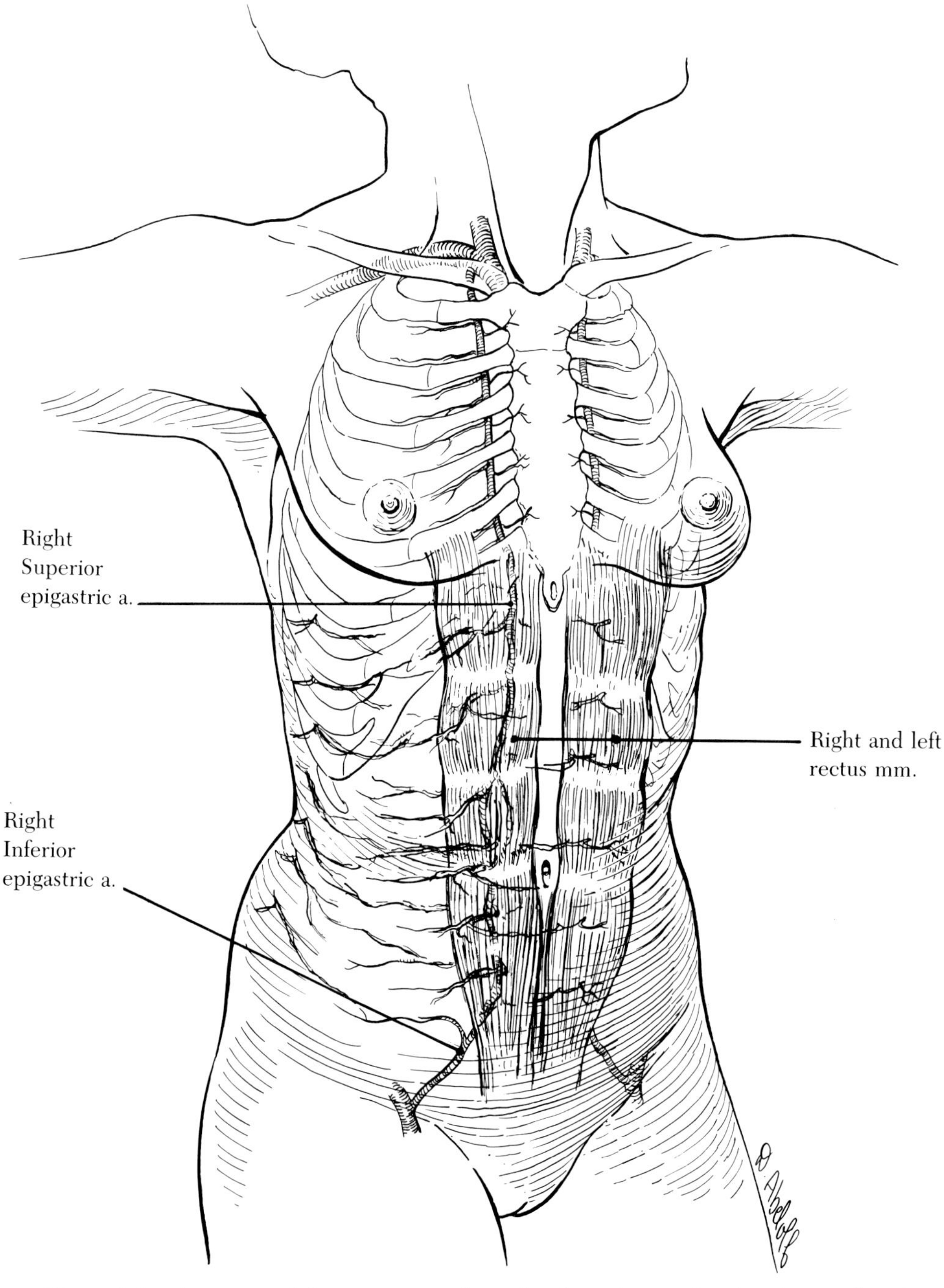

Figure 9.1. Anatomy of the rectus muscle and epigastric arteries showing perforating vessels.

rarely communicate as one large continuous channel but, rather, come together in the substance of the rectus muscle as an arborization of smaller vessels in the region of the umbilicus. A large number of perforators occur in this region just above and below the umbilicus. Arteriography has shown that injection of a contrast medium in the internal thoracic vessels fills the superior epigastric system but does not fill the inferior system unless it has been previously ligated. Similarly, an injection from below does not fill the superior epigastric system in the normal state.

The rectus muscle is a long, strap-like structure inserted superiorly to the lower and anterior borders of the fifth, sixth, and seventh ribs and the xiphoid process. Inferiorly, it originates from the body of the pubis and symphysis. Its medial border is separated from its fellow by the linea alba. Below the umbilicus, the linea alba is narrow and the two recti are practically in contact; but above the umbilicus it is almost 0.5 inch wide. The rectus abdominis is enclosed in an aponeurotic sheath except on the posterior aspect of its lower quarter at the arcuate line, where the sheath is absent, and superiorly where the muscle lies directly on the anterior surface of the costal cartilage.

The rectus muscle is separated into four fairly equal units by transverse tendinous inscriptions. Each unit is individually nourished and innervated in the lateral area from the thoracolumbar vessels and nerves. These tendinous inscriptions are densely adherent to the tough anterior rectus sheath, which covers the entire rectus muscle, but are not adherent to the posterior rectus sheath. Below the arcuate line there is no posterior rectus sheath.

The inferior epigastric vessels originate from the iliac vessels at the inguinal ligament, pass under the internal oblique fascia into the precystic fat, and then course into the posterolateral aspect of the rectus sheath at or about the arcuate line. The vessel then arborizes and enters the substance of the rectus muscle, where it disappears from sight on the posterior aspect of the muscle, usually in the region of the umbilicus. The superior epigastric vessel is a continuation of the internal thoracic vessel and enters the posterior aspect of the superior rectus sheath from the mediastinum in the medial aspect of the muscle. It then courses along the rib to a more central location in the muscle.

Vertical Rectus Abdominus Myocutaneous Flap

J. Michael Drever

The vertical rectus abdominus myocutaneous flap may be the procedure of choice if the latissimus dorsi flap or the lower abdominal transverse rectus abdominus myocutaneous flap cannot be used. Women with spare tissue in the midabdominal region are eligible for this procedure. However, those with flat abdomens or athletes who count on abdominal muscular integrity are not suitable candidates. Neither are those women who object to an abdominal scar, especially if it extends above the umbilicus.

Operative Technique

Preoperatively, with the patient in the erect position, the proposed inframammary crease is marked and the flap outlined (Figure 9.2A). On the contralateral side the distance between the nipple and the true inframammary crease is measured and used as a guide in planning the width of the flap. One advantage of this technique is that the design of the flap need not be finalized until the defect in the chest has been evaluated and the amount of skin and subcutaneous tissue needed has been determined. The length of the flap may be varied according to the needs of the patient. If a radical mastectomy defect is present, the flap is made as long as possible, and the ends are deepithelialized and used to correct the infraclavicular and axillary defect. With a modified radical defect, a shorter flap is adequate.

The flap is incised through skin, subcutaneous tissue, and the anterior rectus sheath. The anterior rectus fascia is incised parallel to the muscle for approximately 4–5 cm above the costal margin to give more mobility to the muscle itself. The umbilicus is carefully circumscribed, to be relocated later (Figure 9.2B). The inferior epigastric vascular pedicle is ligated and cut. The flap is then raised as far as the costal margin (8,9).

As in any other flap procedure, great care should be taken with the pedicle, especially at the costal margin. Sometimes a neurovascular bundle perforates the posterior sheath of the rectus two or three fingerbreadths below the costal margin. This is not the internal mammary. If left, it will tend to pull out the main vascular supply to the pedicle when the pedicle is doubled on itself. Therefore this kind of neurovascular bundle should be sectioned and ligated near the fascia.

A tunnel is made between the superior part of the wound and the inframammary crease incision, and the flap is brought up into position (Figure 9.2C). It may be necessary to detach the superior part of the skin flap from the muscle to allow the flap to be folded in on itself. The tails of the flap are then deepithelialized and are pulled up under the chest wall skin to fill in the infraclavicular defect and develop the breast shape. A silicone implant is usually not needed with this method (Figure 9.2D,E).

If the flap extends below the limit of the arcuate line, a V-shaped defect is left in the rectus sheath to facilitate closure. Alternatively, a more transverse

Figure 9.2. Steps of the operative technique: vertical rectus abdominus myocutaneous flap. **A:** The width of the flap is made equal to the measurement between the nipple and the inframammary crease of the other breast. **B:** The superior part of the skin flap may be detached from the muscle to allow the flap to be folded on itself. **C:** The folded flap is tunneled up into the inframammary crease incision. **D:** The tails of the flap are pulled up under the chest wall to fill in or augment the infraclavicular region. **E:** The flaps are retrieved, and the part to be buried is deepithelialized. The defect below the arcuate line is reinforced with merselene. **F:** The right edge of the wound is undermined and advanced to the left. The umbilicus is relocated, preventing it from being distorted and pulled to the left.

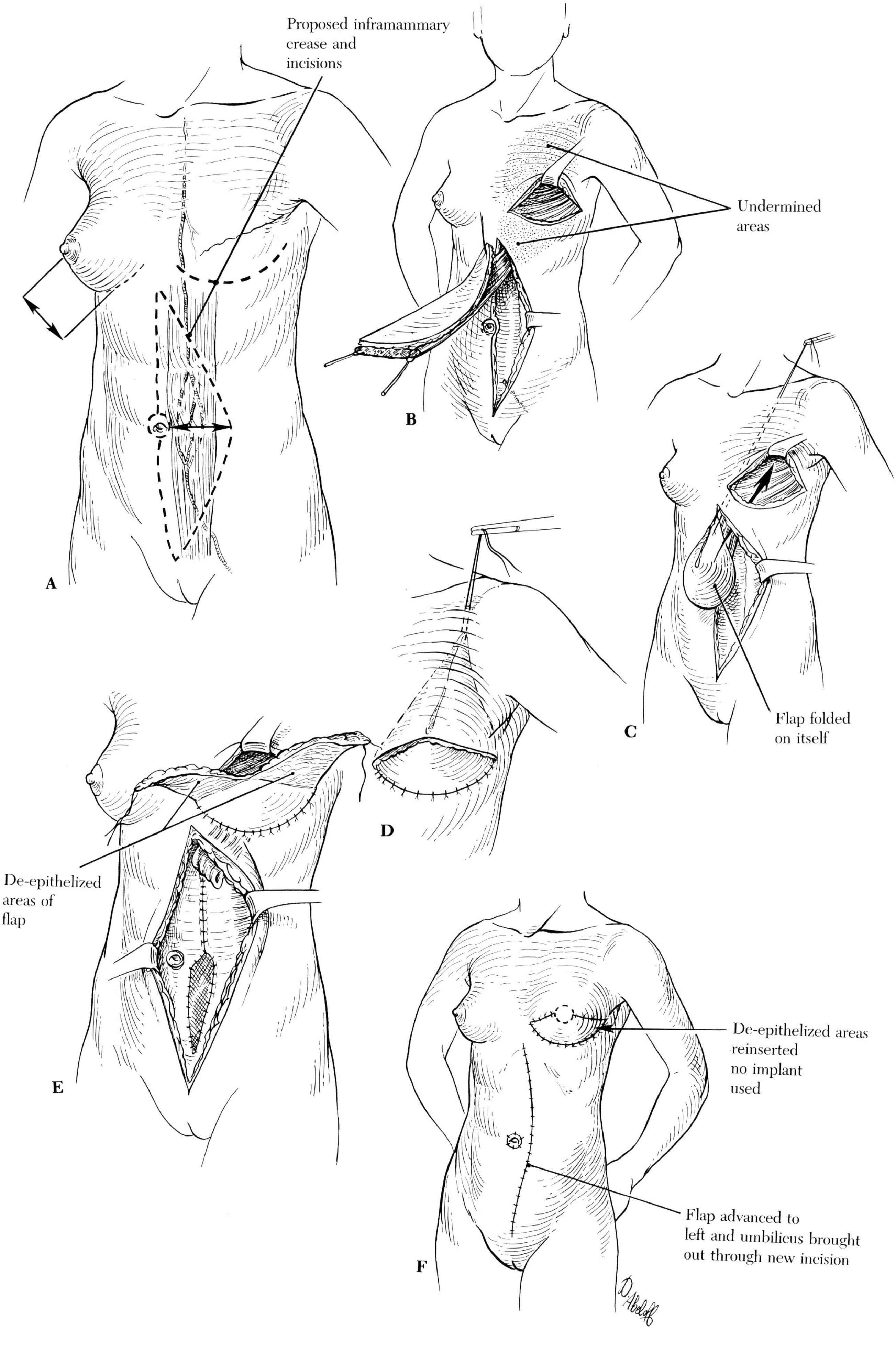
Proposed inframammary
crease and
incisions
Undermined
areas
A
B
C
Flap folded
on itself
D
De-epithelized
areas of
flap
E
De-epithelized areas
reinserted
no implant
used
F
Flap advanced to
left and umbilicus brought
out through new incision

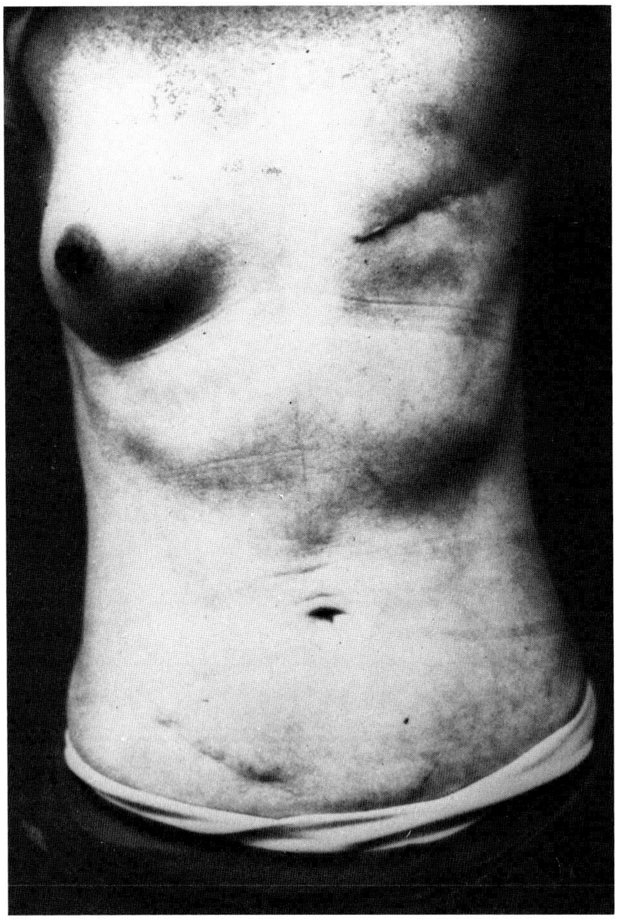

A

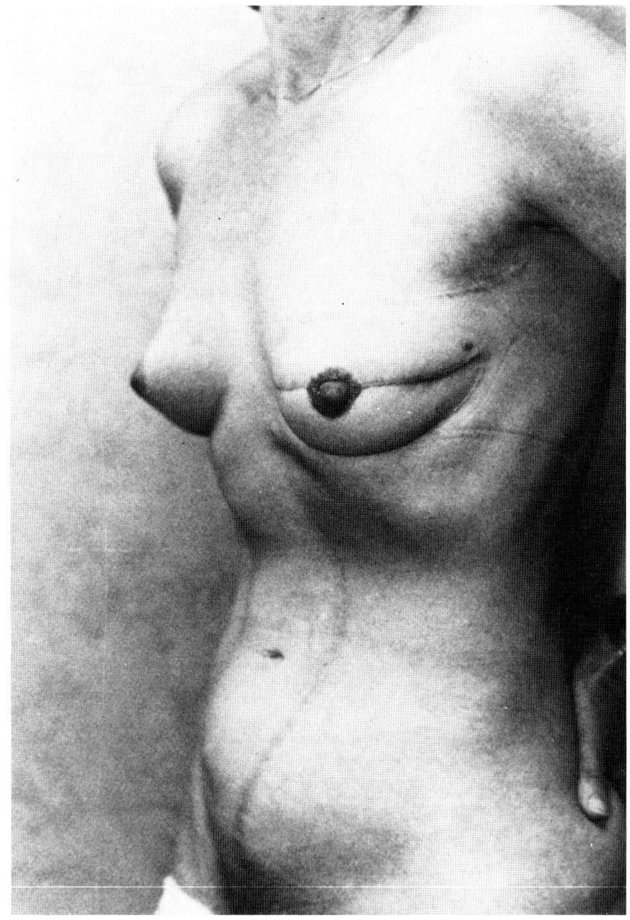

B

Figure 9.3. **A:** Preoperative view of the left modified radical mastectomy defect. **B:** Oblique postoperative views showing good symmetry and a well-healed left paramedian scar. **C:** Oblique view from the contralateral side.

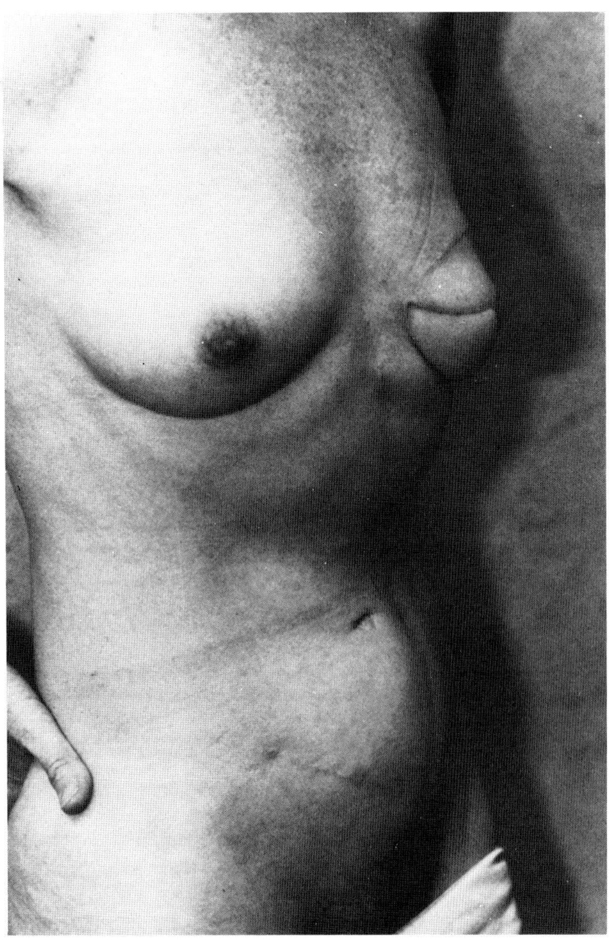

C

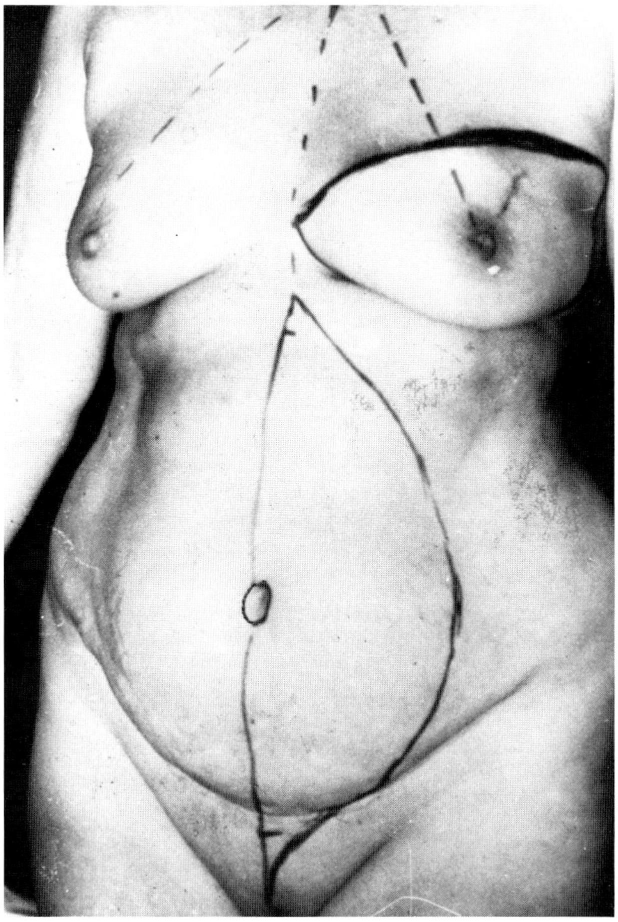

A

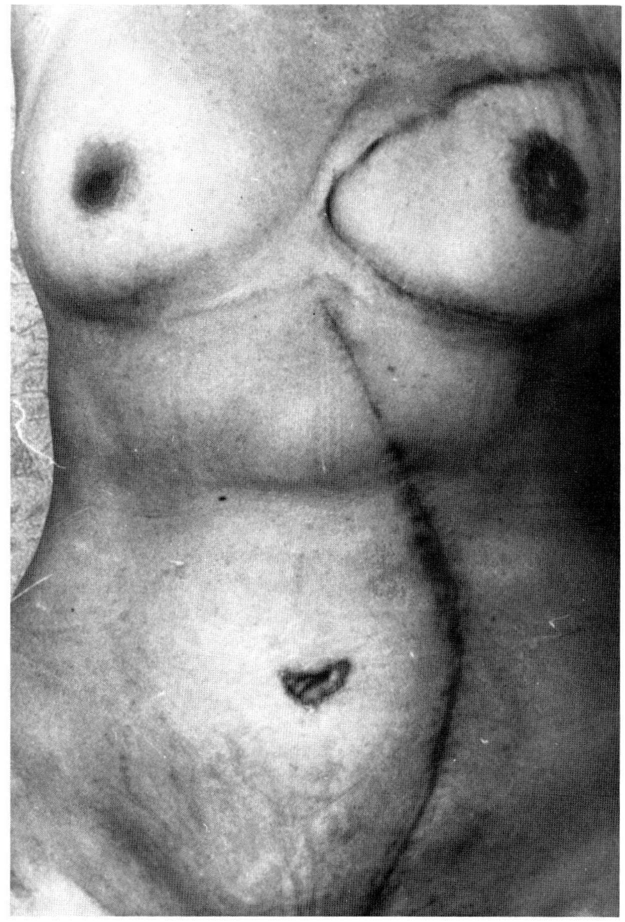

B

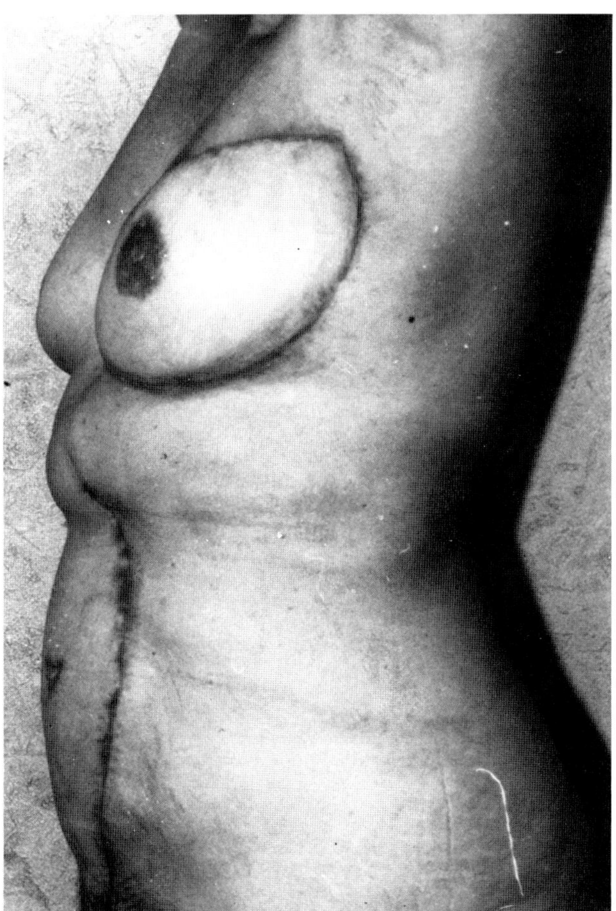

C

Figure 9.4. **A:** Preoperative markings for mastectomy and the flap for immediate reconstruction. **B:** Postoperative AP view. **C:** Postoperative oblique view.

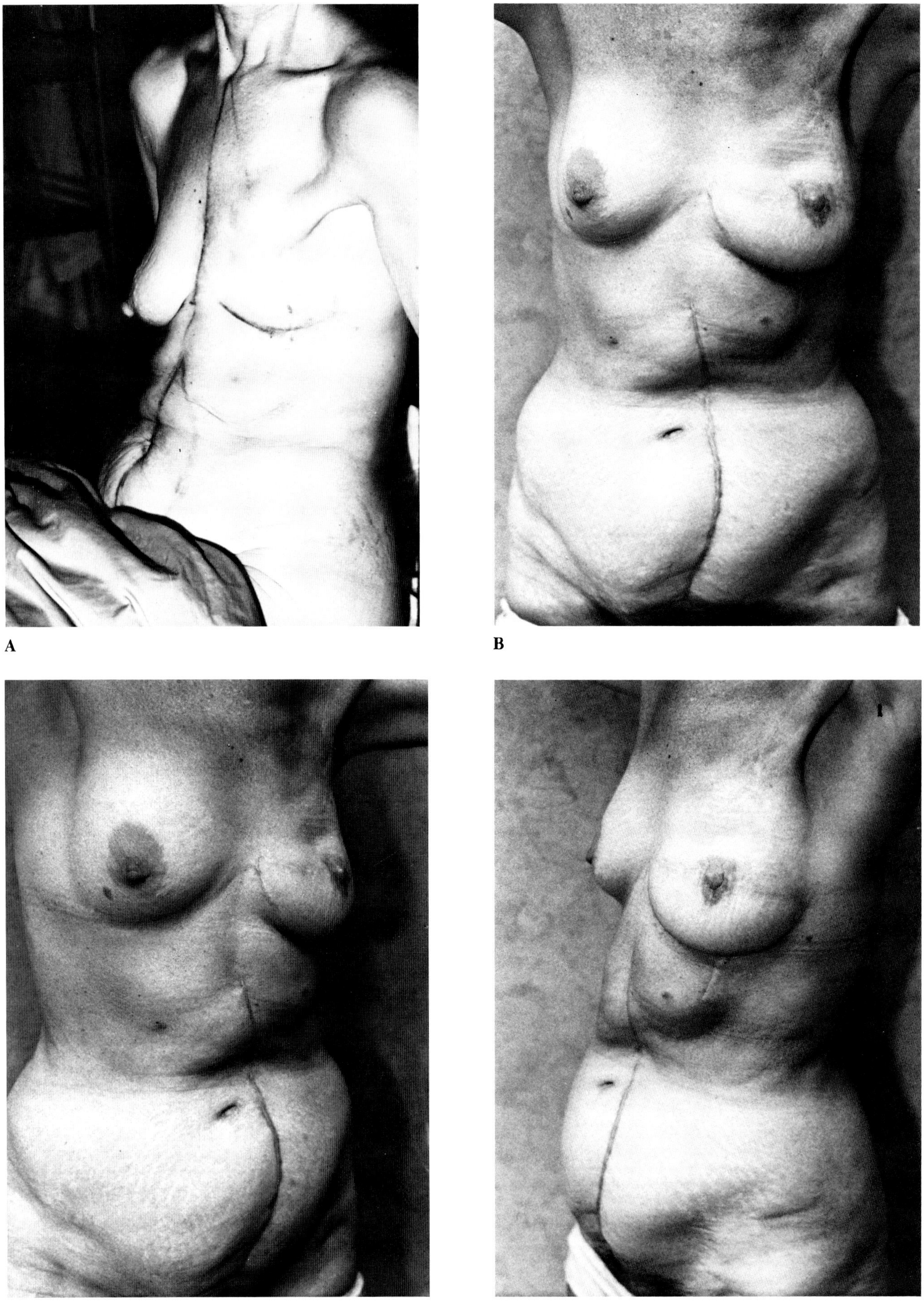

Figure 9.5. **A:** Preoperative oblique view with the proposed incision. **B:** Three-year postoperative AP view. **C:** Three-year postoperative oblique view. **D:** Three-year postoperative oblique view.

incision may be made below the arcuate line, leaving a fascial defect that is repaired with a merselene sheet (Figure 9.2E).

The abdomen is closed by undermining the vertical incision on the contralateral side and advancing it across the midline. The umbilicus is relocated, preventing its position from being distorted off the midline (Figure 9.2F).

Complications

The vertical rectus abdominus flap is a relatively easy procedure to execute and is normally attended by few if any postoperative complications. Fat necrosis, manifested as a hardening under part of the flap, is a rare but occasional complication of this operation. It may be distressing to the patient, who may confuse it with recurrence of her malignancy. This problem is handled by needle biopsy and reassurance. It usually takes 4–6 months for the fat necrosis to soften completely and disappear.

Persistent pain in the costal margin when taking a deep breath, coughing, or straining has also been observed. This may be caused by a stretched intercostal nerve at the base of the muscle pedicle. To avoid this problem, care should be taken to section all of the neurovascular bundles that traverse the posterior sheath of the rectus, as mentioned earlier.

Results

Cosmetically, this procedure results in a more natural appearance than that of the majority of implant operations. It also has the added advantage of thinning the waistline (Figures 9.3–9.8).

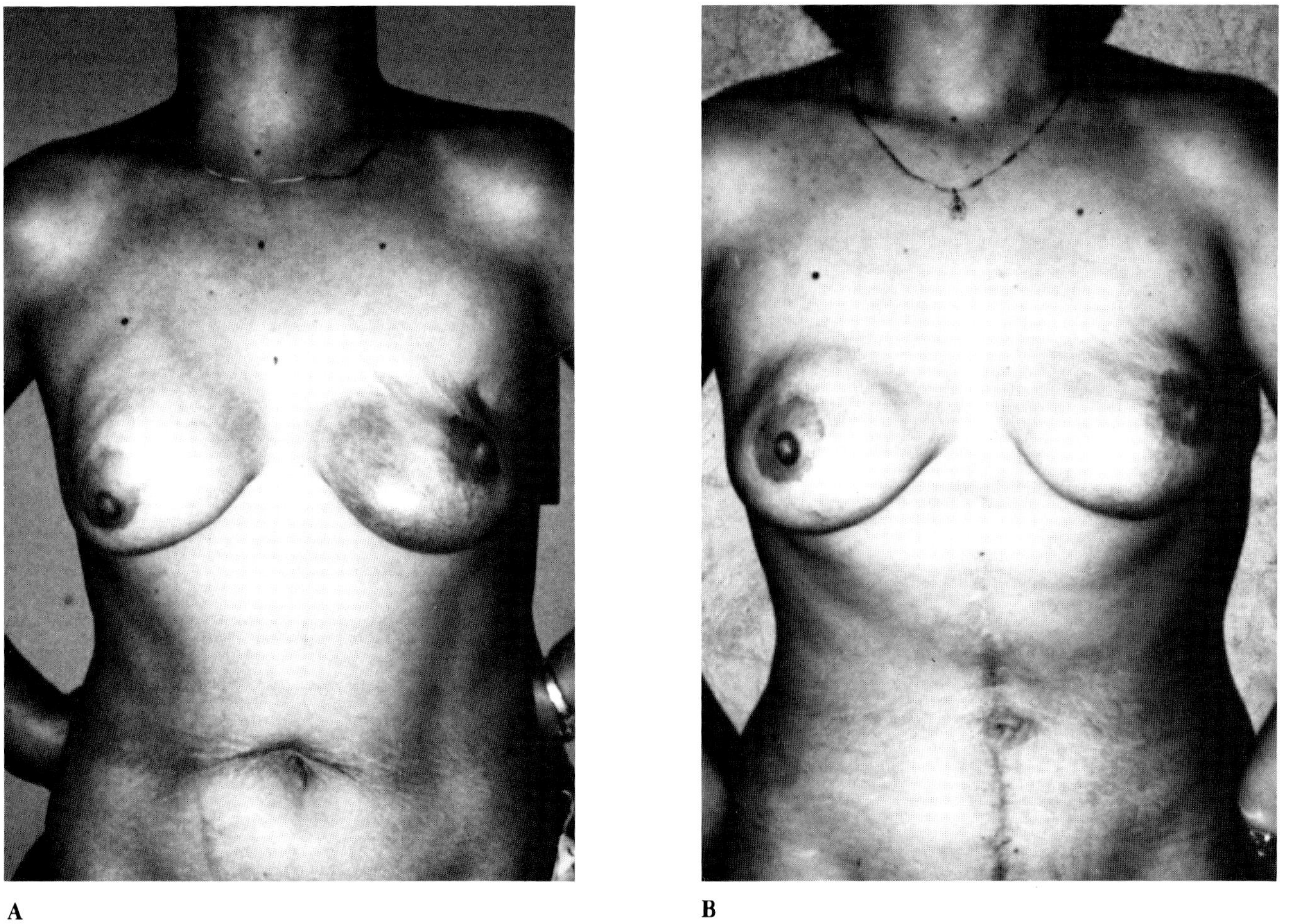

A **B**

Figure 9.6. **A:** Subcutaneous mastectomy cripple (eight previous operations, showing severe skin atrophy with implants about to extrude). **B:** Reconstruction performed with bilateral deepithelialized vertical flaps.

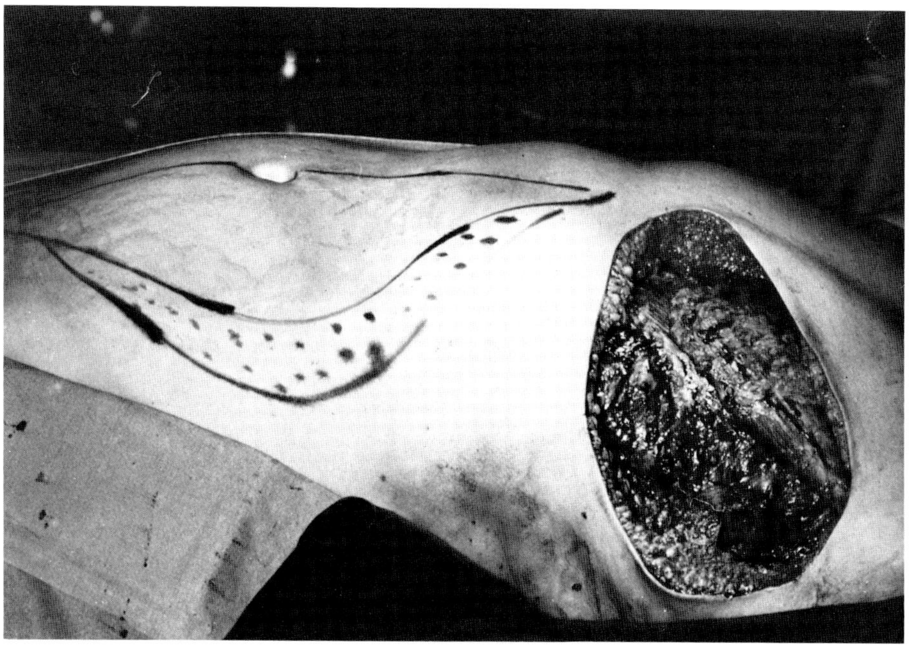

A

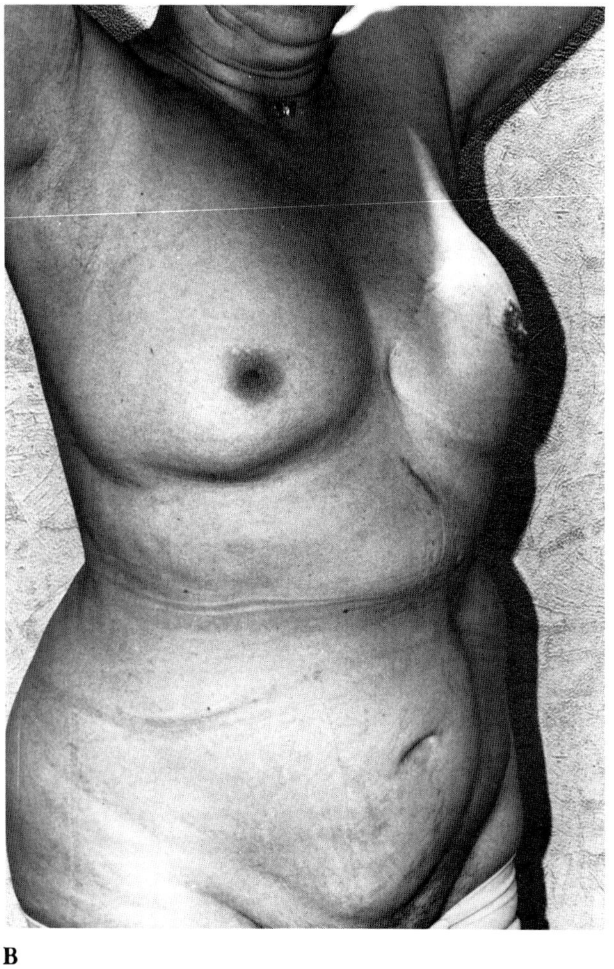

B

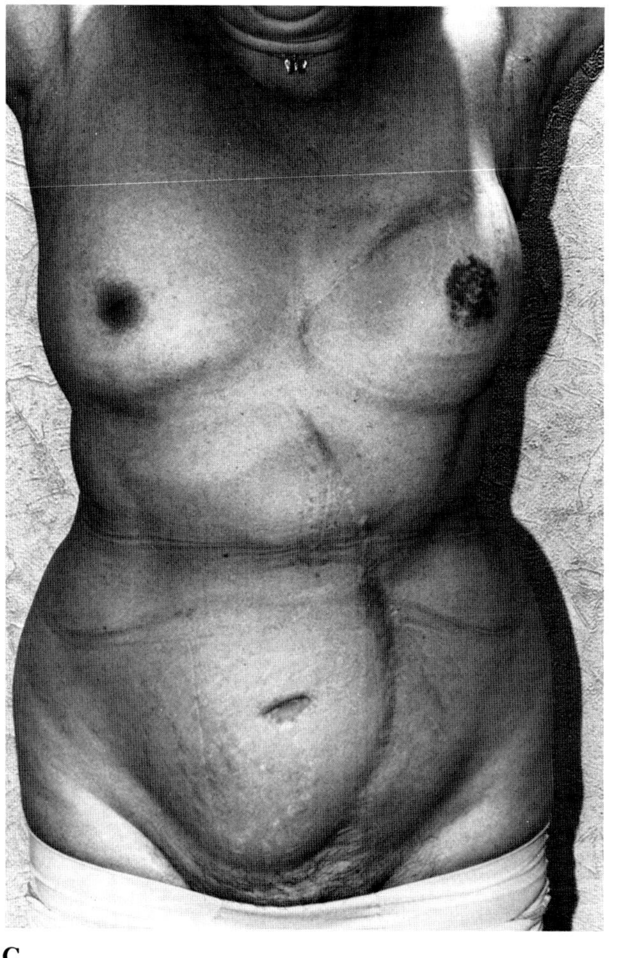

C

Figure 9.7. **A:** Operative view of a mastectomy defect with markings for immediate reconstruction using a left vertical flap. **B:** Two-year postoperative AP view. **C:** Two-year postoperative oblique view.

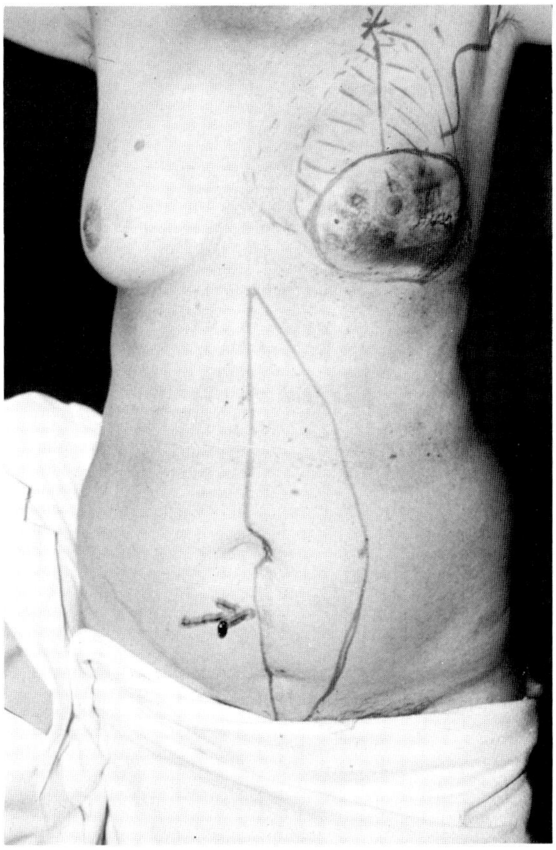

A

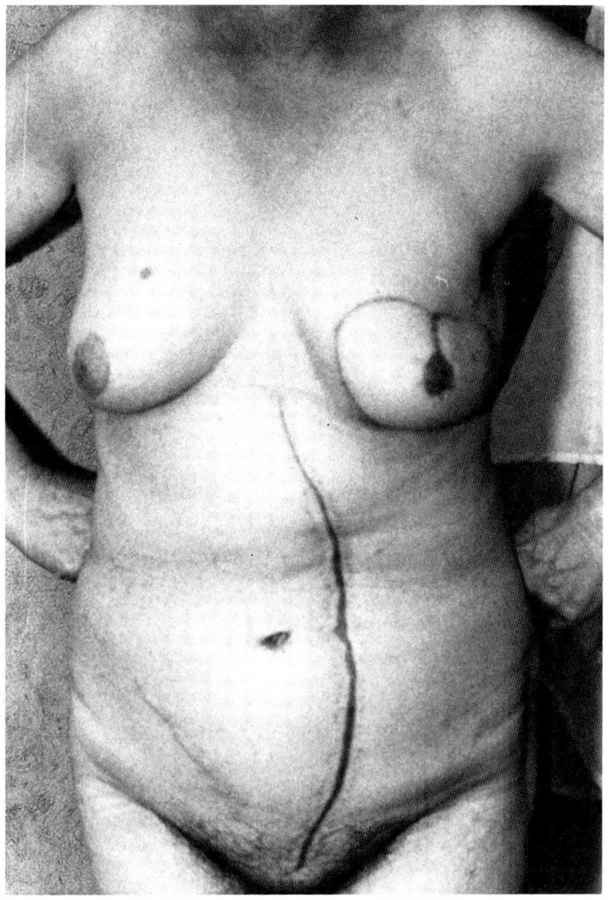

B

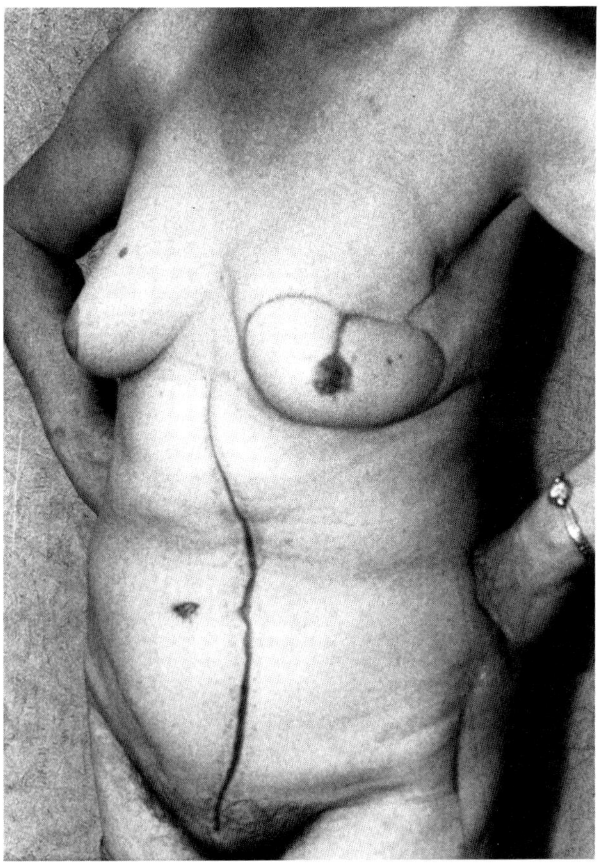

C

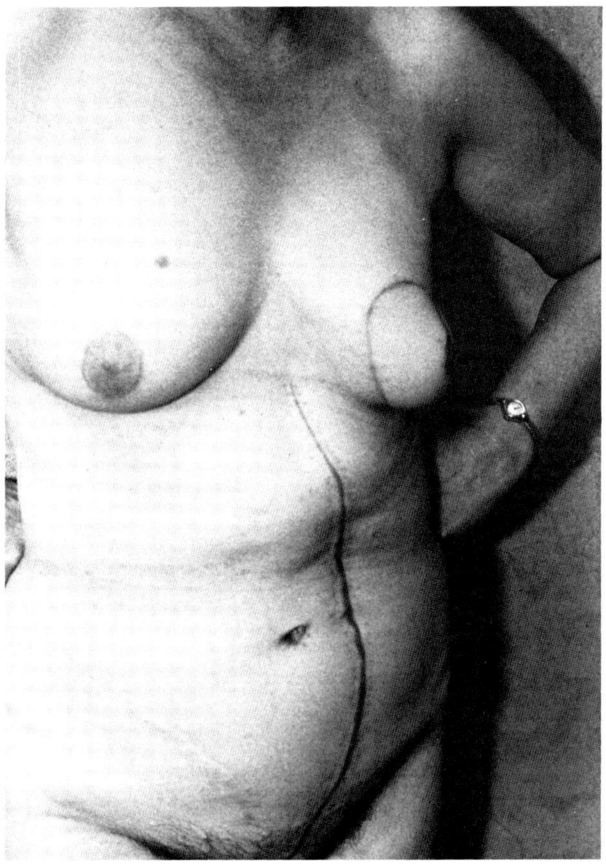

D

Figure 9.8. **A:** Preoperative markings before the mastectomy with immediate reconstruction (note the vertical scar that would hinder a lower transverse flap). **B:** One-year postoperative AP view. **C:** One-year postoperative left oblique view. **D:** One-year postoperative right oblique view.

Contralateral Rectus Abdominus Submammary Flap

Luis O. Vasconez

The woman who has undergone a radical mastectomy has lost breast skin, glandular tissue, the nipple, and muscle. Even with a modified mastectomy, a portion of the pectoralis major muscle may be deficient because of atrophy of the muscle from injury to the medial or lateral pectoral nerves. This loss of tissue usually produces a tightness on the side of the mastectomy.

Although reconstruction of the breast with a latissimus dorsi flap is an excellent method, breast reconstruction is often elected for aesthetic reasons and the creation of a significant scar on the back is unacceptable to some patients. Moreover, removal of the latissimus dorsi muscle may produce an anatomic depression in the back.

When reconstructing the breast, the surgeon should attempt to match the opposite breast, whenever possible, without tampering with it. Therefore the new breast is usually designed with some ptosis. To obtain this effect, the vertical deficit that usually exists on the mastectomized side must be corrected by the addition of extra skin. Most patients have excess skin in the contralateral inframammary region which may be removed and transferred to the mastectomy side (5,14,16). The secondary defect can then be closed with a reversed abdominoplasty, leaving a scar which is easily concealed in the inframammary fold.

The submammary flap is similar to the transverse abdominal flap initially described by Tai and Hasegwa (22). However, with the submammary flap procedure, to ensure that the perforating vessels from the epigastric arcade are kept intact, a portion of the rectus abdominis muscle is included along with the anterior rectus sheath (Figure 9.9E).

As previously described, the superior epigastric artery is a continuation of the internal mammary. It exits approximately 2 cm lateral to the xiphoid and is located deep to the costal margin as it reaches the deep surface of the rectus abdominus muscle. It has a longitudinal course in this muscle and anastomoses with the deep inferior epigastric artery, which is a branch of the femoral artery.

Operative Technique

With the patient in the erect position, the inframammary line is marked both on the intact side and, correspondingly, on the affected side. This line is a constant and cannot be changed despite surgical manipulation, e.g., reduction mammoplasty or procedures for the correction of ptosis. These are the only landmarks that are necessary for the operation other than a marking lateral to the xiphoid to indicate the relative point at which the superior epigastric vessels exit the costal margins.

The transverse contralateral submammary flap is outlined in the form of a "blunt" ellipse or, if possible, that of a sickle, with the upper edge corresponding to the inframammary line (Figure 9.9A). It is extended to the midaxillary line and is made wide enough to provide additional skin for the mastectomized side but not too wide to prevent the defect from being closed primarily by a reverse abdominoplasty.

The pivot point of this flap is relatively high, above the level of the xiphoid, and requires careful dissection underneath the costal margin or actual resection of the seventh costal cartilage subperichondrially.

When the flap is being elevated, the incision is deepened laterally to the fascia level. It is important to include the fascia over the intercostal muscles rather than run the risk of elevating the flap too superficially. The elevation continues medially until the lateral edge of the anterior rectus sheath is identified. This edge is incised vertically below the inferior edge of the island of the skin and superiorly into the costal margins.

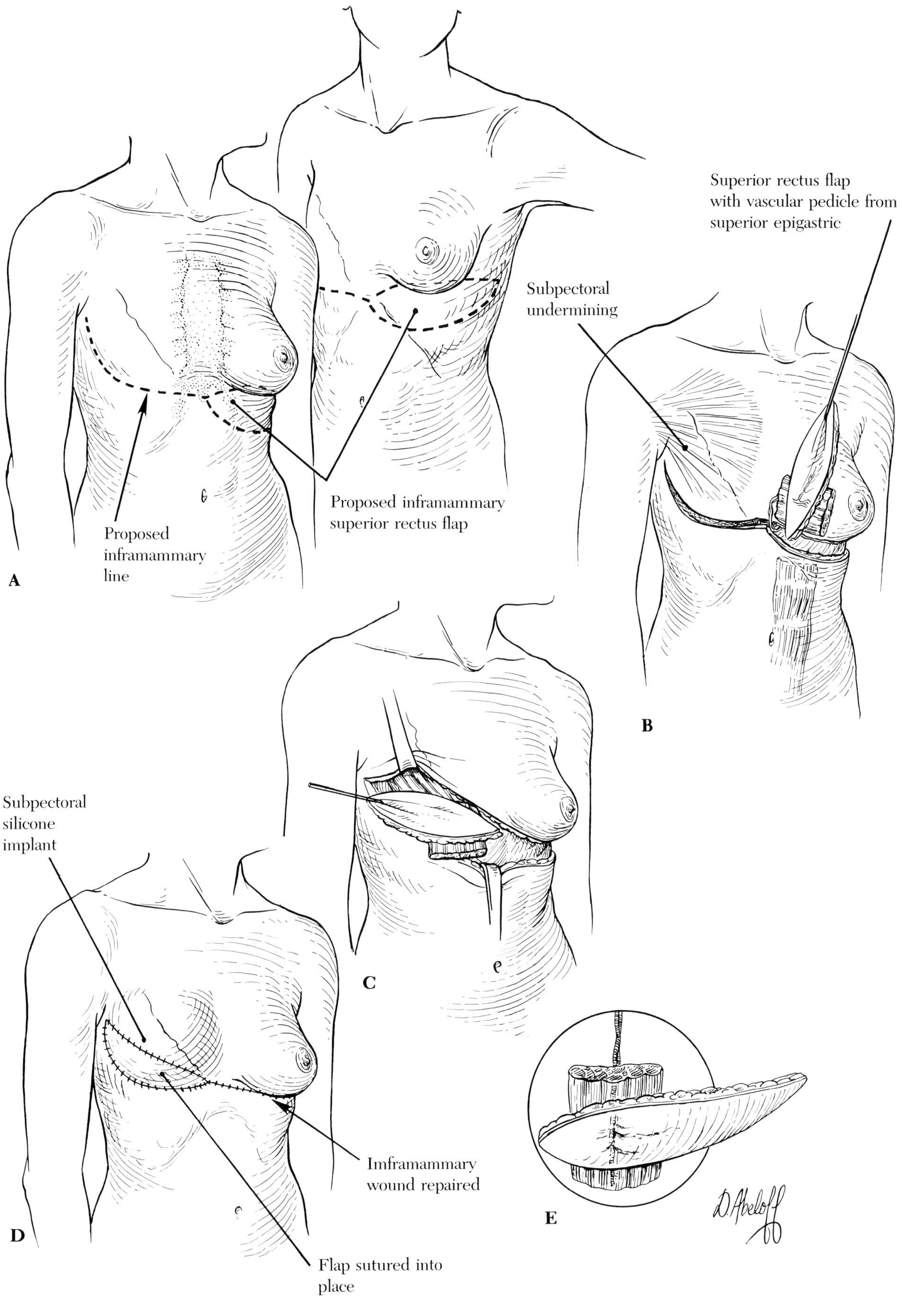

Figure 9.9. Steps of the operative technique: contralateral rectus abdominus submammary flap.

The anterior rectus sheath is then divided transversely, approximately 2–3 cm outside the skin island; the muscle is also divided inferiorly, preferably at one of the intersection tendinea. To facilitate the division of the muscle inferiorly, a longitudinal incision is made in the anterior rectus sheath. Anchoring sutures are placed between the muscle, the anterior rectus sheath, and

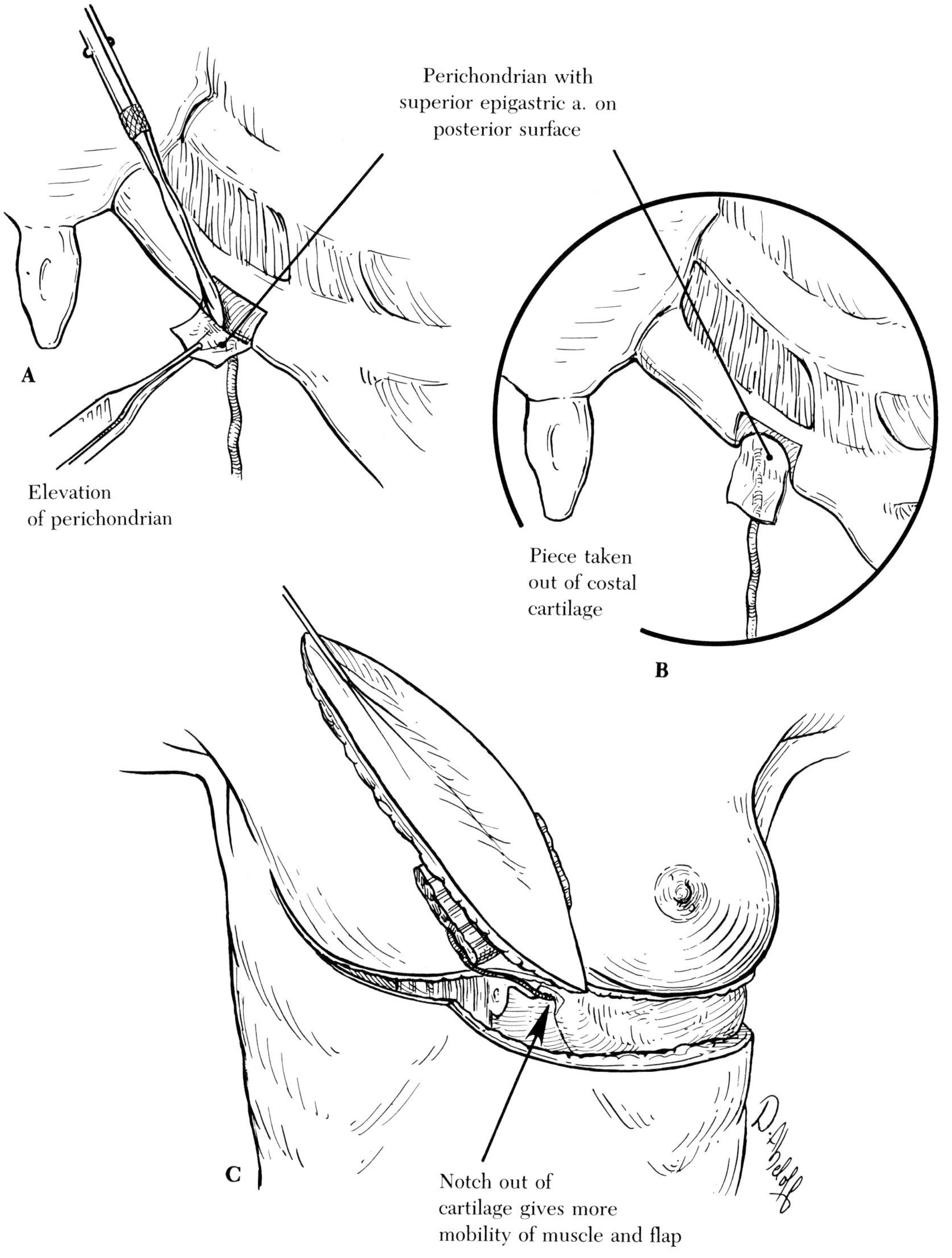

Figure 9.10. Freeing the vascular pedicle.

the island of skin to prevent any shearing forces. The muscle is then elevated bluntly from the posterior rectus sheath. At this point the superior epigastric vessels may be visible.

The origin of the rectus muscle is divided from the costal margin above the level of the xiphoid. It is relatively safe to divide the rectus sheath over the costal margin, but care must be taken when approaching the midline. The flap is then completely circumscribed, with the pivoting point placed sufficiently high that the flap may be transposed without tension into the outlined incision (Figure 9.9B). To do this, the surgeon must dissect underneath the costal margin in the subperichondrial plane or, preferably, remove a portion of the seventh costal cartilage. If an incision is made over the cartilage and the perichondrium is freed with an elevator, the vessels are protected and it is relatively safe to remove some of the cartilage (Figure 9.10A,B). When the vessel is visible the attachments lateral to it can be divided, and dissection can continue superiorly until the pivoting point is high enough to allow transposition without tension (Figure 9.10C).

On the side of the mastectomy, an incision is made in the form of a sickle at the level of the future inframammary crease; above this a subpectoral pocket is developed. The two incisions are connected, and the flap is carefully transposed. The tip of the flap, which originated in the midaxillary line, comes to rest on the most superior part of the opposite anterior axillary line on the side of the reconstruction (Figure 9.9C).

It is very important to minimize any tension on the epigastric vessels. Too much traction produces spasm, which is manifested by extreme pallor of the flap. This may persist and cause considerable distress to the operating team.

The portion of rectus muscle is then sutured to the lower edge of the pectoralis major muscle. An implant of appropriate size is placed in the submuscular plane, and the skin is approximated with fine nylon sutures (Figure 9.9D). Suction catheters are used.

Complications

It must be emphasized that extreme caution be exercised when insetting the flap. The pedicle may appear to be lax, but after the implant is inserted the position of the flap moves laterally, which may cause tension. If tension does occur and spasm develops, the flap should immediately be "taken down" and reinset more medially without tension. Spraying the pedicle with 1% plain Xylocaine often helps to relieve the spasm.

Hematomas are rare but should be evacuated immediately to avoid tension on the pedicle. Complete closure of the defect in the anterior rectus sheath should not be attempted as it may result in strangulation of the pedicle.

Results

The submammary flap is a safe but technically challenging procedure. The dissection is somewhat complex because of the necessary high pivoting point of the flap and the need at times to resect costal cartilage. The results, however, are very satisfactory (Figures 9.11 and 9.12) (23).

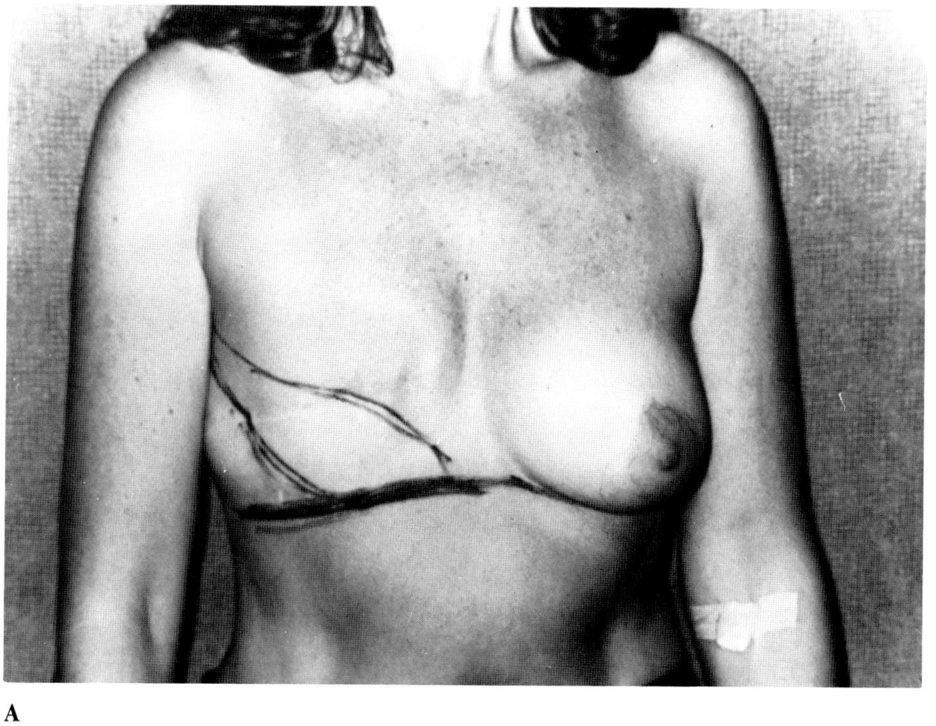

A

Figure 9.11. A: Preoperative view of a right modified radical mastectomy defect with the future inframammary line and position of the flap marked.

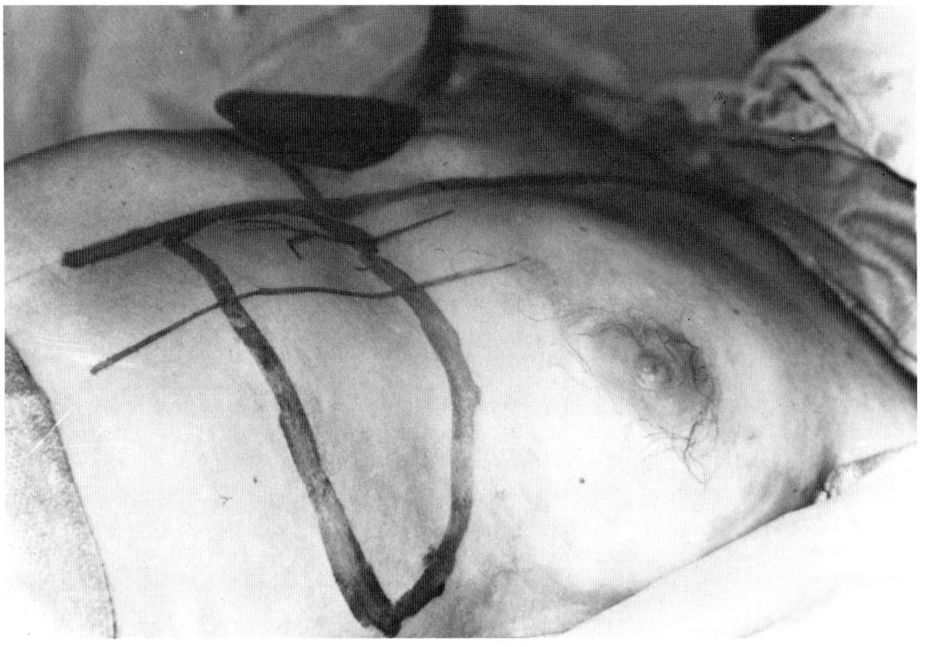

B

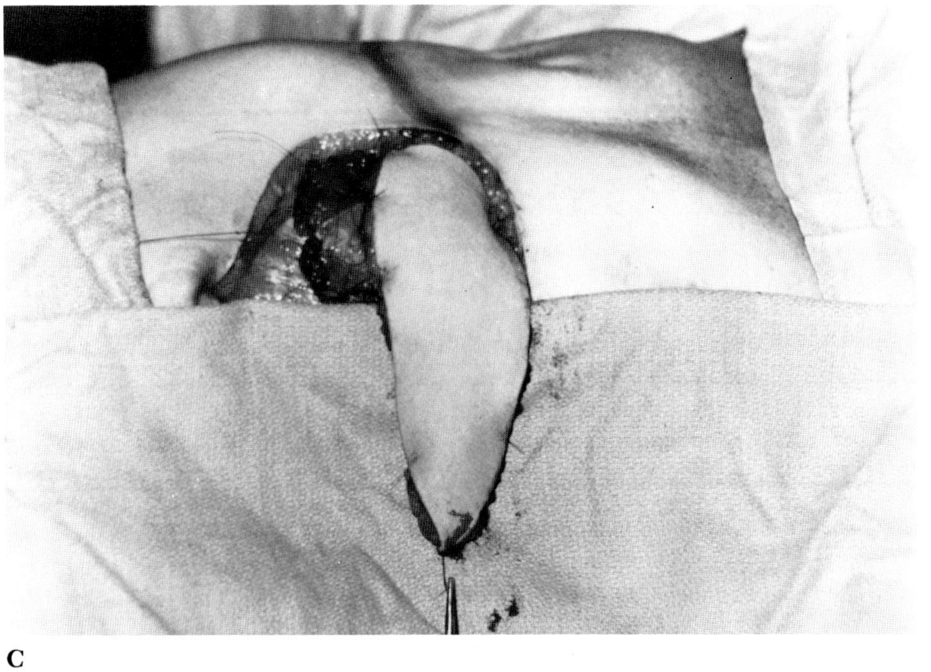

C

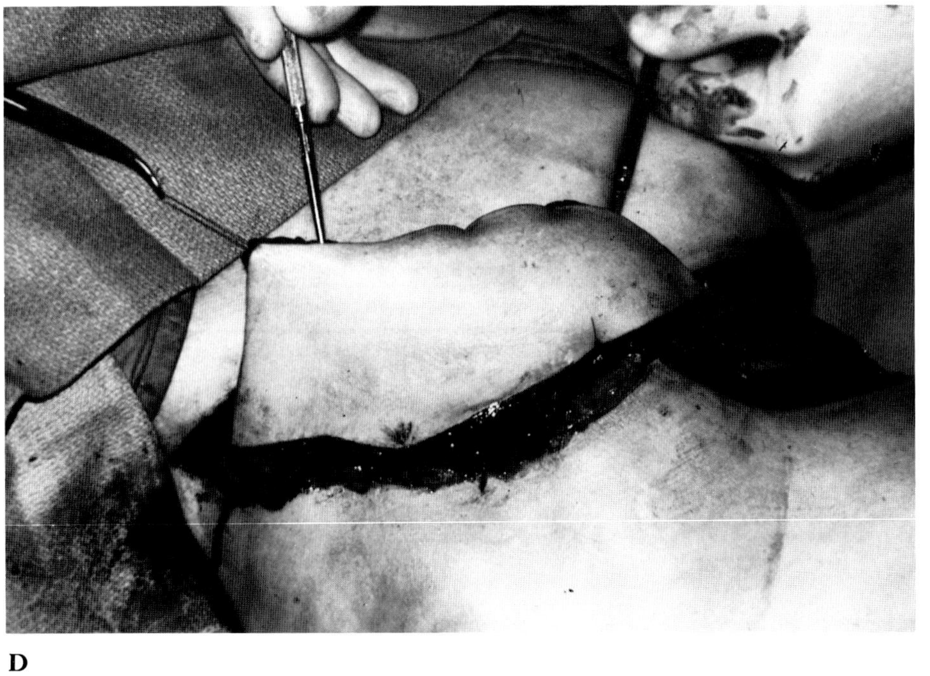

D

B: Marking the contralateral submammary flap. **C:** Intraoperative view of the contralateral flap elevated showing a segment of rectus muscle. **D:** Flap very carefully rotated into position without tension on the pedicle.

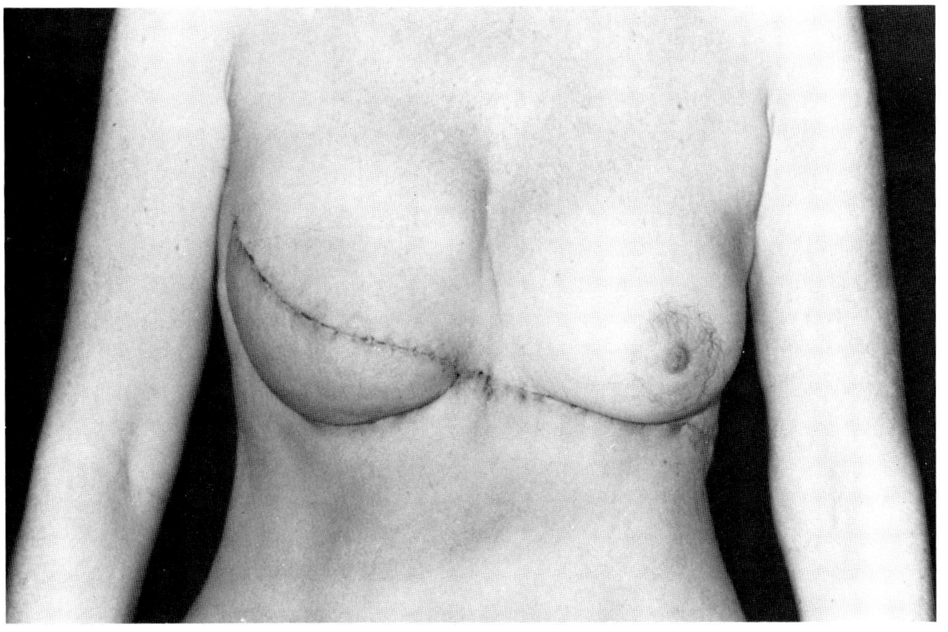

E

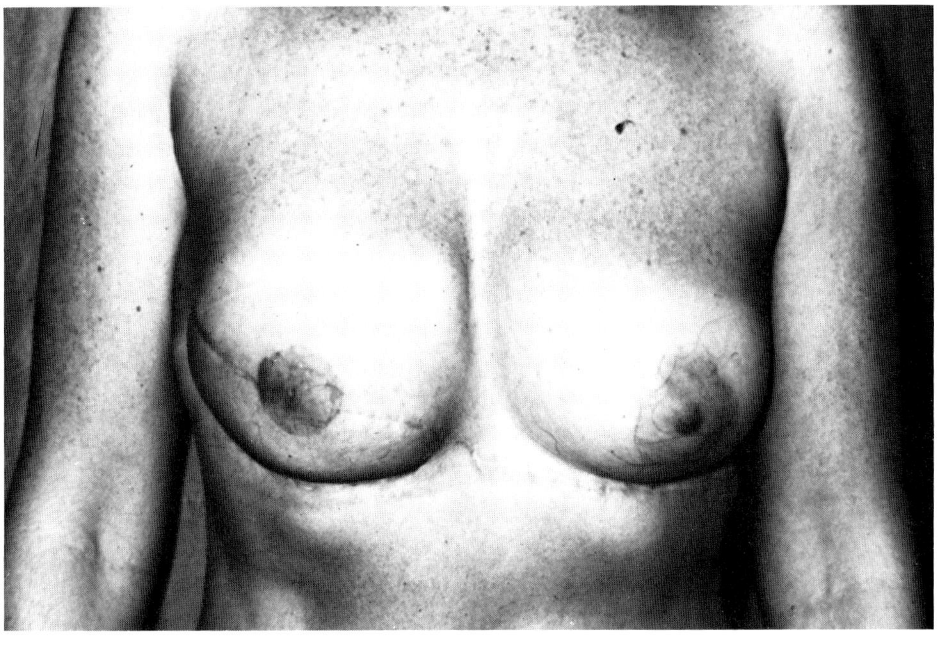

F

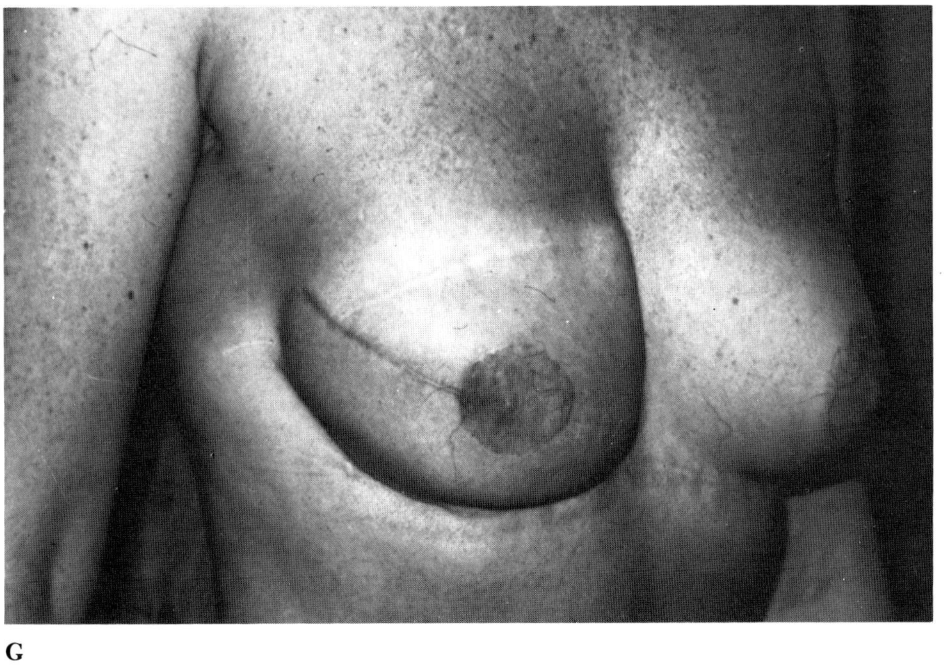

G

E: Postoperative result showing good symmetry of the breast mound. A silicone gel implant was used. **F:** Final postoperative result, AP view, after nipple reconstruction. **G:** Final postoperative result, oblique view, after nipple reconstruction.

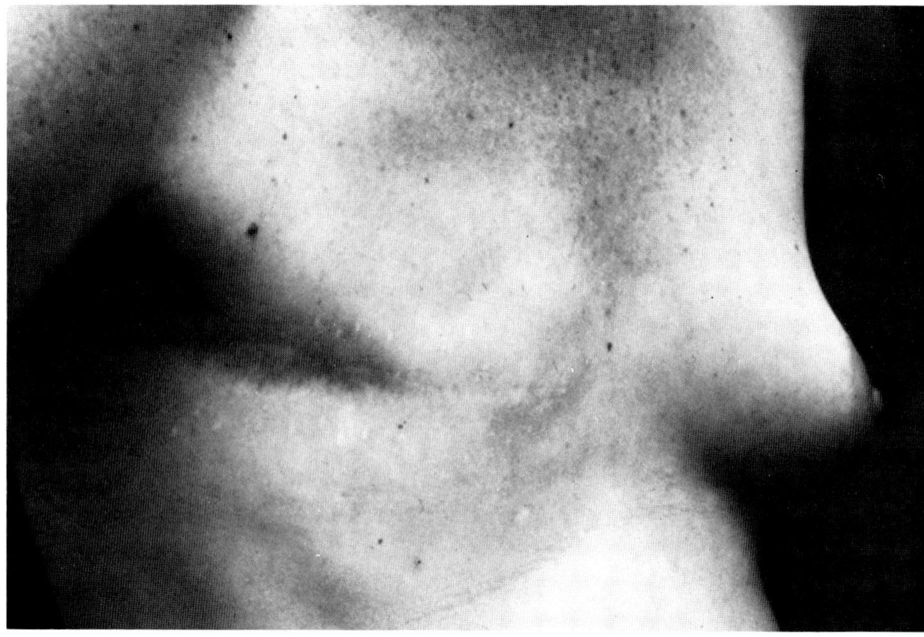

A

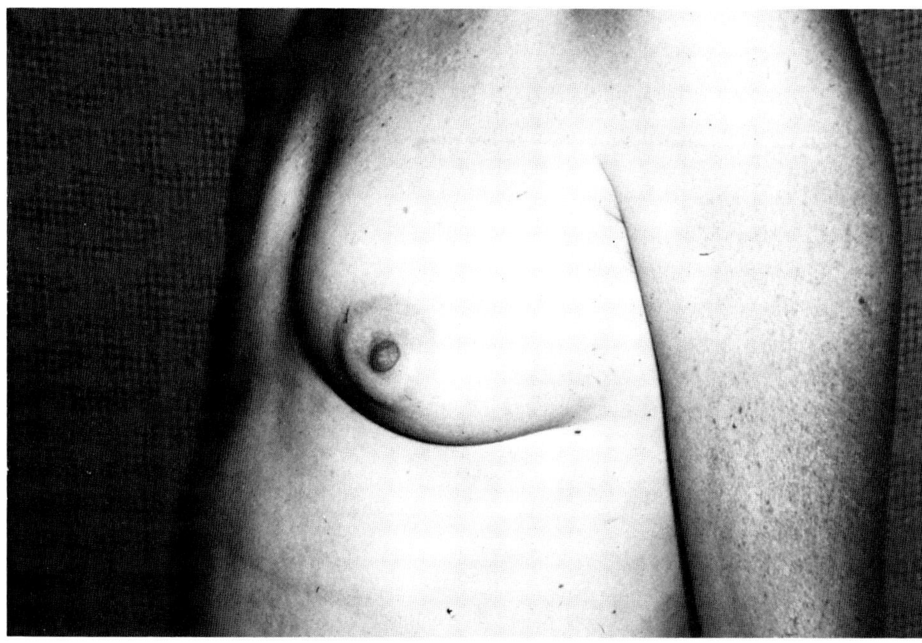

B

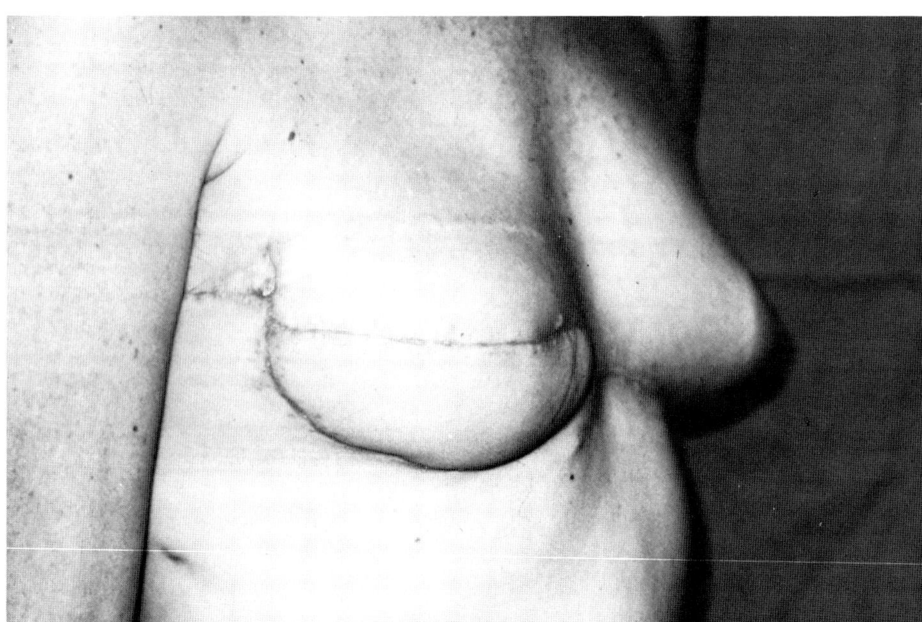

C

Figure 9.12. **A:** Preoperative right oblique mastectomy defect **B:** Preoperative left oblique view. **C:** Postoperative right oblique view with flap inset and silicone implant in place **D:** Postoperative left oblique view of breast mound **E:** AP view with nipple reconstruction

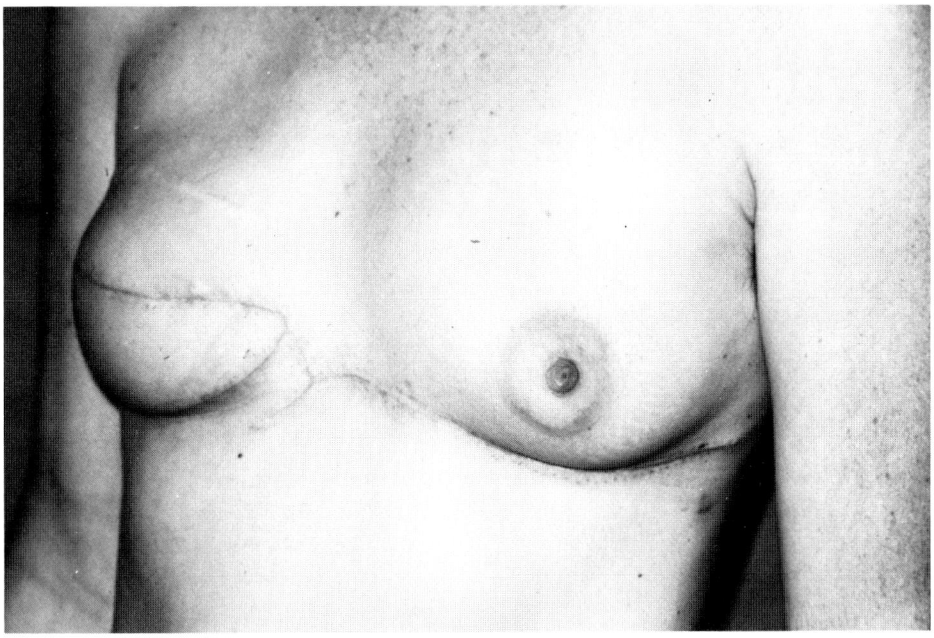

D

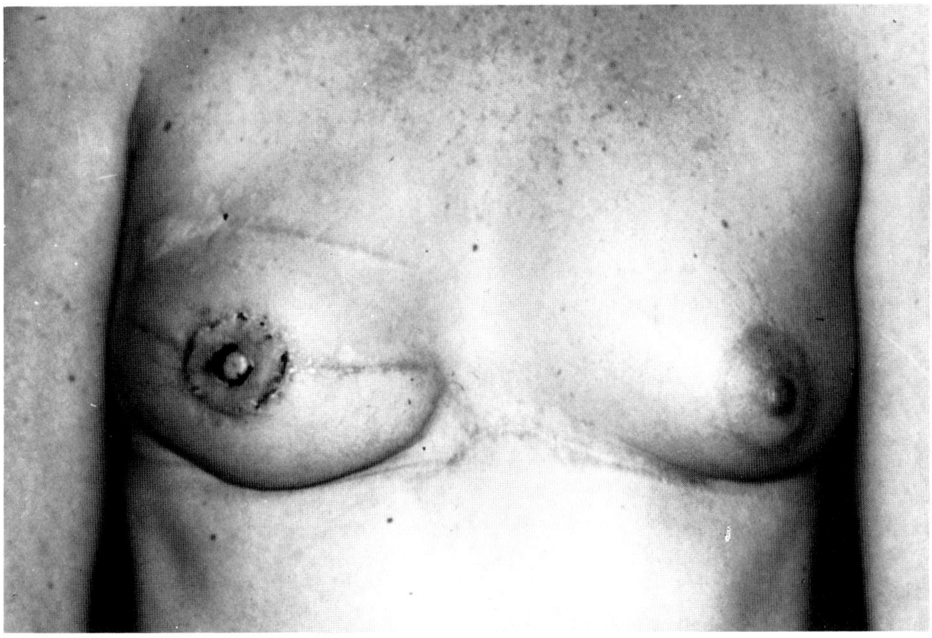

E

Unilateral Transverse Abdominal Island Flap

Carl R. Hartrampf, Jr.

Most mastectomy defects can be reconstructed using the transverse abdominal island flap technique. It may be the procedure of choice for women who have undergone a radical Halsted mastectomy where the resulting infraclavicular hollow and the anterior axillary fold can be filled with soft, natural material.

Contraindications

A previous abdominoplasty with disruption of the rectus perforators or abdominal scars that disrupt both superior epigastric vessels naturally preclude the success of this method of breast reconstruction. However, if the patency of the superior epigastric vessels is merely in doubt, this may be determined by preoperative arteriograms or by dividing the inferior epigastric artery at the beginning of the operation (21). Abdominal scarring per se is not a contraindication, although it may make mapping out the area of the flap more challenging. A paramedian abdominal scar excludes the use of the underlying ipsilateral rectus muscle, but the contralateral one can be used. Similarly a Kocher cholecystectomy scar means that the right superior epigastric vessels have been divided, but the left side can be used. If no scarring is present either side of the abdomen may be used.

This involved operation is naturally not recommended when the patient requests another technique or prefers a scar on her back to a scar on her abdomen. It is also contraindicated in individuals with severe systemic illness, e.g., diabetes, uncontrolled hypertension, or chronic respiratory or severe cardiac disease. It is usually not recommended for heavy smokers.

Preoperative Planning

With the patient erect, the exact limits of the mastectomy defect are marked, and the expected level of the inframammary crease is drawn. Generally, the inframammary crease is pulled down more on the mastectomy side during closure of the abdominal defect, and allowance must be made for this by marking the crease an inch or more above the contralateral side or the reconstructed breast will be too low.

The longitudinal and transverse dimensions of the proposed breast are determined by measuring the same points on the opposite breast in a curvilinear fashion across the nipple point (Figure 9.13). The transverse dimension *AB* is equal to the measurement from the parasternal line across the nipple to the anterior axillary line. The longitudinal dimension *CD* is equal to the measurement from the uppermost point of the mastectomy defect across the nipple to the inframammary line and should be as generous as possible to allow the new breast a normal projection and a natural ptosis comparable to that of the opposite breast. These measurements are now transferred to the abdomen.

In the absence of abdominal scarring, measurement *CD* can extend across the midline to approximately the lateral edge of the contralateral rectus muscle. Abdominal scarring, however, decreases the supply of tissue in this area, and it may be necessary to harvest additional tissue above the umbilicus. The amount of tissue needed is balanced with the amount of tissue available.

Operative Technique

The patient is placed on the operating table in a supine position with arms abducted and knees slightly flexed for future ease of closure of the abdominal wound. The upper marking of the transverse abdominal island flap is incised

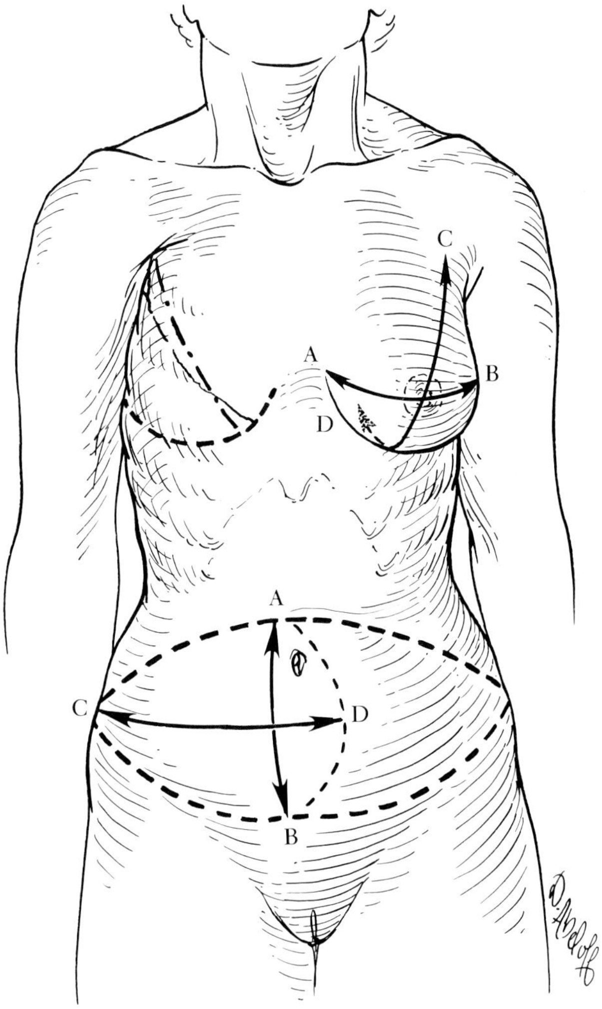

Figure 9.13. Measuring out the abdominal flap using the ipsilateral pedicle.

down to the fascia and undermining is performed to above the rib cage. The mastectomy scar is excised and the chest flaps are elevated to the limits of the mastectomy defect, often to the clavicle and humerus in the case of an extreme radical. All limiting scar in the axilla and elsewhere is released. A tunnel is made between the chest wound and the epigastric abdominal wound, large enough to admit a fist (Figure 9.14B).

The undermined upper abdominal flap is then pulled down as far as possible towards the pubis. At the same time, the pubic skin is pushed upward. This maneuver permits the future lower incision of the island flap to be determined more accurately, so that the greatest dimension of flap can be obtained that would allow easy closure of the abdominal wound. The inferior incision is then made across the abdomen in a concave direction, to meet the superior incision at its lateral extent on each side.

The contralateral flap is elevated first, with the dissection carried out exactly on the external oblique fascia to prevent damage to the smaller vessels in the abdominal flap. As the midline is approached, the position of the lateral edge of the rectus sheath and the number and location of vessel perforators are noted (Figure 9.14C). The ipsilateral side of the flap is now elevated to the lateral edge of the rectus sheath.

A vertical incision is made in the lateral rectus sheath half way between the umbilicus and the pubis. The muscle is split bluntly and the location of the inferior epigastric pedicle entering the posterolateral surface is located (Figure 9.14D). The pedicle is clamped, divided and ligated. The incision in the lateral edge of the rectus sheath is extended upwards to the top of the flap, leaving approximately 1 cm cuff of rectus sheath and a lateral segment of rectus muscle. Sutures are placed securing the subcutaneous fat of the flap to the fascia and muscle to prevent any shearing or separation during maneuvering of the flap.

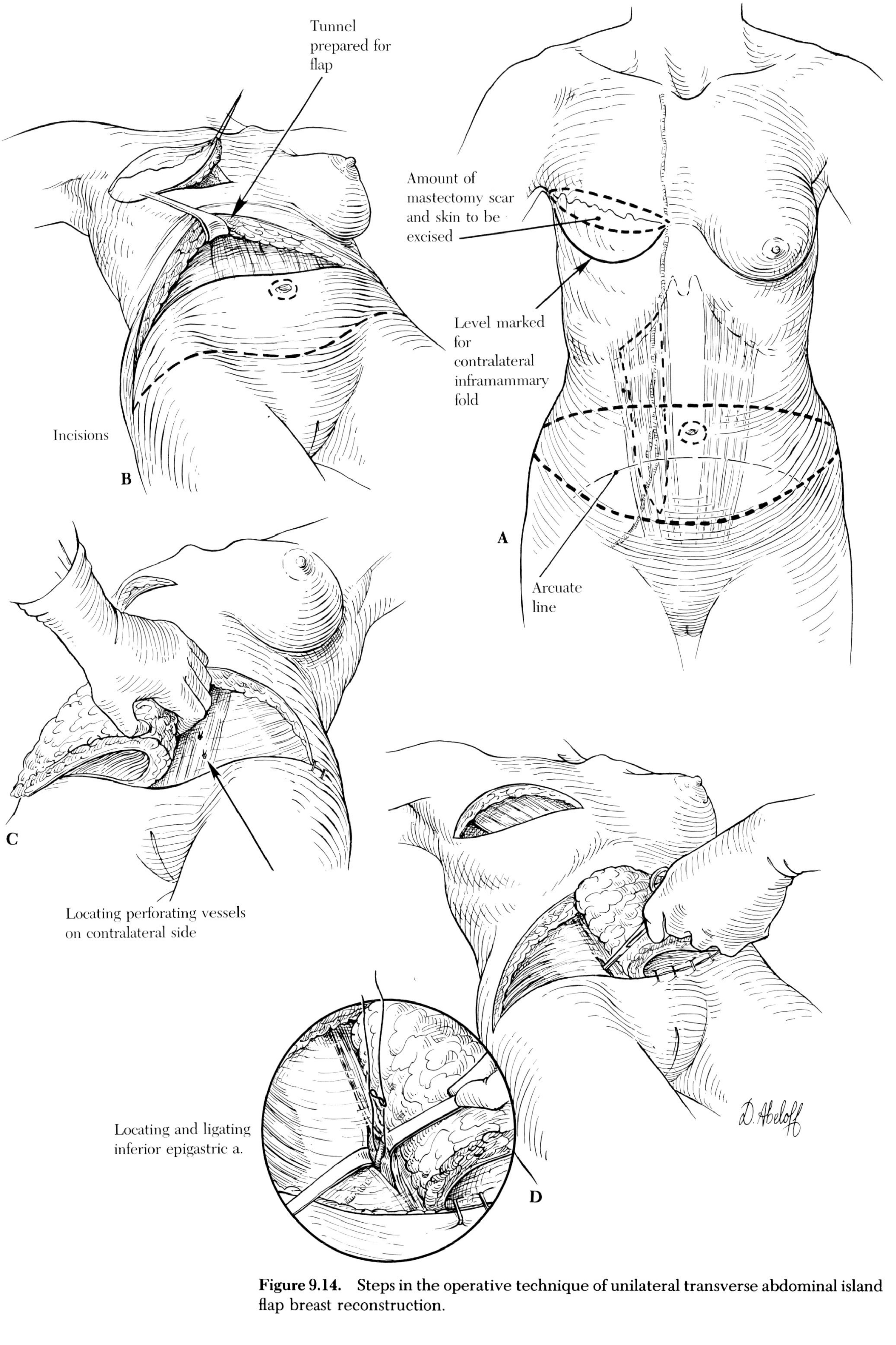

Figure 9.14. Steps in the operative technique of unilateral transverse abdominal island flap breast reconstruction.

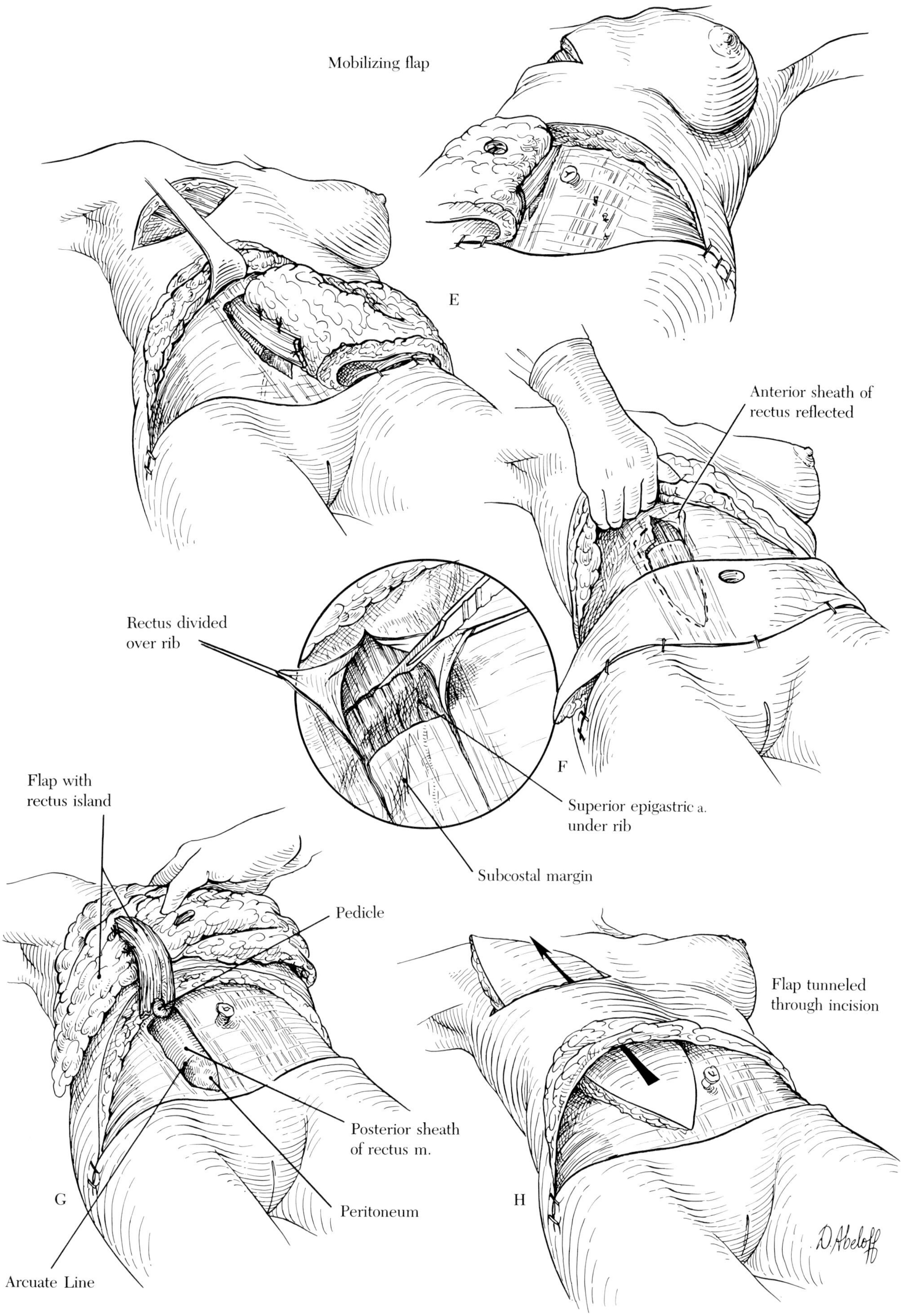
Mobilizing flap
E
Anterior sheath of rectus reflected
Rectus divided over rib
F
Superior epigastric a. under rib
Subcostal margin
Flap with rectus island
Pedicle
Posterior sheath of rectus m.
Peritoneum
G
Arcuate Line
Flap tunneled through incision
H
D. Abeloff

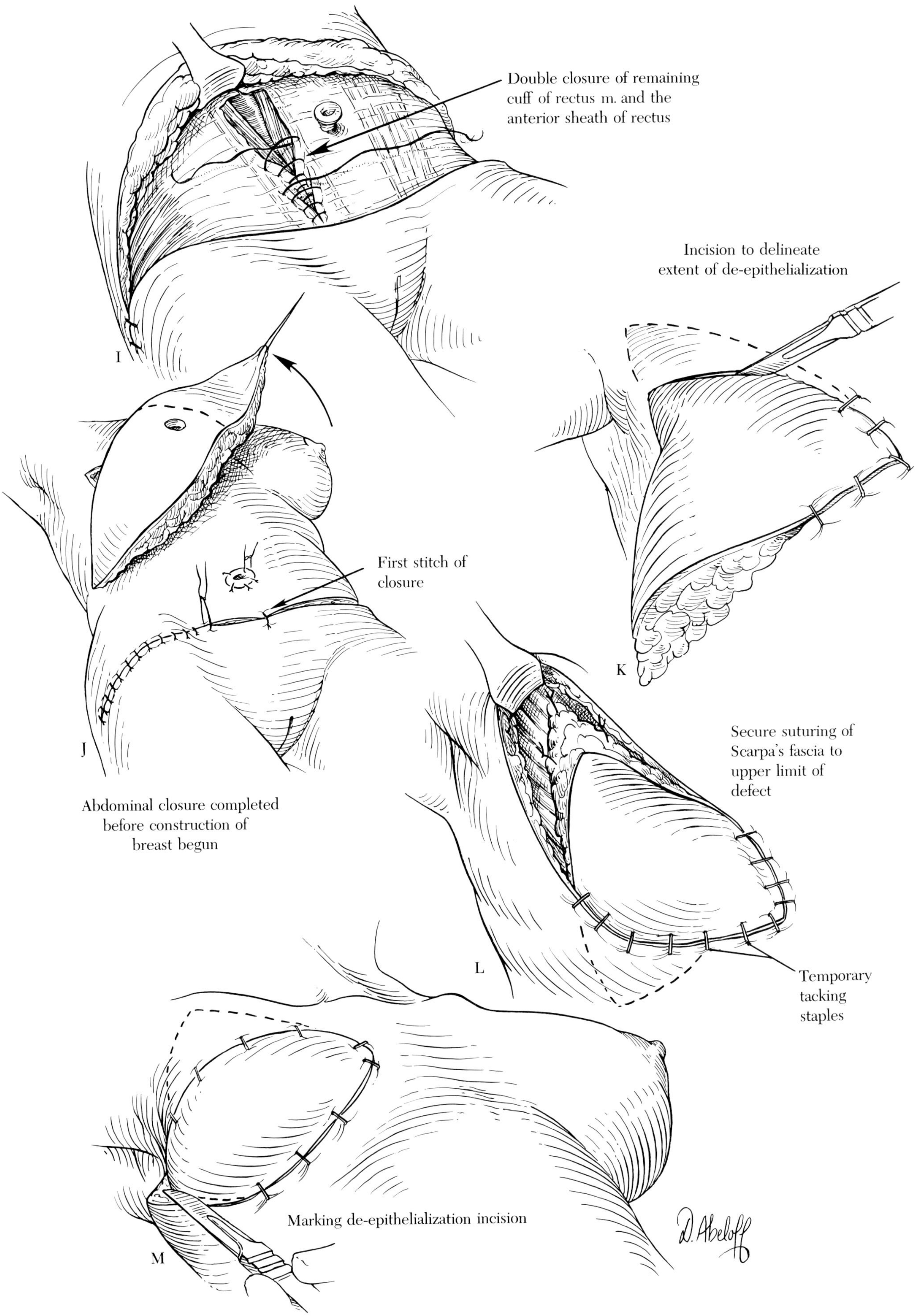
Double closure of remaining cuff of rectus m. and the anterior sheath of rectus
I
Incision to delineate extent of de-epithelialization
First stitch of closure
K
J
Secure suturing of Scarpa's fascia to upper limit of defect
Abdominal closure completed before construction of breast begun
L
Temporary tacking staples
Marking de-epithelialization incision
M
D. Abeloff

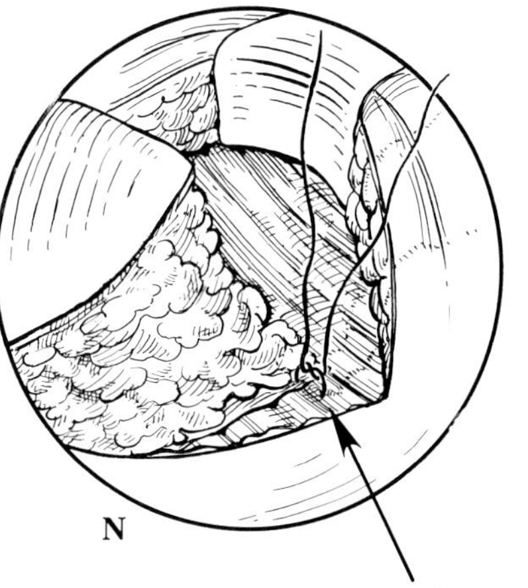

N

Tacking Scarpa's fascia to body wall

Placing skin stitches

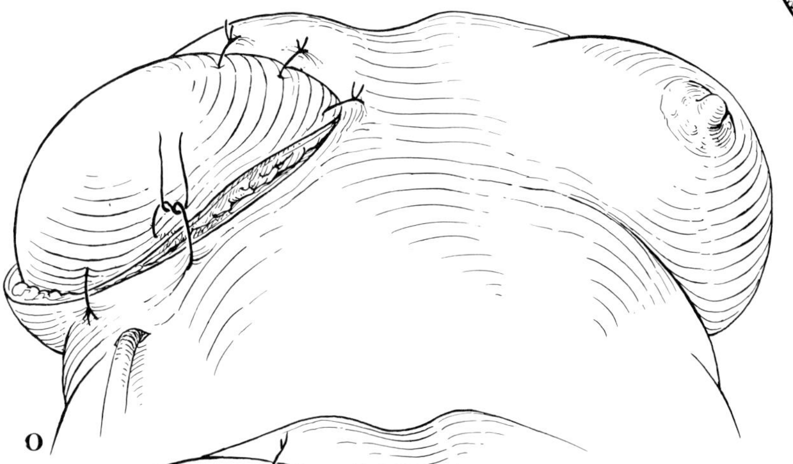

O

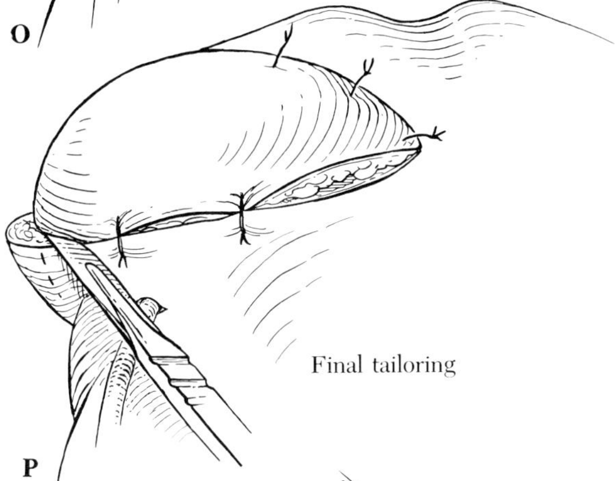

Final tailoring

P

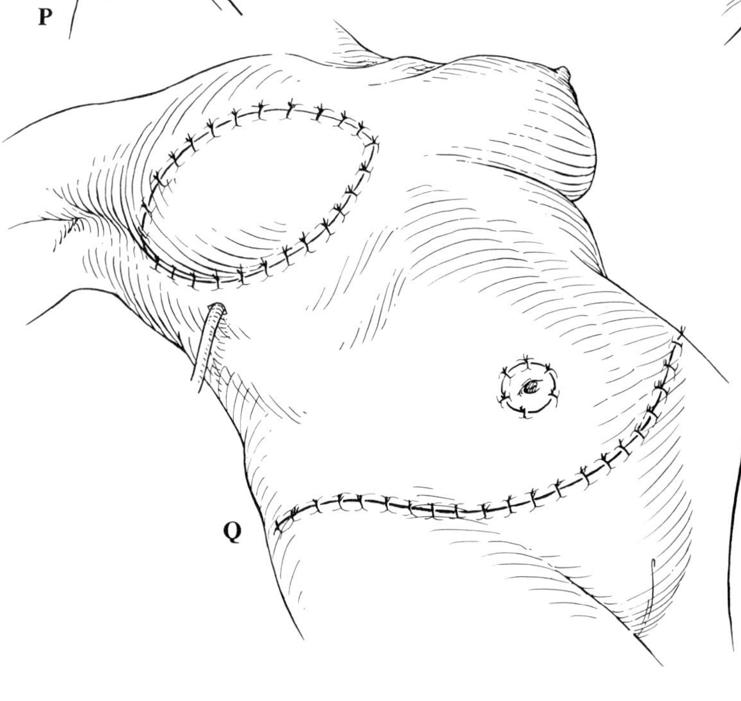

Q

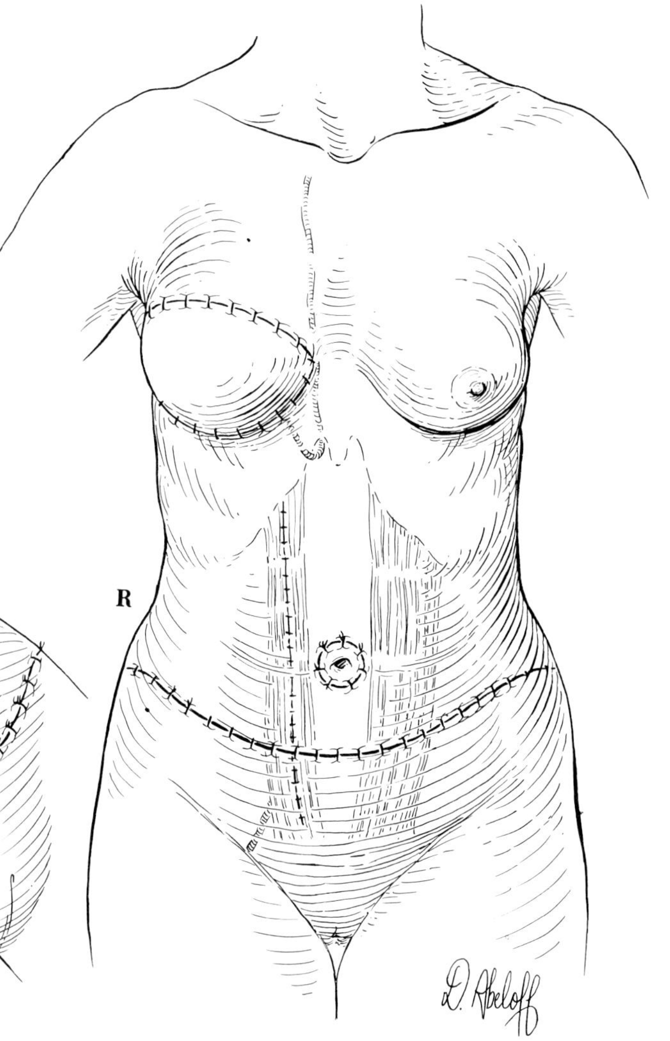

R

The central portion of the rectus sheath inferiorly is incised in a V shape. The medial edge of the rectus sheath beneath the flap is incised upwards towards the umbilicus, leaving approximately 1 cm of cuff rectus sheath. At the level of the V cut in the fascia, the rectus muscle is divided transversely (Figure 9.14E). The rectus muscle, with the large flap attached is carefully delivered upwards. The arcuate line, which demonstrates the lowest extent of the posterior rectus sheath, is noted. Below this line the peritineum is seen (Figure 9.14G). Inferior epigastric vessels are usually present on the posterior surface of the rectus muscle. As the rectus muscle is freed up the inferior epigastric vessels usually disappear into the muscle to arborize in a rich network with branches of the superior epigastric vessels at the level of the umbilicus. The umbilicus may be circumscribed and left as an apple core on the posterior rectus sheath (Figure 9.14G) or it may be excised and sutured back later as a full thickness graft.

The rectus sheath above the flap may be left on the muscle. The rectus sheath is incised at the medial and lateral border of the muscle. The muscle pedicle above the flap then has anterior rectus sheath attached when it is elevated up on the chest. As an alternative, the rectus sheath superior to the flap can be split vertically upwards in the midline and the two halves of the sheath are peeled back from the muscle (Figure 9.14F). The dissection can be difficult and may cause damage to the rectus muscle because of the adherent tendinous intersections. As the flap and muscle pedicle is elevated up to the costal margin, some communicating laterally placed nerves and vessels may be encountered. These are segmental nerves and vessels from the thoraco-lumbar complex and they have to be divided to free the pedicle. This is particularly important immediately below the costal margin. If these nerves and vessels are not divided, they will restrict the upward mobilization of the pedicle. In addition, atrophy of the muscle may not occur and sometimes the patients may complain of subcostal discomfort. The superior epigastric vessels may or may not be seen on the posterior surface, but the plane of dissection should be directly on the posterior rectus sheath and away from the muscle. The undermining of the skin in the epigastrium should have reached to the level of the fifth rib, the anterior rectus sheath should be opened to that point and the bulk of the rectus muscle can now be divided transversely, well above the anterior surface of the seventh rib, to facilitate rotation of the pedicle (Figure 9.14F). The muscular pedicle can be narrowed at this point again to facilitate rotation. Great care is taken to avoid injury to the superior epigastric pedicle as it emerges beneath the rib cage, approximately 2 cm from the sternum. The entire transverse abdominal island flap is now supported by a small segment of rectus muscle containing the superior epigastric vessels (Figure 9.14G).

The transverse abdominal island flap and its pedicle is then delivered through the "tunnel" into the mastectomy defect (Figure 9.14H).

The operating table is flexed and the patient's knees are brought further towards the chest. The abdominal wound is closed before the future inframammary line is finally decided. If the inframammary line is incised before closure of the abdomen, there is a tendency for the final inframammary line to be too low. A double layer running permanent suture closure of the remaining rectus muscle and rectus fascia is performed (Figure 9.14I).

After the abdomen has been closed, attention is turned to the sculpturing or shaping of the abdominal flap into the new breast mound (Figure 9.14J). Skin staples are useful in holding the flap in a temporary position on the chest wall while the final plans for tailoring the flap to be inset are made. During this maneuvering, one should be very aware of the folding of the underlying rectus muscle. It is very important to avoid any acute kinking that could impede the vascular flow. If possible, it is best to position the muscle pedicle in a lazy S form so that no acute kinks occur. The medial and superior part of the flap is usually going to be de-epithelialized and inset underneath the chest skin flaps to produce "fill" and contour to the upper part of the breast and chest (Figure 9.14K). Time spent at this point of the operation is well used and the difference between a good or an only fair result is often decided at this point. The de-epithelialized part of the flap is sutured to the underlying chest wall and not to the chest skin flap (Figure 9.14L).

Final tailoring and closure is then performed with drains being inserted behind the flap and brought out through stab wounds in the axilla (Figure 9.14 0,P,Q).

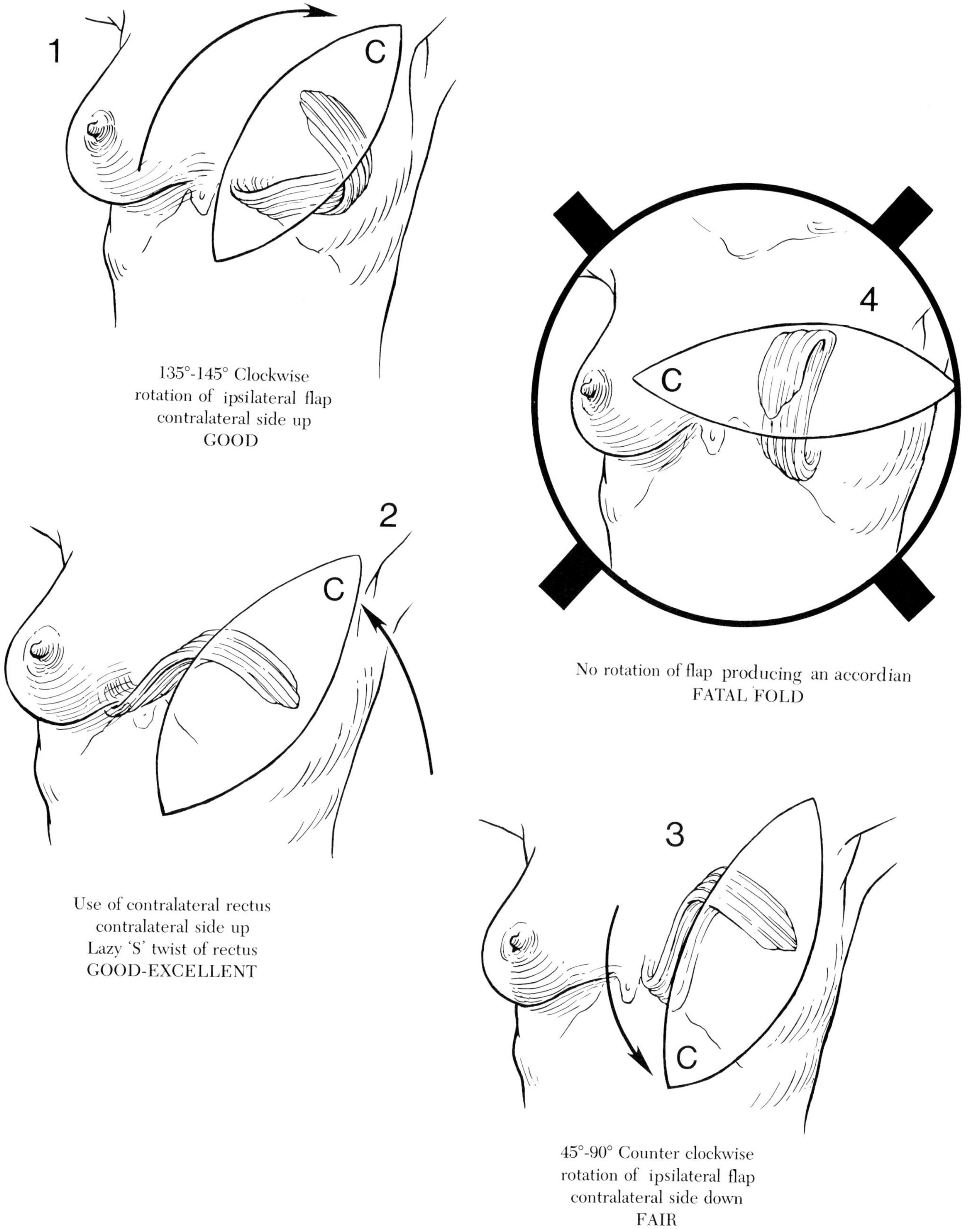

Figure 9.15. Combinations of flap rotation.

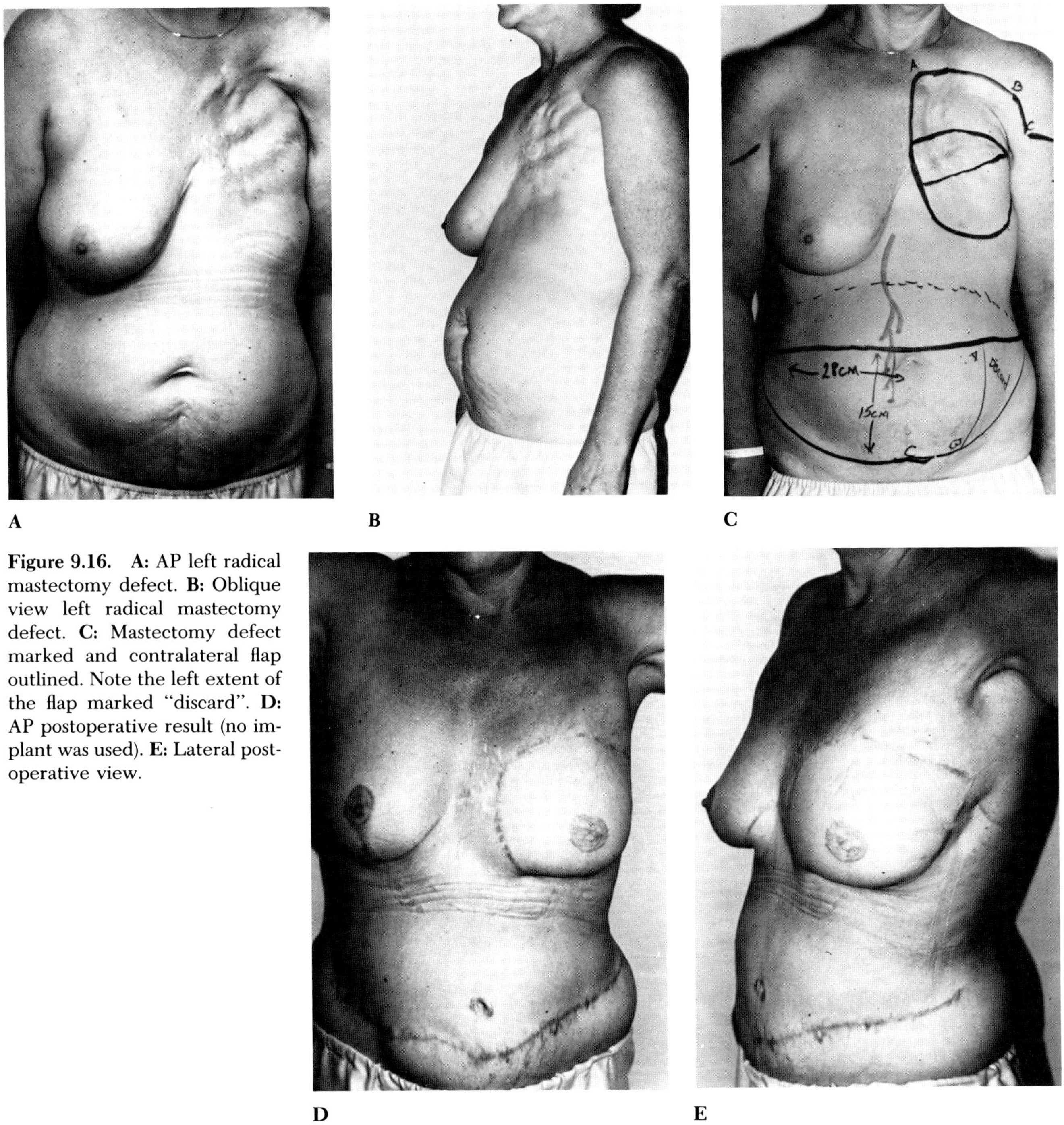

Figure 9.16. **A:** AP left radical mastectomy defect. **B:** Oblique view left radical mastectomy defect. **C:** Mastectomy defect marked and contralateral flap outlined. Note the left extent of the flap marked "discard". **D:** AP postoperative result (no implant was used). **E:** Lateral postoperative view.

Points of Caution

Adequate time and attention should be paid to shaping the new breast in order to maximize the benefits of this transverse flap operation.

The upper edge of the flap dermis of Scarpa's fascia should be secured to the upper limits of the mastectomy defect (clavicle, muscle, humerus, etc.) with permanent suture material (Figure 9.14L,N). Tissue under the upper skin flap should be deepithelialized or thinned as necessary to give a normal shape to the upper breast. The lower portion of the flap should be allowed to "hang out" and be fixed to the inframammary skin line only with skin or dermal sutures (Figure 9.14K,M). Deep fixation in the lower breast area is not necessary and could jeopardize the venous return by "bridling" the vascular pedicle. Temporary staple fixation aids in maneuvering this flap tissue into its final form (Figure 9.14 O–R). The breast pocket should be drained.

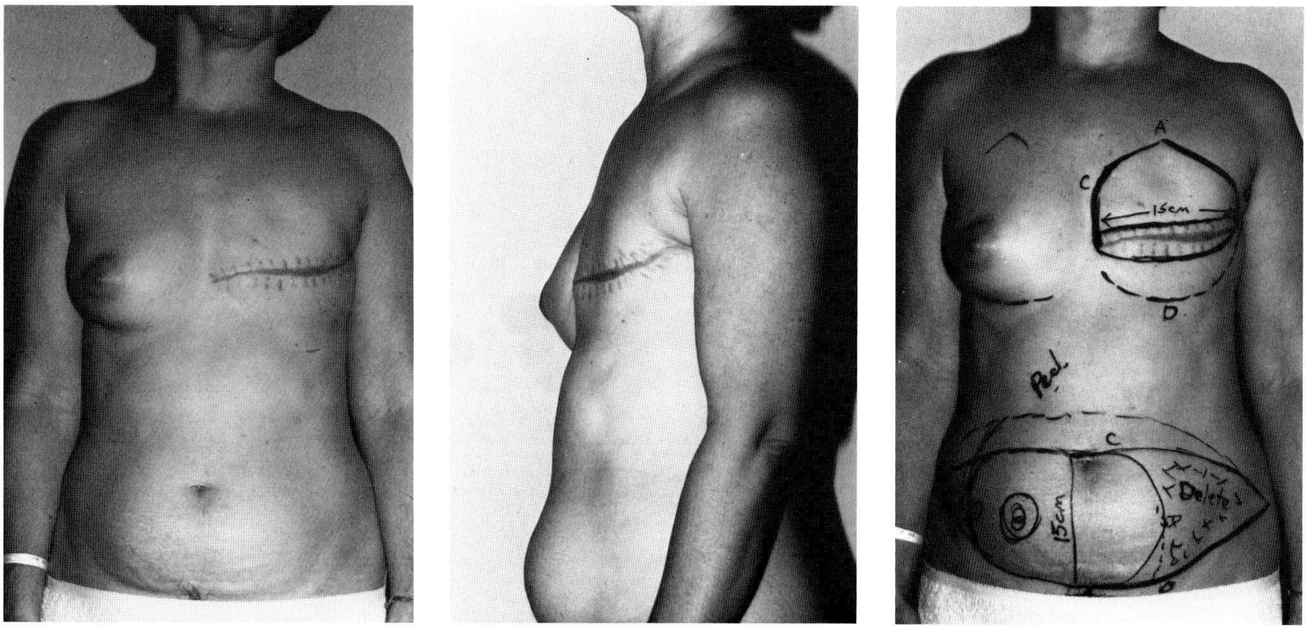

A B C

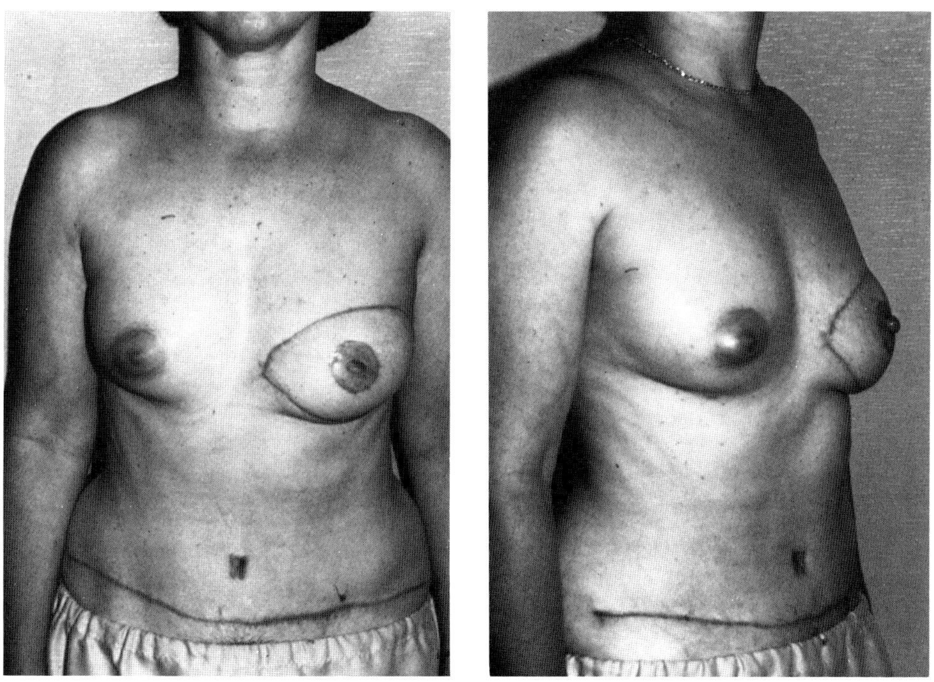

D E

Figure 9.17. **A:** AP left modified radical mastectomy defect. **B:** Lateral view. **C:** Mastectomy defect marked and contralateral flap outlined. **D:** AP postoperative view (no implant was used). **E:** Oblique postoperative view.

The possible combination of flap rotations and molding maneuvers is unlimited. In any fixation or shaping effort, the underlying vascular pedicle must be considered (Figure 9.15). Arterial input has not been a problem with this flap, but venous return can be severely compromised by either a double accordion "fatal fold" or excess tension on the muscular pedicle. Because obstruction of venous drainage is usually not apparent until several hours after completion of the operation, potential problems should be sought out and corrected at the shaping stage of the procedure.

It is very important to maintain adequate perfusion through the flap by avoiding hypovolemia (6). Blood transfusions are usually necessary.

Postoperative monitoring of the color and warmth of the flap is essential during the first few hours to allow correction of vascular problems before irreversible tissue damage occurs. A flap that appears mottled and cool and does not respond to therapeutic measures should be reexplored and the offending "kink" or tight pedicle corrected. Figures 9.16–9.18 represent this technique.

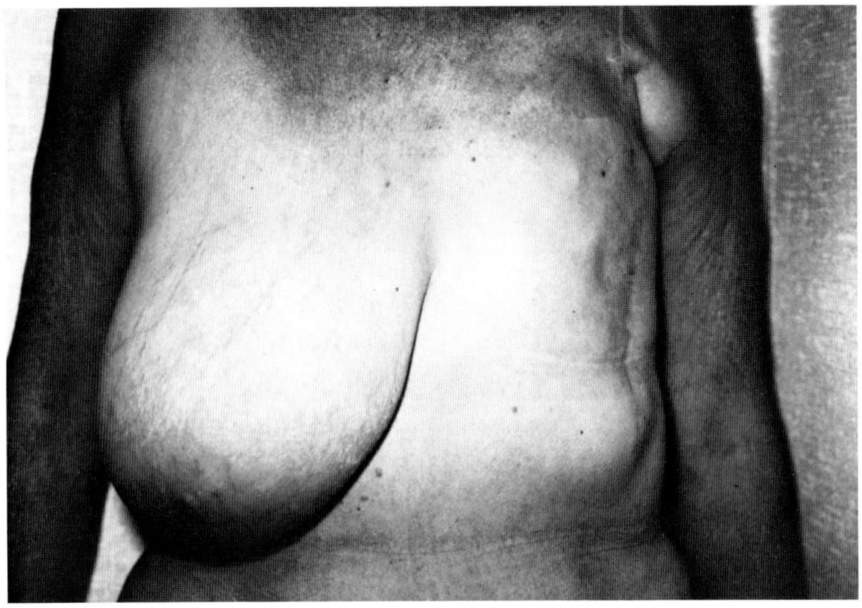

A

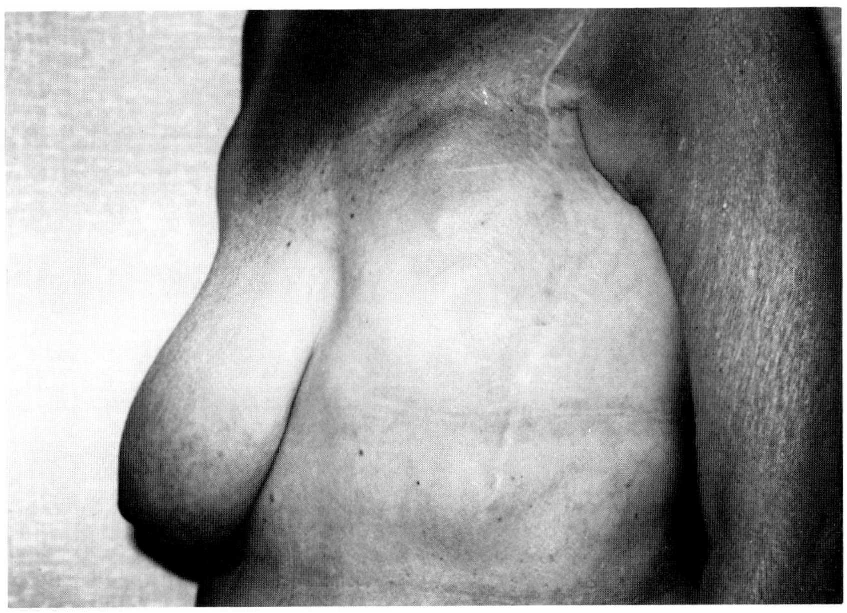

B

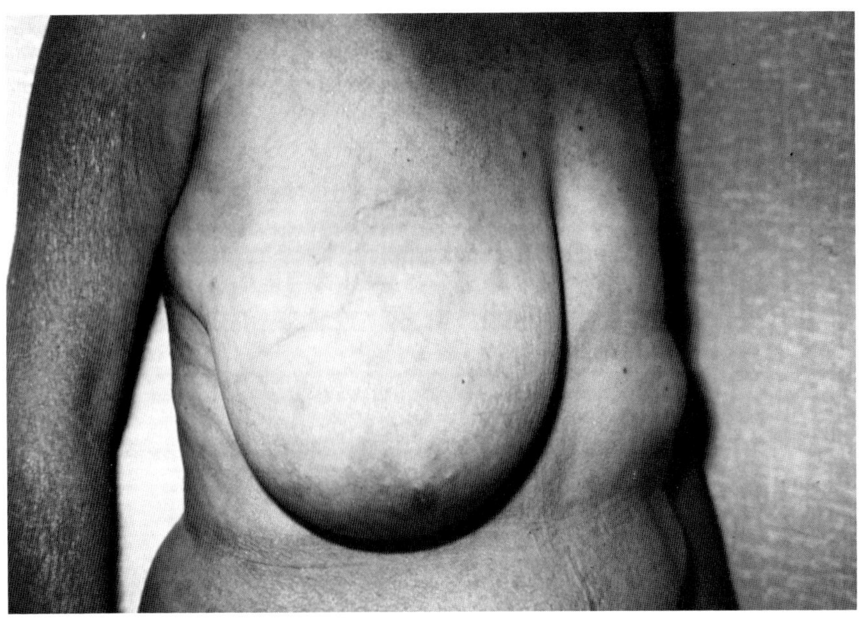

C

Figure 9.18. Salvage procedure. **A:** AP left radical mastectomy defect **B:** Left oblique view **C:** Right oblique view.

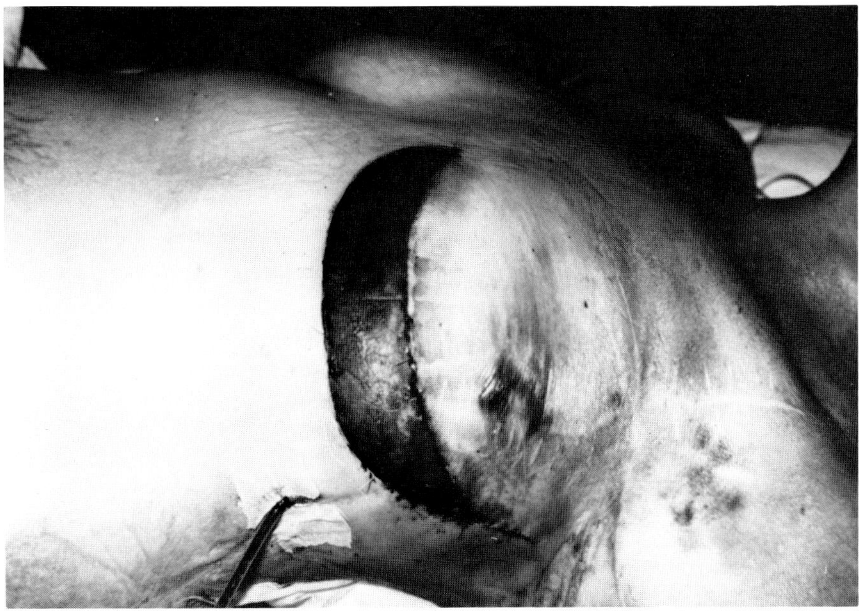

D

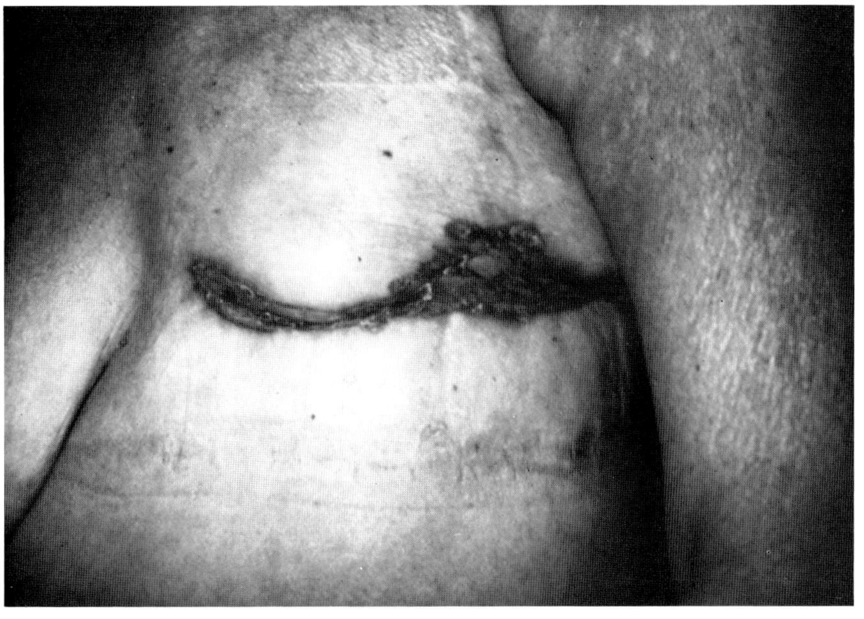

E

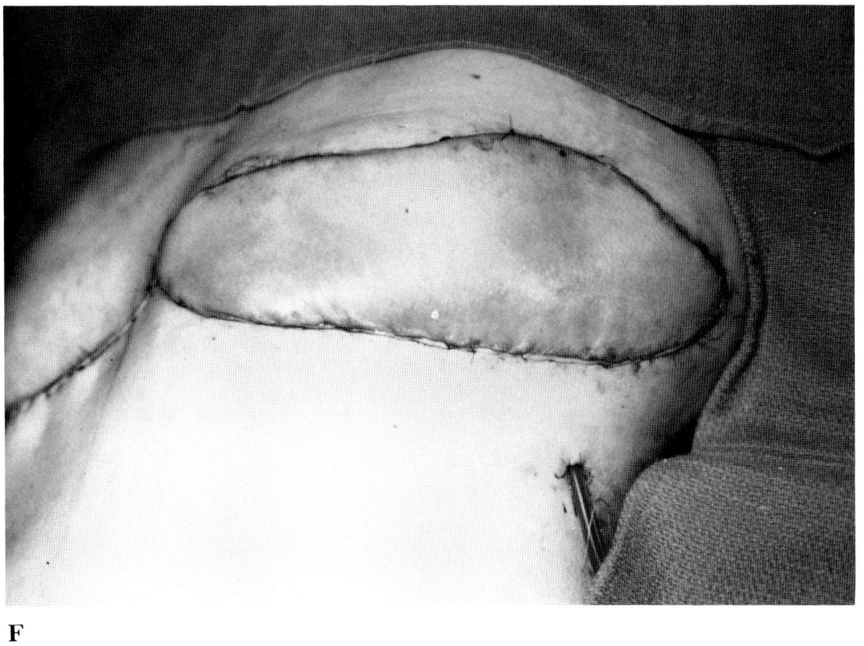

F

First attempt at reconstruction using left latissimus dorsi musculocutaneous flap. **D:** Necrotic latissimus dorsi musculocutaneous flap resulting from inadvertent division of collateral circulation. The thoraco-doral artery had been divided at the time of the mastectomy, but this fact was not realized at the time of reconstruction. **E:** Skin grafted defect after debridement of dead flap. *Second attempt at reconstruction using the contralateral rectus abdominus submammary flap.* **F:** Congested contralateral rectus abdominus submammary flap. Cause unknown. Further congestion occurred and flap died.

G: Dead contralateral rectus abdominus submammary flap. This flap was also debrided and the resulting defect skin grafted. This patient was presented to Dr. Hartrampf for a possible salvage procedure. **H:** An ipsilateral transverse abdominal island flap was used. **I:** AP final postoperative result after reduction mammoplasty to right side, augmentation mammoplasty under transverse abdominal flap left side and bilateral nipple reconstruction. **J:** Left oblique postoperative result. **K:** Right oblique postoperative result.

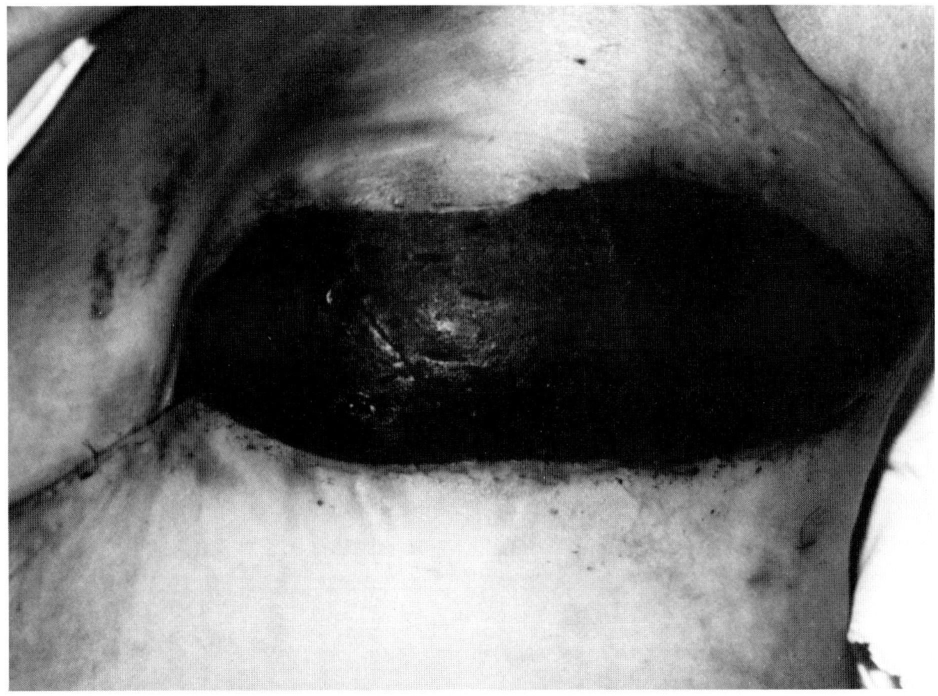

G

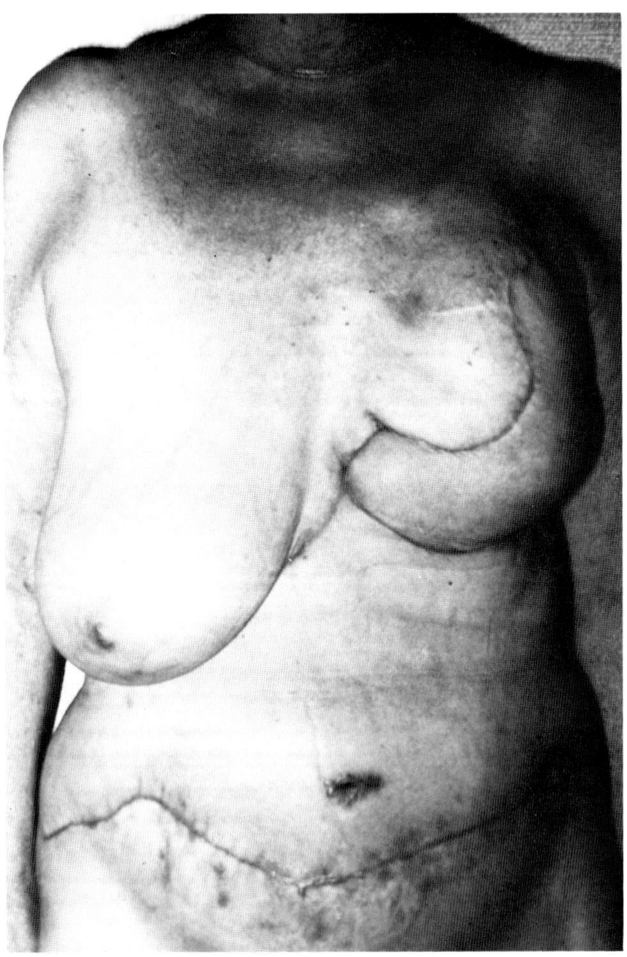

H

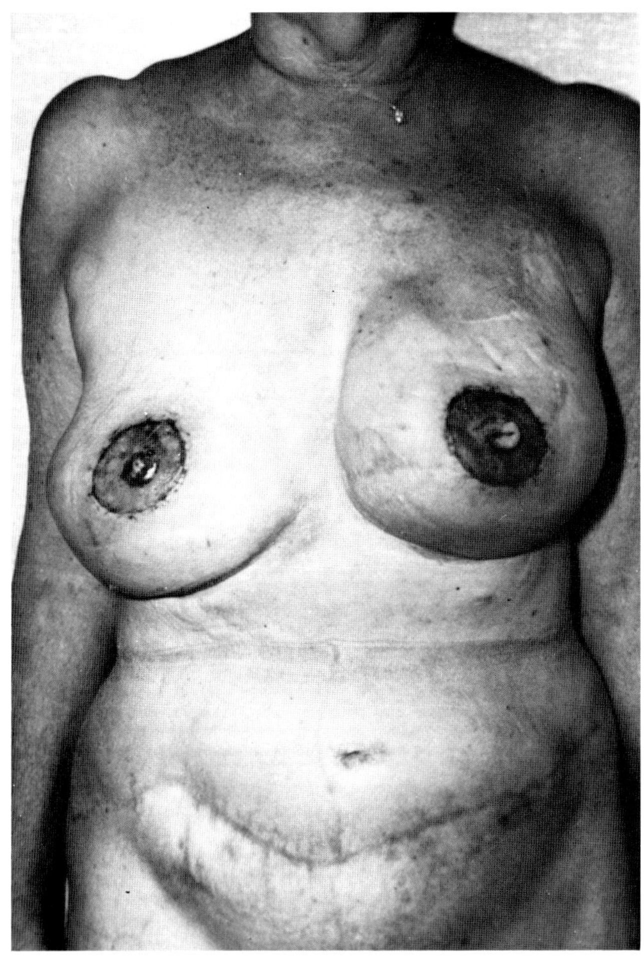

I

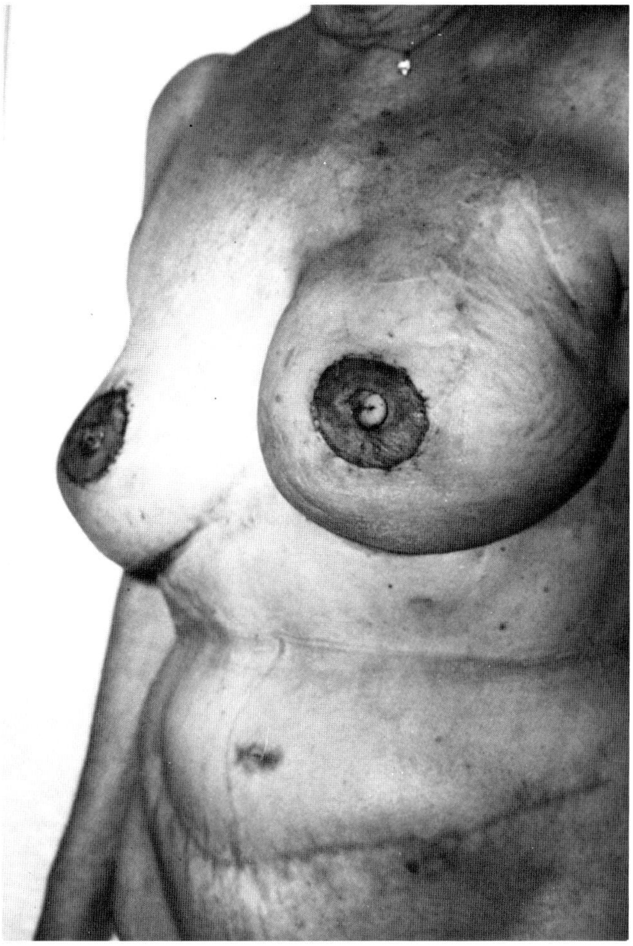

J

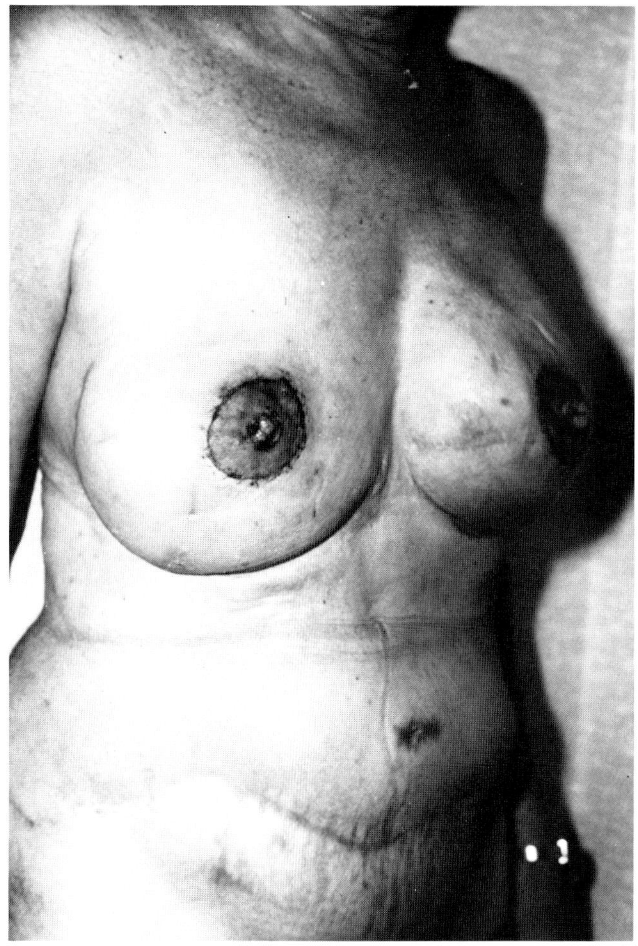

K

Bilateral Transverse Abdominal Island Flap

Bernard M. McGibbon

The bilateral transverse abdominal island flap is ideal for reconstruction of bilateral radical or modified radical mastectomy defects.

Basically the operation is identical to the unilateral procedure except that in the bilateral technique no tissue is discarded. The abdominal flap is divided vertically in the midline, and each half is raised on the ipsilateral rectus muscle.

There are, however, a few points in technique that require elaboration. After the flaps have been outlined but not yet elevated laterally, the inferior flap margin should be incised across the midline down to the rectus sheath to reveal the position and width of the recti muscle. This avoids inadvertent separation of the flap from the muscle and is particularly important if there is a diastasis of the recti muscles and they are placed more laterally than normal. A tunnel is made behind each rectus muscle using the index finger. The muscle is then transected and the inferior epigastric vessels can be identified, clamped, divided and tied. The inferior cut edge of the rectus muscle is suture ligatured.

Unlike the unilateral flap reconstruction, where the umbilicus may be excised and reapplied later as a graft, in the bilateral reconstruction the umbilicus is less likely to be pulled to one side and is therefore usually circumscribed and left behind (Figure 9.19B).

V-shaped incisions are made on each side of the inferior rectus sheath during elevation of the flaps (Figure 9.19D). These incisions can usually be closed to ensure strength below the arcuate line. Closure of the remaining rectus sheath superiorly is usually not possible, and marlex mesh or merselene is used to strengthen the abdominal wall (Figures 9.19E and 9.20).

As in the unilateral technique, the inframammary crease incision on each side is decided after the abdominal wound is closed. The level is equivalent to the midpoint of the inner upper arm or the sixth rib.

It has not been found necessary to skeletonize the pedicle completely at the costal margin. The strap-like muscle is folded around the rib cage. If the lower subcostal nerves are sectioned meticulously, the muscle will atrophy later and the bulge sometimes seen will disappear with time.

Because of the resulting weakness of the abdominal wall, a narrowed abdominal Velcro binder is placed over the transverse incision postoperatively to give support. Later, when the wounds have fully healed, a program of abdominal exercises is prescribed.

Blood transfusions are always required. Because this is an elective procedure, it is the ideal situation for autologous transfusions. Volumetric replacement is important to ensure adequate perfusion through the flaps.

Complications of Unilateral and Bilateral Transverse Abdominal Island Flap

The transverse abdominal island flap is a straightforward but somewhat lengthy procedure. Unilateral reconstruction takes an average of 4.5 hr and the bilateral procedure an average of 6.5 hr. Careful preoperative planning is essential.

Figure 9.19. *Bilateral breast reconstruction using the transverse abdominal island flap.* **A:** Outline of proposed incisions, lower abdominal incision is not made until upper abdominal flap has been elevated and mastectomy scars have been excised. At that time, the operating table is flexed and the abdominal flap is pulled down like a "window blind". The lower incision of the abdominal flap can then be determined accurately by pushing up on the supra-pubic skin and at the same time pulling down on the flap. This allows the greatest dimension of flap to be harvested and at the same time easy closure of the abdominal wound is made possible. **B:** The upper incision is made

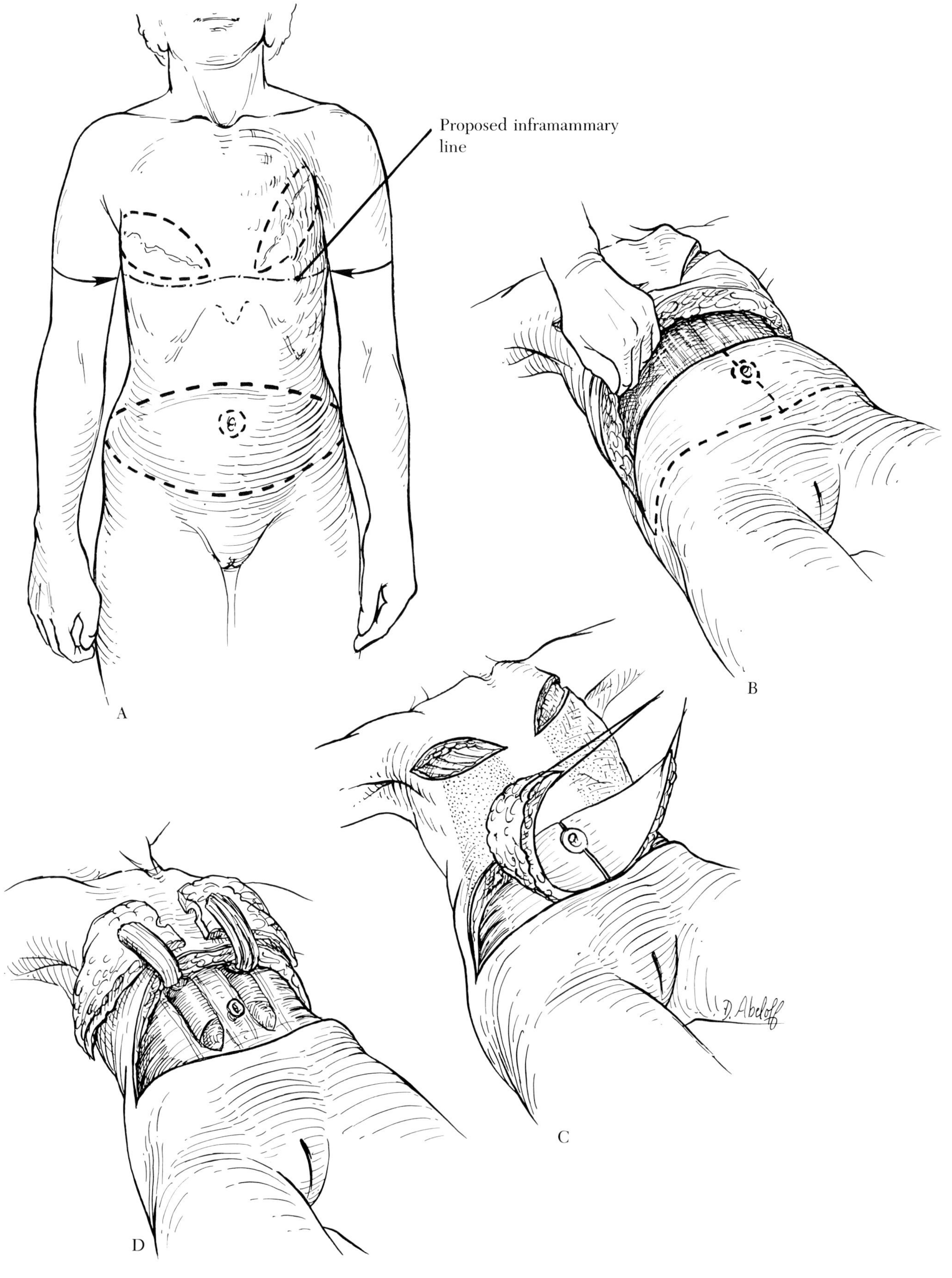

and undermining is performed up onto the lower rib cage. The mastectomy scars are excised and tunnels are made from the epigastric wound into the medial part of the mastectomy wounds. The tunnels are made large enough to permit a fist to pass through. **C:** The umbilicus is circumscribed and the flap is divided in the midline. The flaps are elevated to the lateral edge of the rectus sheath. **D:** The rectus sheath is divided as a V on each side inferiorly. The rectus muscle is transected, the inferior epigastric arteries are identified, ligated and divided and the inferior rectus muscle

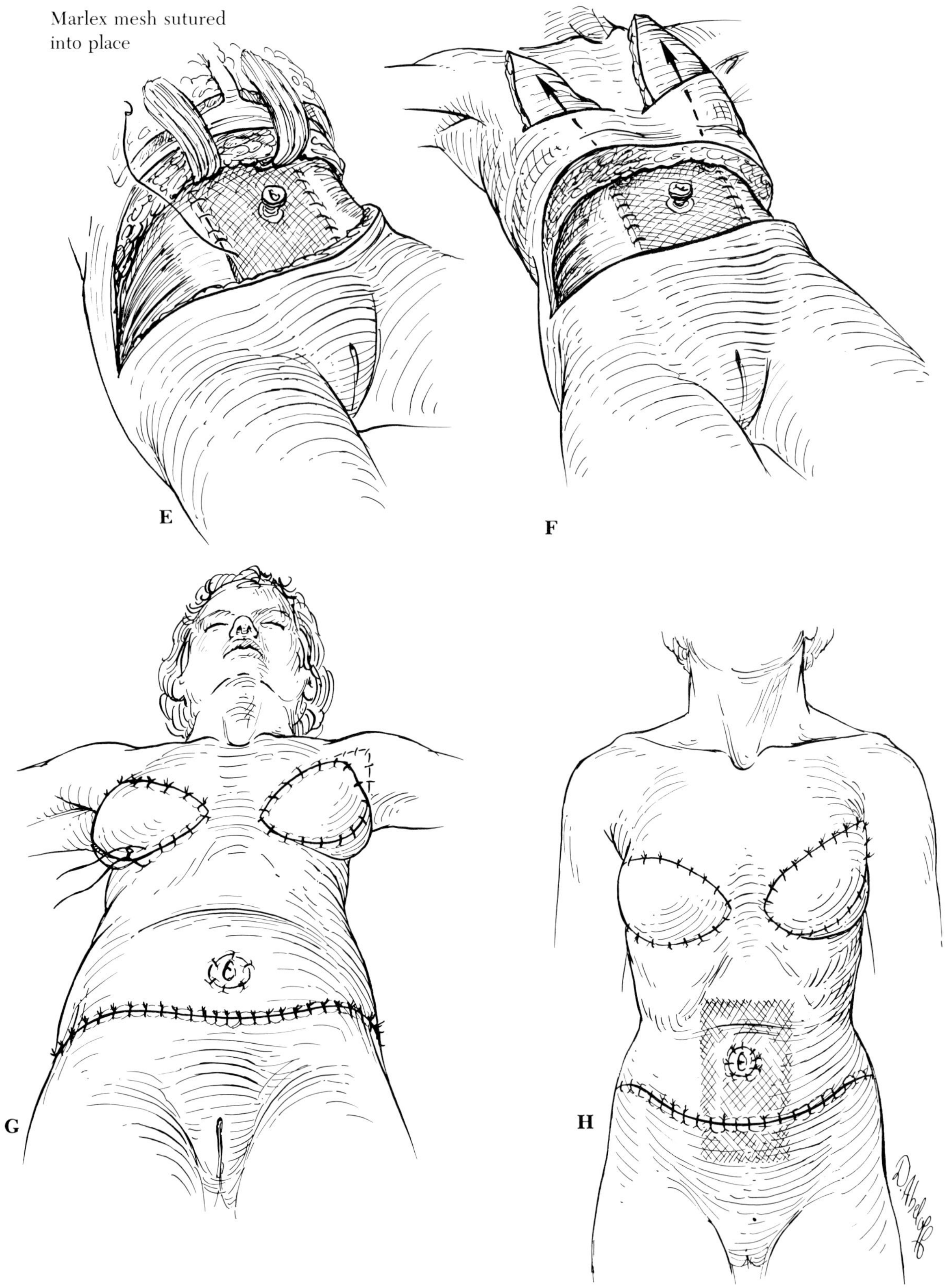

is then elevated in a cephalad direction with the attached cutaneous and fat flap. **E:** The V shaped defect in the rectus sheath is closed superiorly as far as possible with every attempt being made to repair the defect up to or above the arcuate line. The remaining rectus sheath above this is closed as much as possible. Marlex or merselene mesh is used to overlay the rectus area and is sutured into position. An opening is made for the umbilicus. **F:** The flaps are passed up the tunnels and the abdomen is closed with subcutaneous and subcuticular sutures. The umbilicus is brought out through a T shaped incision in the midline of the flap. **G:** After closure of the abdomen, the location of the final inframammary incision is made. **H:** Final wound closure is then performed. Part of the transverse flap is deepithelialized and is used to "fill out" the anatomical defect above, lateral and medial to the mastectomy scar, which is excised. To get the most symmetrical result it is helpful to try and make the chest incisions themselves symmetrical even though the mastectomy scars may not have been.

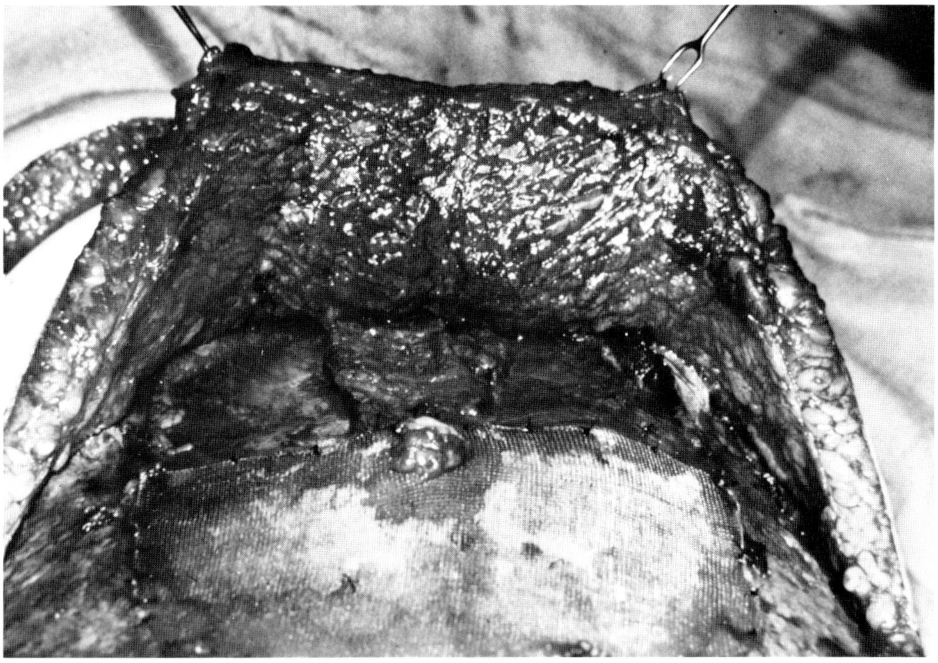

Figure 9.20. Abdominal wall strengthened by marlex mesh.

Subcostal scars should be viewed with suspicion, and knowledge of the patency of the superior epigastric arteries is essential. Preoperative arteriograms are helpful but are not without associated morbidity.

Many of the complications of the transverse abdominal island flap technique are those that accompany any extensive surgical procedure. There are, however, a few specific problems that need to be addressed. With an operative wound of this magnitude, heat and fluid loss can be excessive if precautions are not taken. Both of these factors have deleterious effects on the flap. Heating pads and adequate preheated intravenous fluids are recommended together with intraoperative hourly urine monitoring and recording the core temperature using esophageal thermometer probes. The flaps often remain pale and cool for some hours after the operation, and a fluorescein test may be inconclusive. Usually this means that a peripheral spasm is present which disappears later. A more ominous sign is mottling or frank congestion with excessive hyperemia and very rapid blanching and refill. This indicates venous congestion caused by kinking of the pedicle, and unless it is relieved flap loss will occur. Total flap loss is rare, but occasionally tip loss occurs if the flap is extremely large and part of the flap is random rather than axial.

Careful "sculpturing" of the flap is time-consuming but essential. There is a tendency to make the flaps too large and bulky superiorly. "What you see is what you get" is a good axiom to remember at the operating table. Very little flap shrinkage and ptosis occur postoperatively. Secondary debulking procedures can be done at the time of nipple reconstruction. It is important to start closing the abdominal defect before defining the inframammary crease; otherwise the reconstructed breast will be too low.

Occasionally a patient complains of a bulge in the subcostal region. This is caused by the rectus muscle as it folds around the costal margin. If the muscle has been adequately denervated, it will atrophy and the bulge will disappear.

As mentioned by Drever in his discussion of the vertical rectus abdominus flap, pain at the costal margin may be caused by a stretched intercostal nerve at the base of the muscle pedicle. This problem can also occur with the transverse island flap technique and may likewise be corrected by sectioning the nerve.

The concern of a ventral hernia developing after this procedure is justified. However, with careful closure of the rectus sheath, particularly below the arcuate line, the risk is reduced. In the bilateral procedure marlex mesh or merselene is recommended.

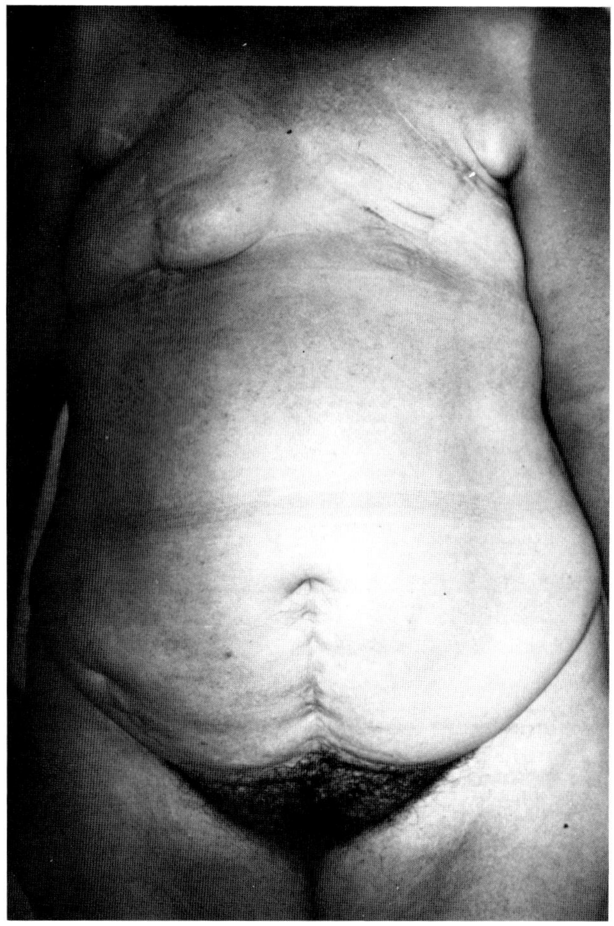

A

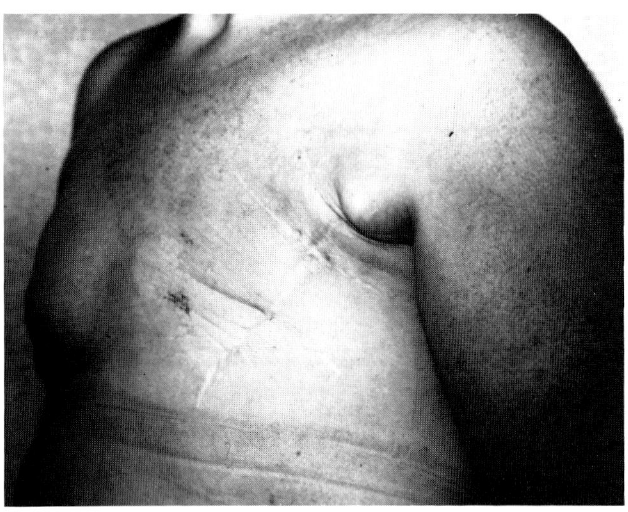

B

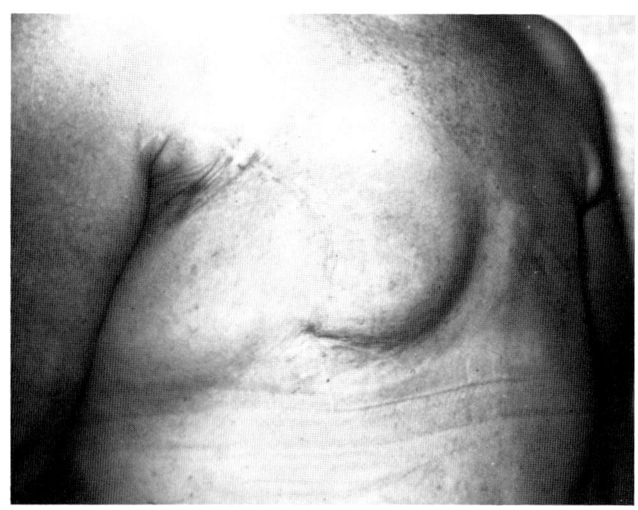

C

Figure 9.21. **A:** AP bilateral radical mastectomy defect, preoperative view. **B:** Left oblique preoperative view. **C:** Right oblique preoperative view. **D:** AP post-operative view. Bilateral transverse abdominal island flap reconstruction (no implants used). The deformity over the left flap was caused by wound breakdown in an area previously irradiated. Full thickness skin grafts from the upper inner thighs were used for areolae. Nipple reconstruction was performed using quadrapod flaps. **E:** Post-operative left oblique view after deformity caused by irradiation had been revised. **F:** Postoperative AP view. **G:** Postoperative right oblique view.

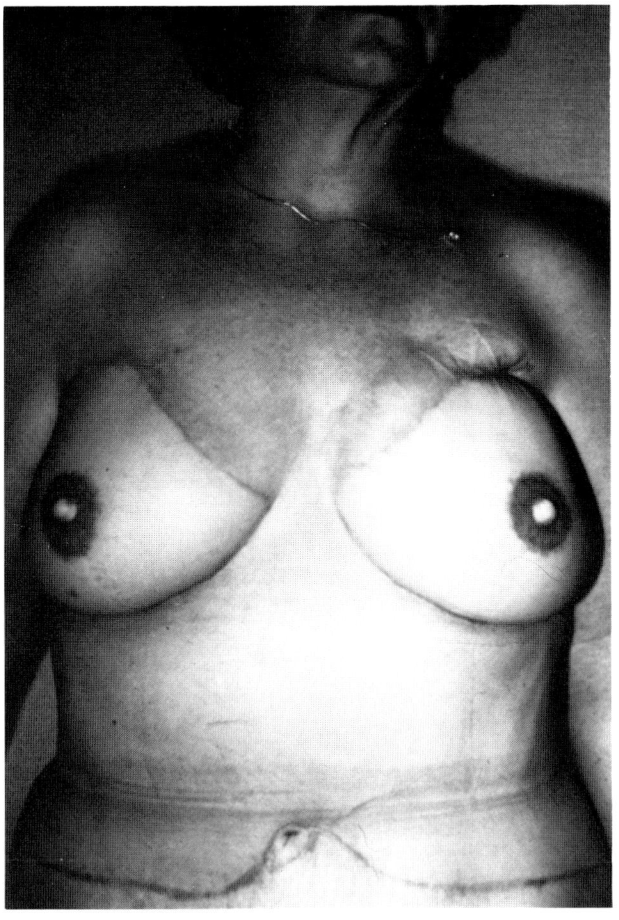

D

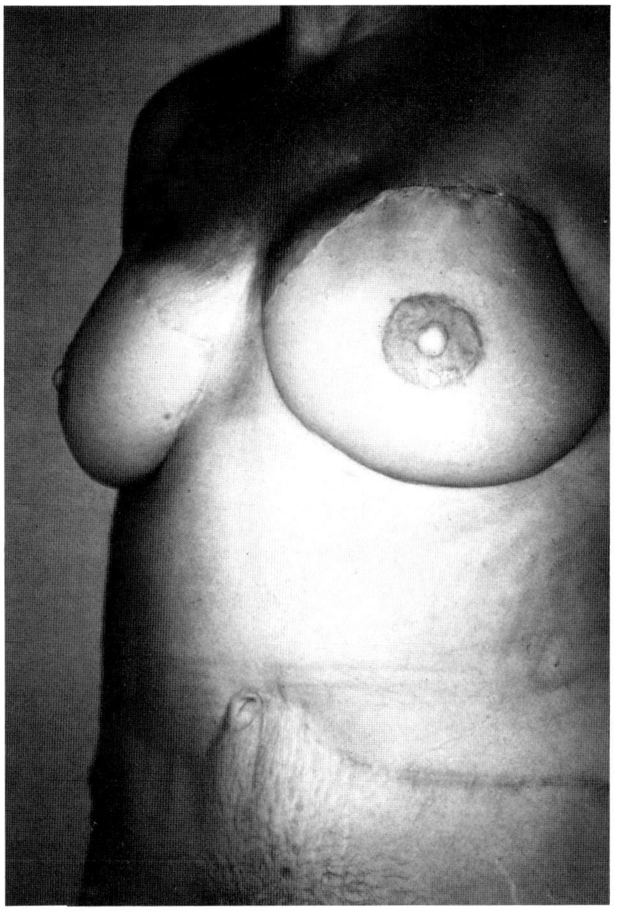

E

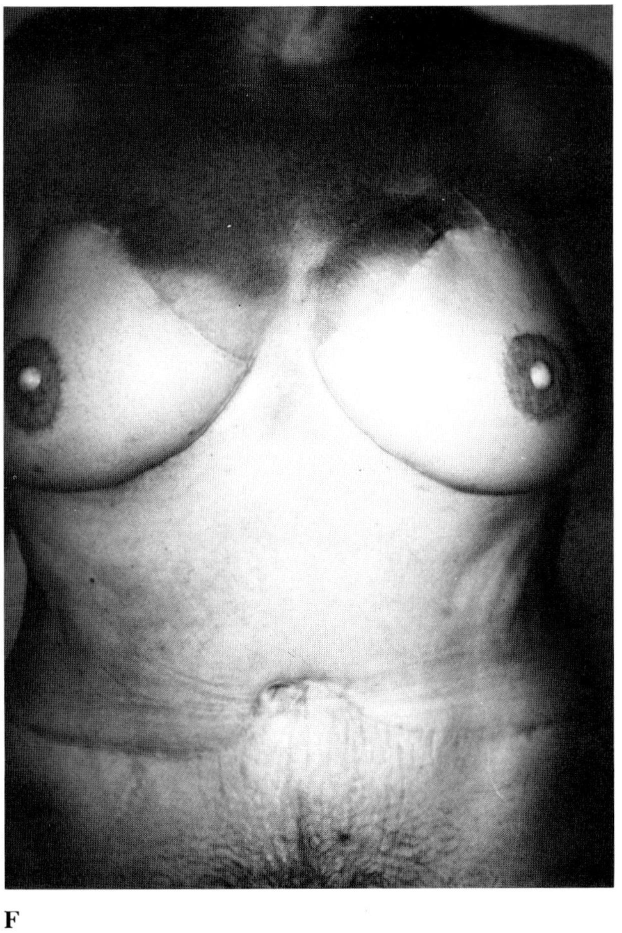

F

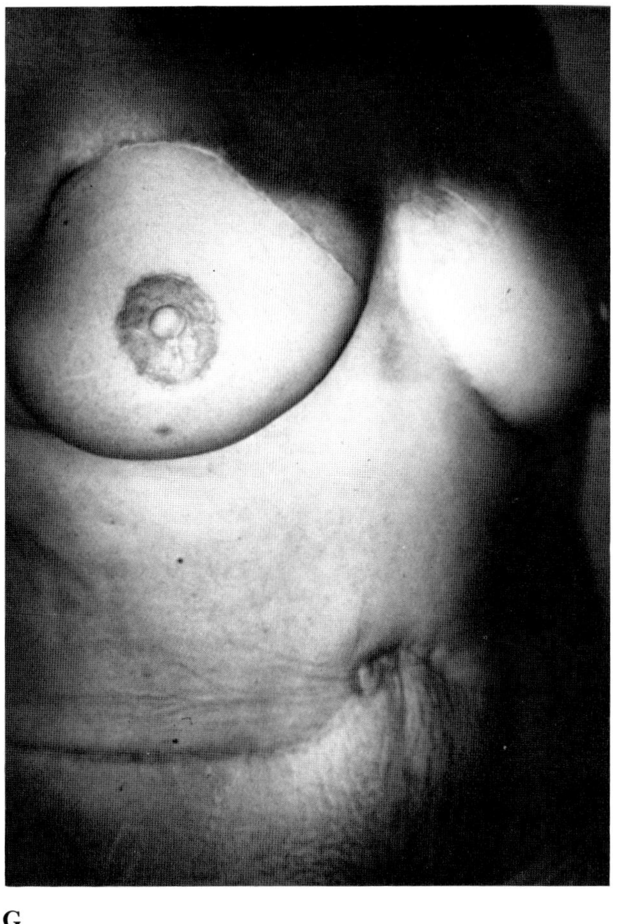

G

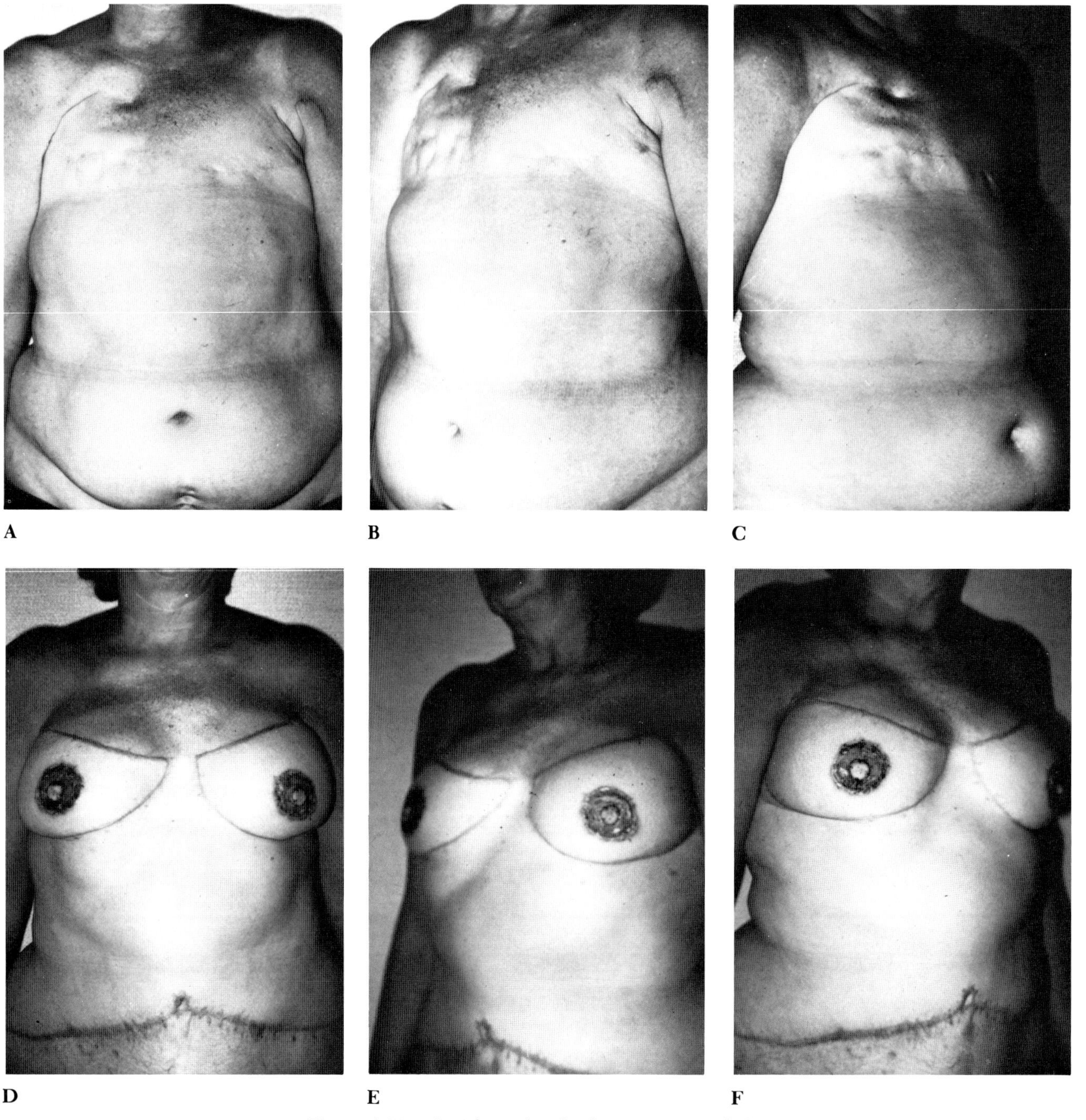

Figure 9.22. **A:** Bilateral radical mastectomy defect, AP view with a deep anatomic depression of the right upper chest. **B:** Preoperative left oblique view. **C:** Preoperative right oblique view. **D:** Postoperative AP view with successful correction of the anatomic depression using a deepithelialized part of the flap. (No implant used.) **E:** Postoperative left oblique view. **F:** Postoperative right oblique view.

Figure 9.23. **A:** Bilateral modified radical mastectomy defect, AP view. **B:** Preoperative left oblique view. **C:** Preoperative right oblique view. **D:** Postoperative AP view without implants. Nipples were reconstructed from local quadrapod flaps and the areolae from inner thighs skin graft. **E:** Postoperative left oblique view. **F:** Postoperative right oblique view.

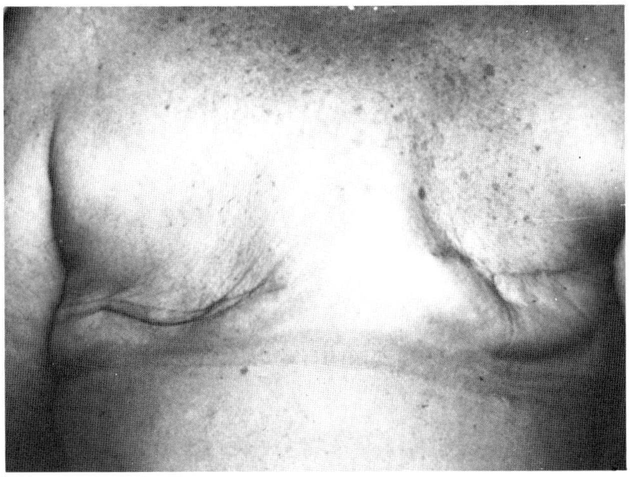

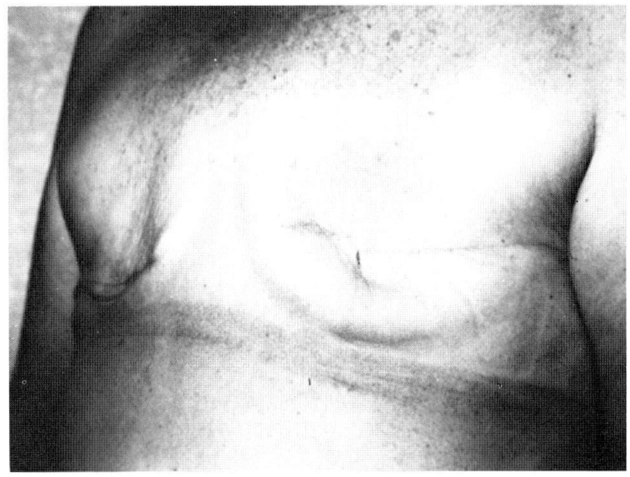

A **B**

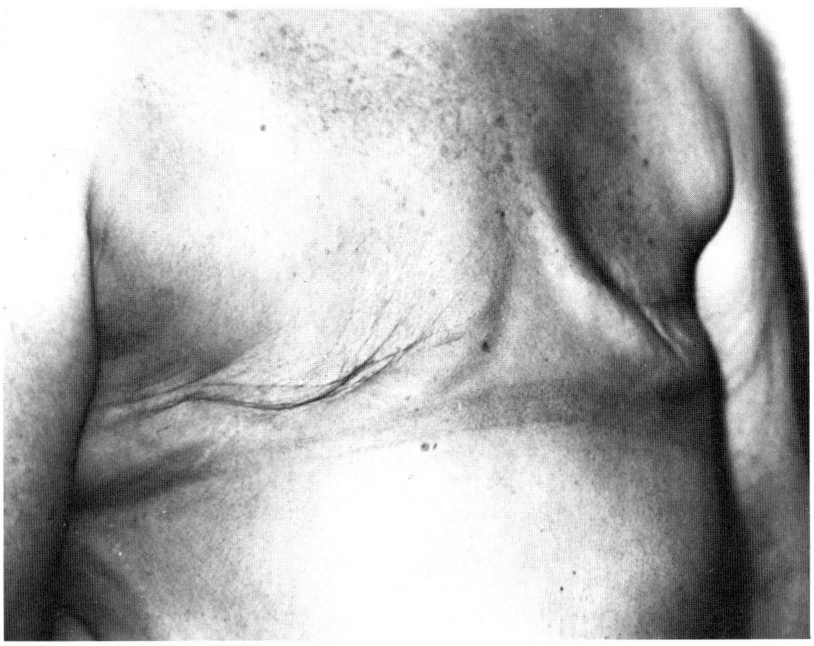

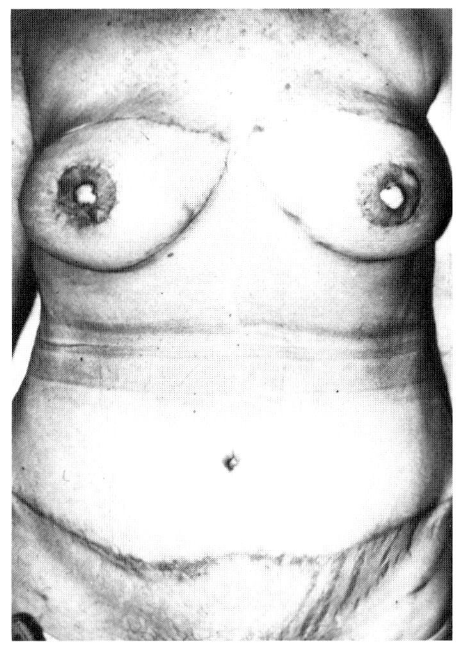

C **D**

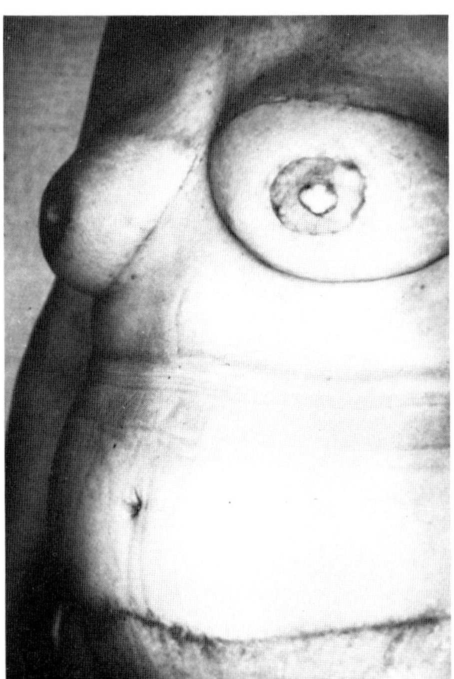

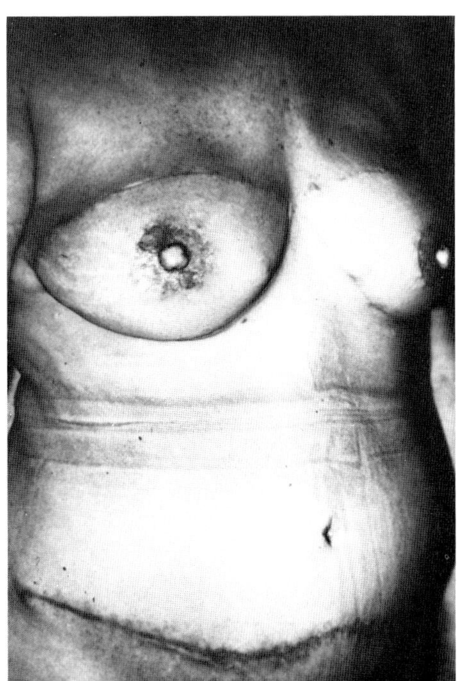

E **F**

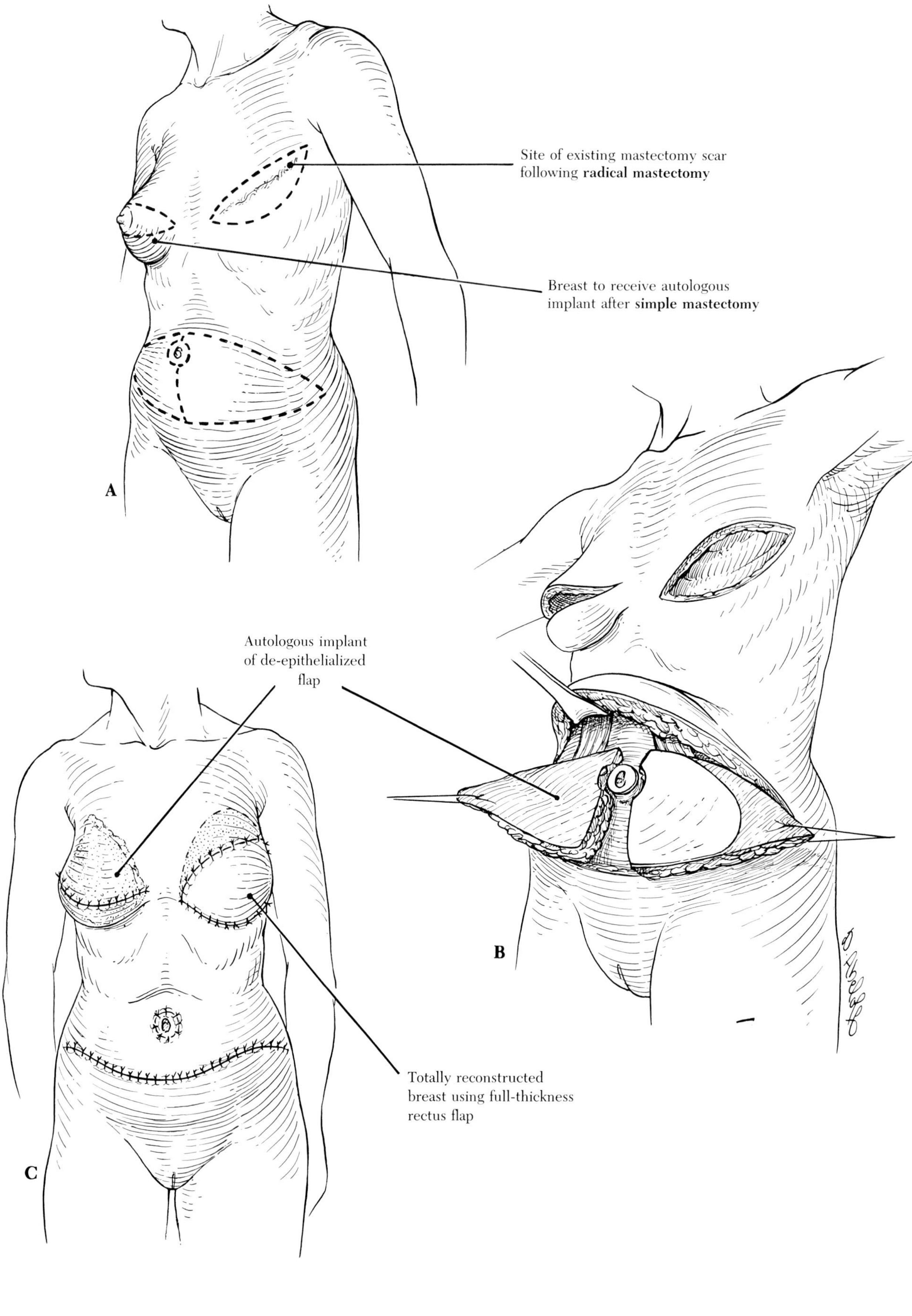

Figure 9.24. Bilateral transverse abdominal island flap using one-half of flap to reconstruct ipsilateral breast and the other half of flap to use as "fill" for opposite breast that requires reconstruction after a prophylactic subcutaneous or simple mastectomy. The flap has been deepithelialized and is used instead of an implant.

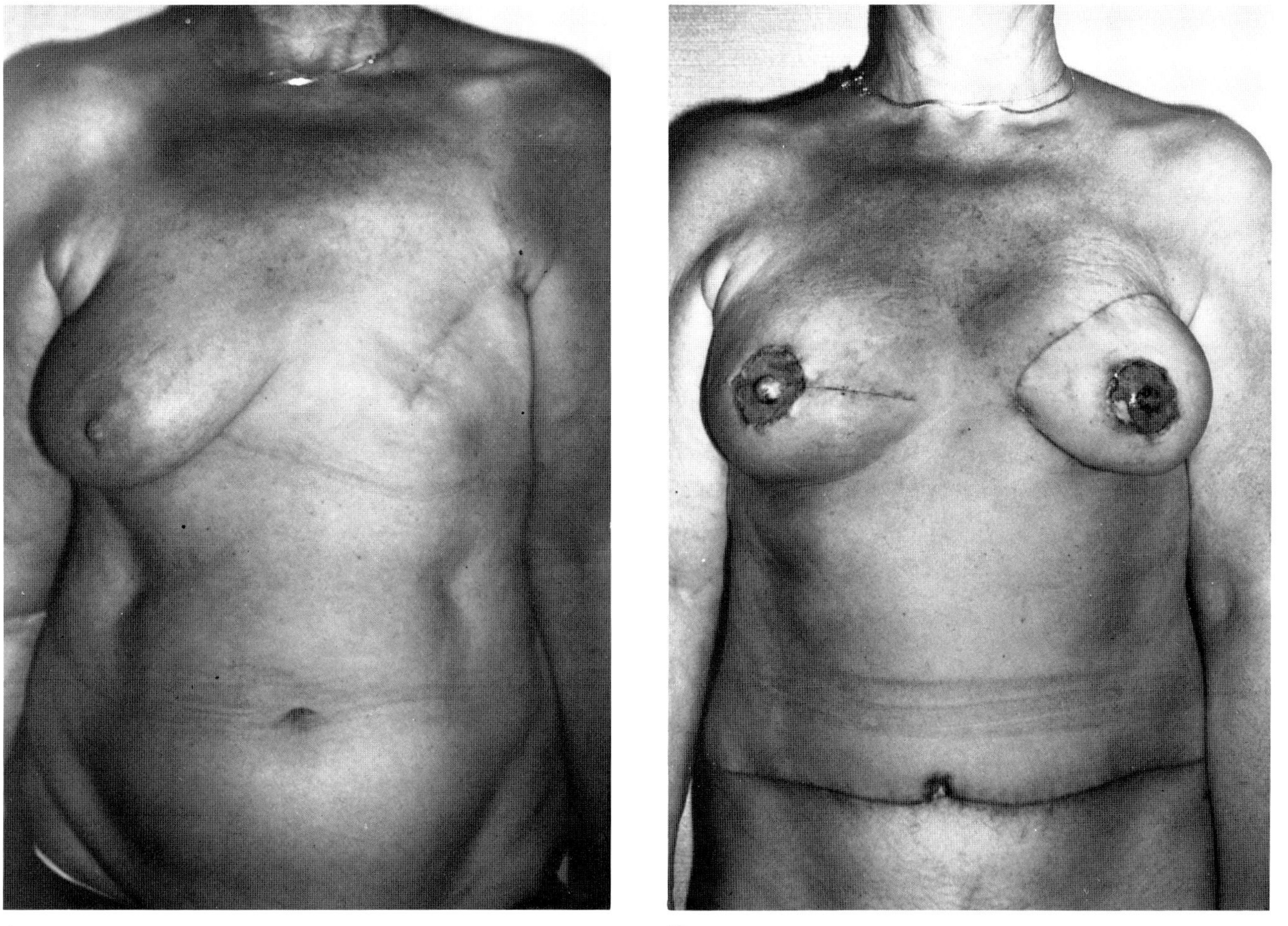

A B

Figure 9.25. **A:** Preoperative left modified radical mastectomy defect with fibrocystic disease of right breast and strong family history of breast carcinoma. To have left breast reconstruction and right simple mastectomy and reconstruction. **B:** Postoperative left breast reconstruction using left half of transverse abdominal island flap. The right half has been deepithelialized and used as "fill" for the simple mastectomy defect.

Lower abdominal swelling and a "loss of waist" may cause concern for a few months postoperatively. Both of these problems become less obvious with time. Abdominal muscle exercises are recommended after the wounds have fully healed. Seroma formation occurs on occasion.

As was noted by Drever, fat necrosis may occur. This is recognized by a hardness that softens within a few months.

Results

The fact that breast reconstruction can frequently be performed using only autogenous tissue makes the transverse abdominal island flap an attractive procedure. With careful "sculpturing" of the flap, very acceptable results can be achieved. This operation is particularly suitable for bilateral reconstruction because good symmetry can usually be obtained (Figures 9.21–9.23).

The bilateral transverse abdominal island flap may also be used to good advantage for the unilateral mastectomy defect when the opposite breast requires augmentation or reconstruction, e.g., after a prophylactic subcutaneous mastectomy when a deepithelialized flap is used instead of an implant (Figure 9.24, 9.25A,B.)

References

1. Bohmert H, 1975: Eine neue Methode zur reconstruktion der Weiblichen Brust nach radikaler Mastektomie. In: Plastiche Chirugie des Kopf und Hals Bereiche und der Weiblichen Brust, edited by H Bohmert. Georg Thieme Verlag, Stuttgart.
2. Bohmert H, 1980: Experience in breast reconstruction with thoraco-epigastric and advancement flaps. Acta Chir Belg 79:105–110.
3. Brown GR, Vasconez LO, Jurkiewicz MJ, 1975: Transverse abdominal flaps and the deep epigastric arcade. Plast Reconstr Surg 55:416–421.
4. Cronin TD, Upton J, McDonough JM, 1977: Reconstruction of the breast after mastectomy. Plast Reconstr Surg 59:1–14.
5. DeLa Plaza R, 1981: Post-mastectomy reconstruction by a contralateral abdomino-mammary flap. Ann Plast Surg 6:97–102.
6. Dell PC, Seaber AV, Urbaniak JR, 1980: Effect of hypovolemia on perfusion after digit replacement. Am Coll Surg Surg Forum 31:503–504.
7. Dinner MI, Labandter HP, Dowden RV, 1982: The role of the rectus abdominus myocutaneous flap in breast reconstruction. Plast Reconstr Surg 69:209–214.
8. Drever JM, 1977: The epigastric island flap. Plast Reconstr Surg 59:343–346.
9. Drever JM, 1981: Total breast reconstruction. Ann Plast Surg 7:54–61.
10. Drever JM, 1983: The lower abdominal transverse rectus abdominus myocutaneous flap for breast reconstruction. Ann Plast Surg 10:179–185.
11. Drever JM, Hodson-Walker N, 1983: Breast reconstruction using the lower abdominal transverse rectus abdominus myocutaneous flap. Breast 9:7–12.
12. Fugino T, 1967: Contribution of the axial and perforator vasculature to circulation in flaps. Plast Reconstr Surg 39:125–137.
13. Hartrampf CR, Scheflan M, Black PW, 1982: Breast reconstruction with a transverse abdominal island flap. Plast Reconstr Surg 69:216–224.
14. Lejour M, 1982: Reconstruction of the breast with a contralateral epigastric rectus myocutaneous flap. Chir Plast 6:181.
15. McCraw JB, Dibbell DG, Carraway JH, 1977: Clinical definition of independent myocutaneous vascular territories. Plast Reconstr Surg 60:341–352.
16. Millard DR Jr, 1981: Reconstruction mammoplasty using an economical flap from the opposite breast. Ann Plast Surg 6:374.
17. Robbins TH, 1979: Rectus abdominus myocutaneous flap for breast reconstruction. Aust NZ J Surg 49:527–530.
18. Scheflan M, Dinner MI, 1983: The transverse abdominal island flap. I. Indications, contraindications, results and complications. Ann Plast Surg 10:24–35.
19. Scheflan M, Dinner MI, 1983: The transverse abdominal island flap. II. Surgical technique. Ann Plast Surg 10:120–129.
20. Shaw DT, Payne RL, 1946: One stage tubed abdominal flaps. Surg Gynecol Obstet 83:205–209.
21. Slavin SA, 1983: The rectus abdominus myocutaneous flap: observation and refinements (correspondence and brief communications). Plast Reconstr Surg 71:280–281.
22. Tai Y, Hasegwa H, 1974: A transverse abdominal flap for reconstruction after radical operations for recurrent breast cancer. Plast Reconstr Surg 53:52–54.
23. Vasconez LO, Psillakis J, Johnson-Gieberk R, 1983: Breast reconstruction with contralateral rectus abdominus myocutaneous flap. Plast Reconstr Surg 71:668–675.
24. Webster JP, 1937: Thoraco-epigastric tubed pedicles. Surg Clin North Am 17:145.

10

Contralateral Breast

Bernard M. McGibbon

Management of the contralateral breast in a mastectomy patient is a controversial issue and one which must be decided individually in every case. The woman who has a carcinoma of one breast has a 15% chance of developing one on the other side. Depending on the circumstances, treatment may range from extensive preventive surgery to necessary cosmetic adjustment (10,14,19).

Subcutaneous Mastectomy and Simple Mastectomy

Subcutaneous mastectomy or simple mastectomy should be considered for the contralateral breast in high-risk cases, e.g., lobular carcinoma (on the mastectomy side), extensive fibrocystic disease, sclerosing adenosis, and a history of breast cancer in first-order relatives. Surgeons differ strongly in their views as to whether one of these procedures should be performed in such cases and, if so, which one (5,6,10). Each patient requires separate evaluation.

If the contralateral breast is normal in size or only mildly ptotic, the technique described by Jarrett et al. is suitable (13). A subcutaneous mastectomy is followed by immediate reconstruction with submuscular placement of the implant (Figures 10.1–10.13).

When the breasts are larger or more ptotic, a skin reduction with repositioning of the nipple must be accomplished. The method used by Spira (26) and Rubin (25) is particularly applicable and is shown in Figures 10.14–10.16. The breast parenchyma is excised and the nipple removed. The lower edge of the detached pectoralis major muscle is sutured to the upper edge of the deepithelialized inferior skin flap to form a submuscular-dermal pocket for the implant. The breast skin flaps are brought down over the breast mound to form a skin brassiere.

Another technique, shown in Figures 10.17–10.19, is useful in patients with lesser degrees of ptosis. This method is a modification of Rubin's "cushion augmentation" where the deepithelialized superior flap is folded upward (24).

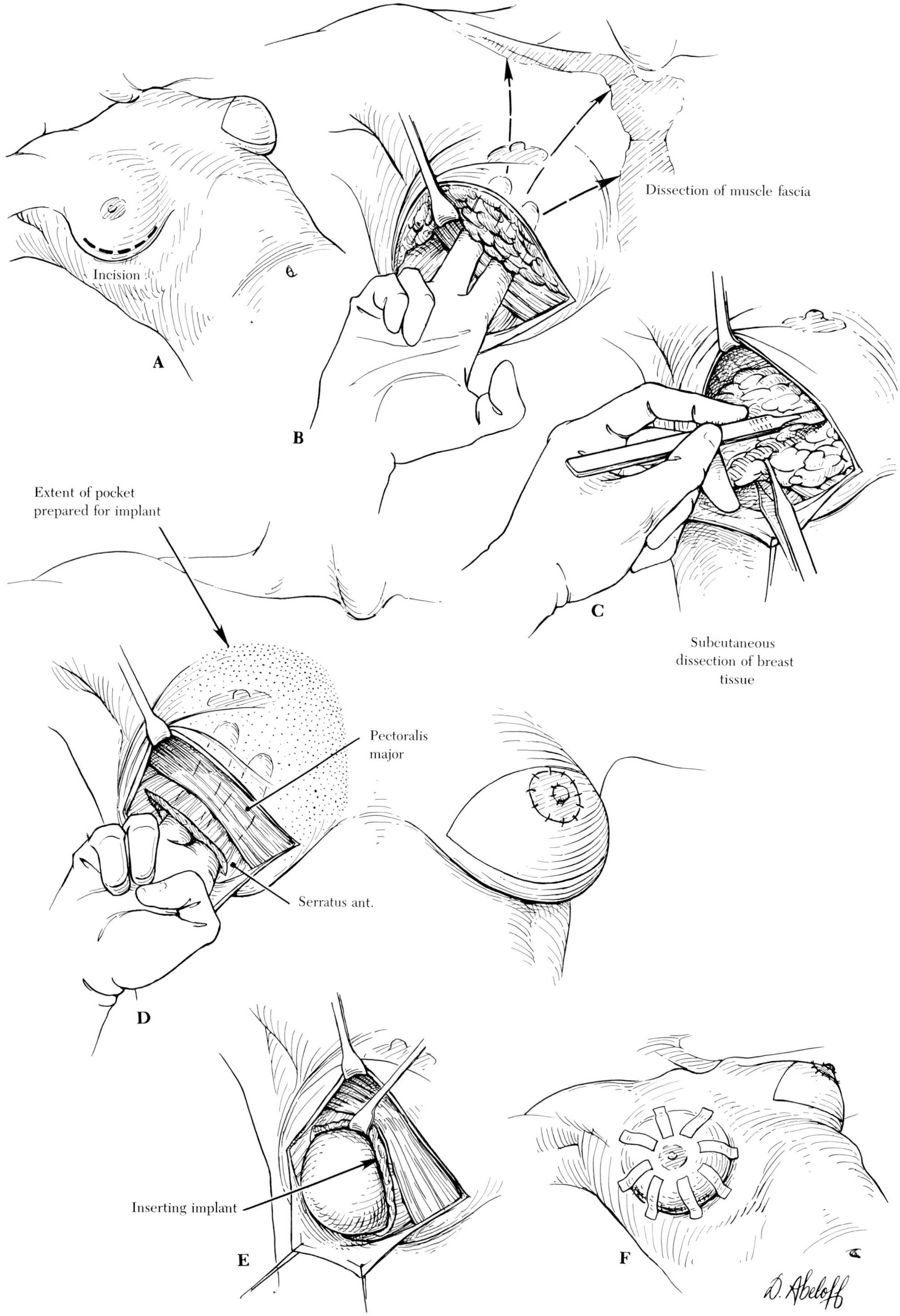
Dissection of muscle fascia
Incision
A
B
Extent of pocket prepared for implant
C
Subcutaneous dissection of breast tissue
Pectoralis major
Serratus ant.
D
Inserting implant
E
F
D. Abeloff

Figure 10.1. Subcutaneous mastectomy in a normal-sized or mildly ptotic breast followed by immediate reconstruction (Jarret technique). **A:** The proposed incision, 9 cm long, is placed 1–2 cm above the inframammary fold so that the scar will be on the undersurface of the breast. **B:** Dissection is performed on the muscular fascia from the sixth interspace to the clavicle and from the sternum to the midaxillary line. **C:** Subcutaneous sharp dissection of the breast parenchyma over the same area leaving thin skin flaps. **D:** A 7-cm incision is made through the serratus anterior fibers directly over the sixth rib. Careful dissection lifts the muscle off the fifth and sixth ribs and the interspace until the edge of the pectoralis major muscle is reached. A subpectoral pocket is then developed by blunt dissection. **E:** Submuscular insertion of a silicone gel implant. **F:** Taping the skin maintains the nipple in position while redundant skin contracts.

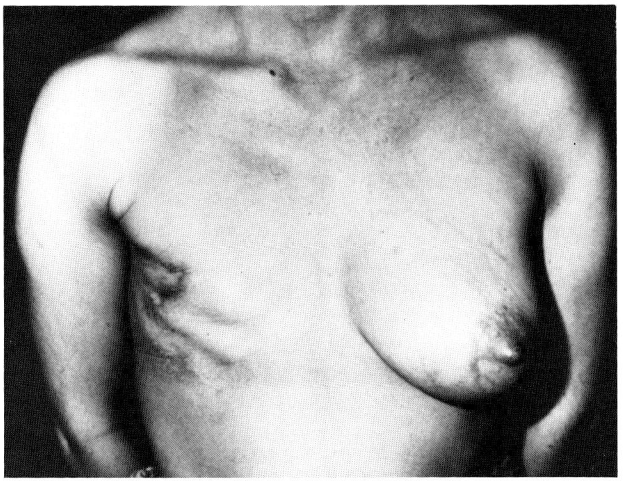

Figure 10.2. AP right modified radical mastectomy deformity.

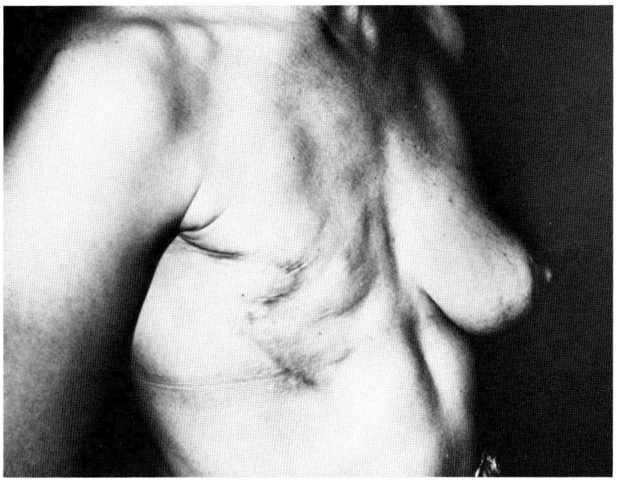

Figure 10.3. Oblique view of the patient in Figure 10.2.

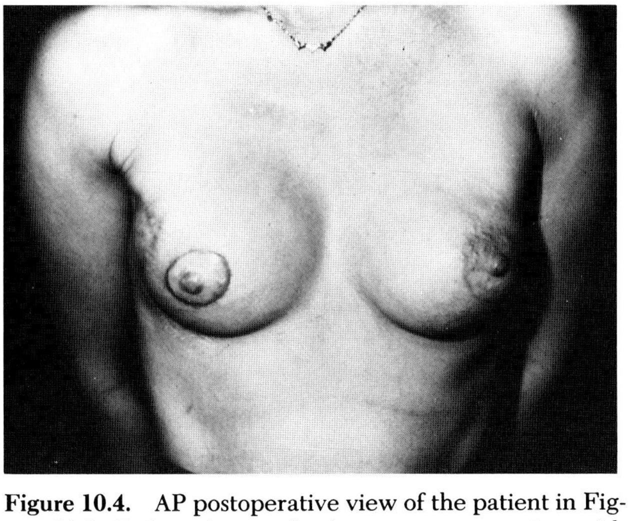

Figure 10.4. AP postoperative view of the patient in Figure 10.2. Right submuscular breast reconstruction with simultaneous left subcutaneous mastectomy and immediate submuscular reconstruction using 250-cc bilumen implants on each side. The nipple-areola had been banked on the abdomen at the time of mastectomy several years ago (a procedure no longer done), it was retrieved and regrafted 3 months after the breast mound reconstruction, giving an excellent result.

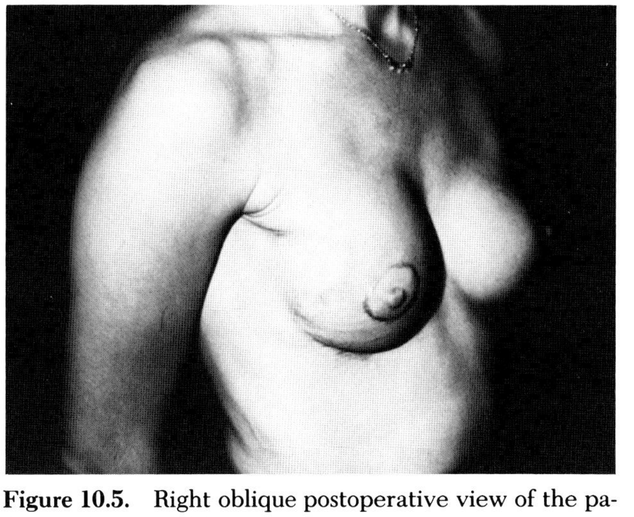

Figure 10.5. Right oblique postoperative view of the patient in Figure 10.4.

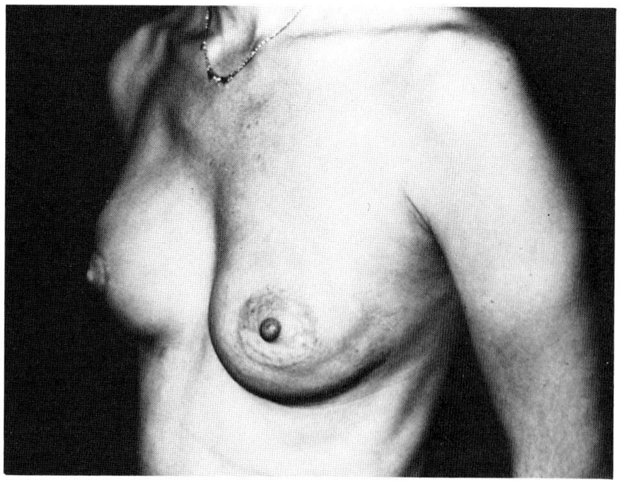

Figure 10.6. Left oblique postoperative view of the patient in Figure 10.4.

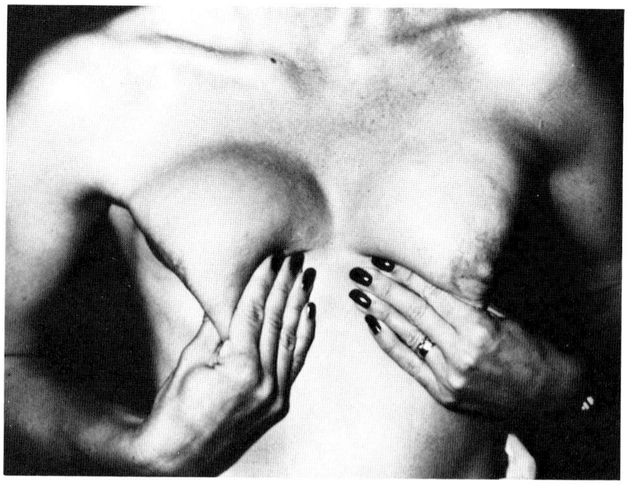

Figure 10.7. Patient demonstrating softness of the breasts.

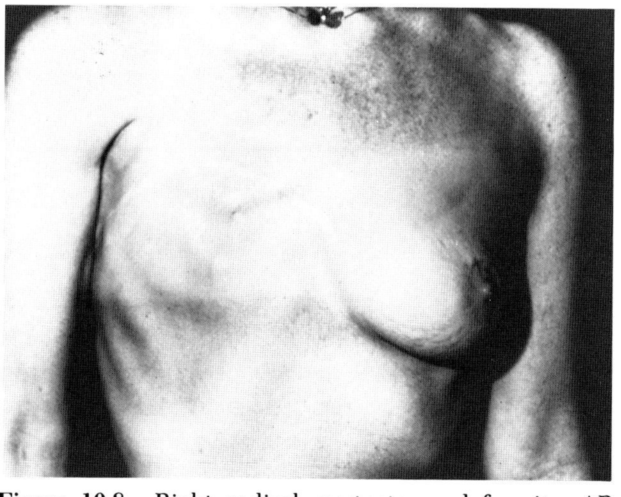

Figure 10.8. Right radical mastectomy deformity, AP view.

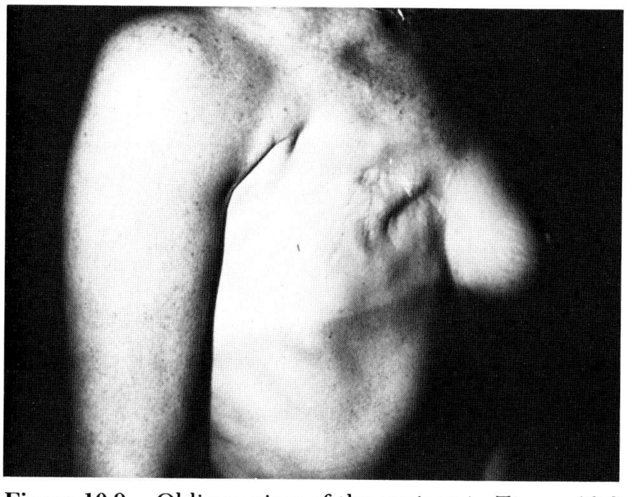

Figure 10.9. Oblique view of the patient in Figure 10.8.

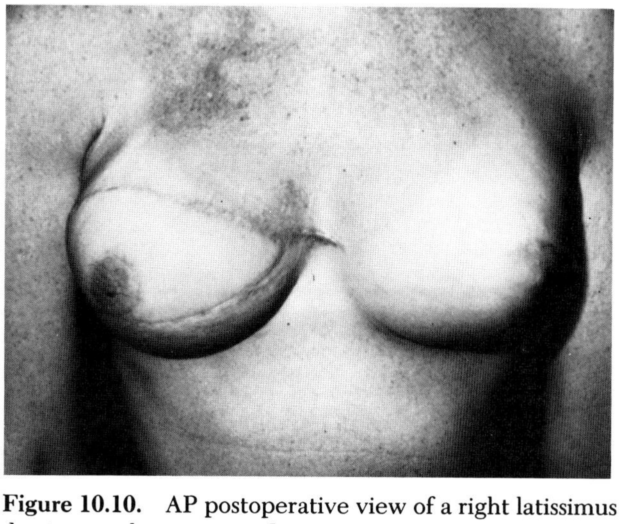

Figure 10.10. AP postoperative view of a right latissimus dorsi musculocutaneous flap reconstruction with a 275-cc bilumen implant. Three months later a left subcutaneous mastectomy with submuscular reconstruction was done using a 275-cc bilumen implant, at the same time an upper thigh graft and half the opposite nipple was used for the nipple-areola reconstruction.

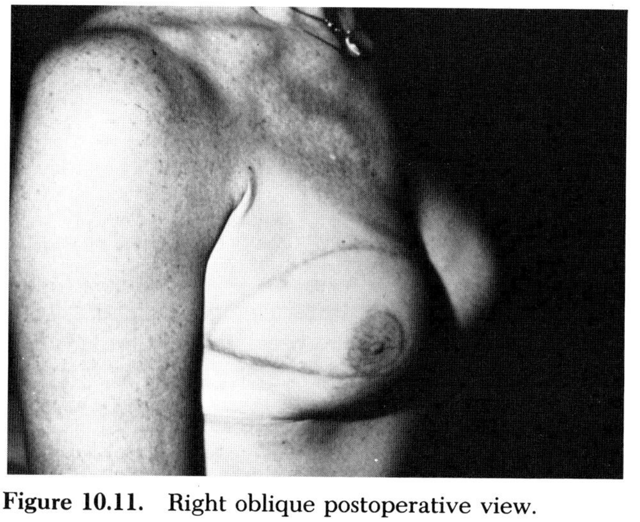

Figure 10.11. Right oblique postoperative view.

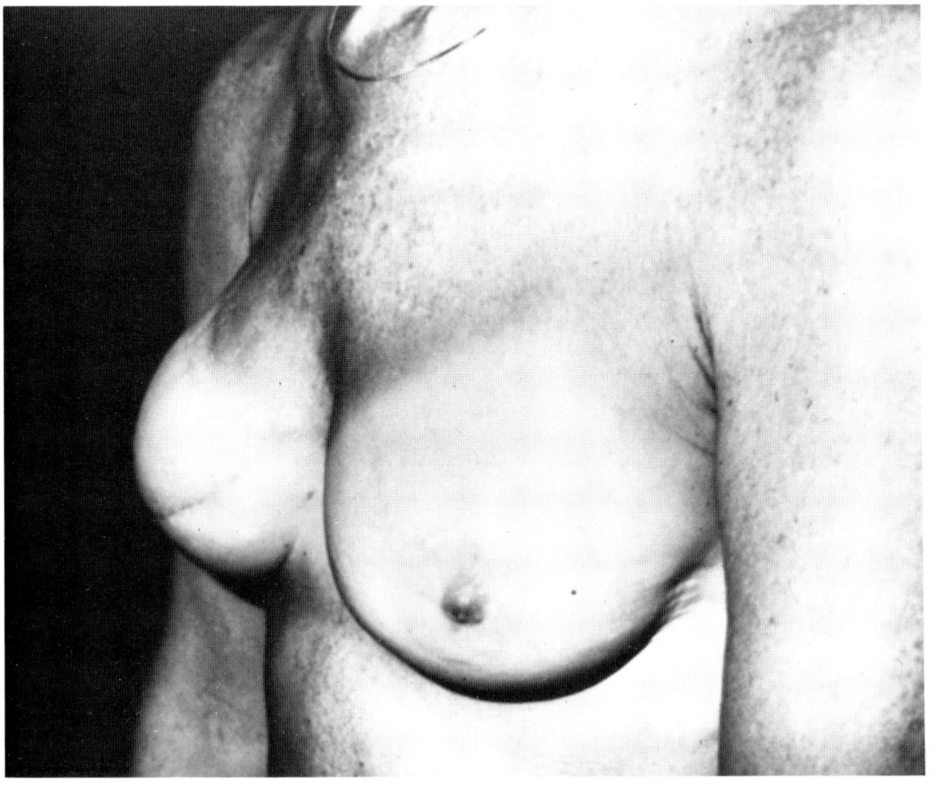

Figure 10.12. Left oblique postoperative view of the patient in Figure 10.10.

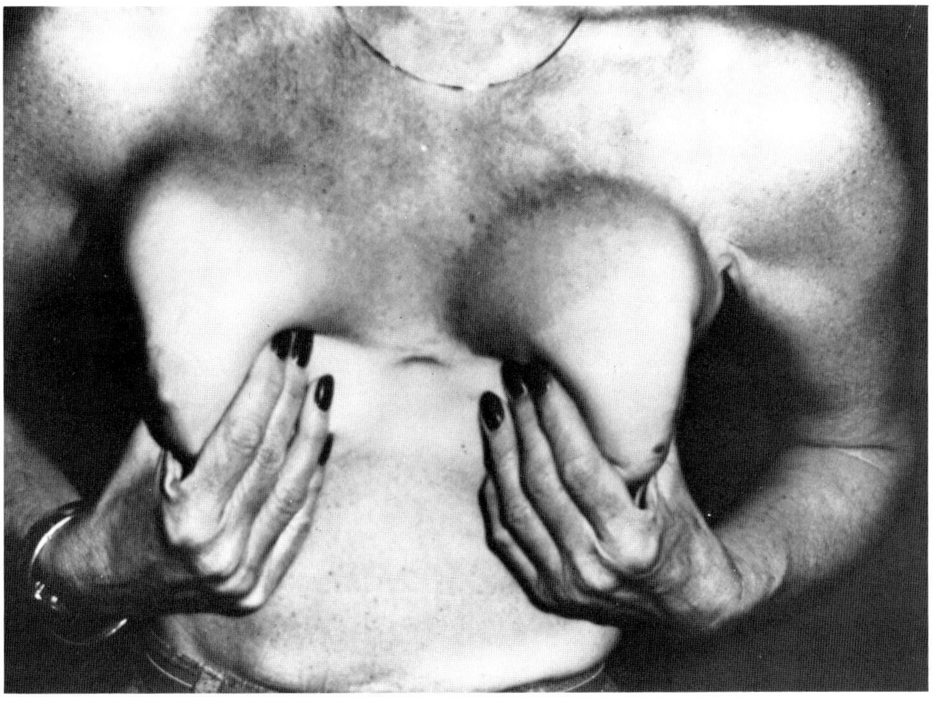

Figure 10.13. Patient demonstrating softness of the breasts. (Photographs in Figures 10.2–10.13 were kindly supplied by Dr. J. J. Jarrett, Oregon.)

Both of these techniques have the advantage of good exposure (a criticism of other methods of subcutaneous mastectomy), which enables more complete removal of the breast tissue. It also allows a reduction in the breast skin and provides a double layer of protection over the prosthesis.

A simple mastectomy, as advocated by Horton et al., can be used for breasts of all shapes and sizes (11,12). In small breasts the nipple-areola complex

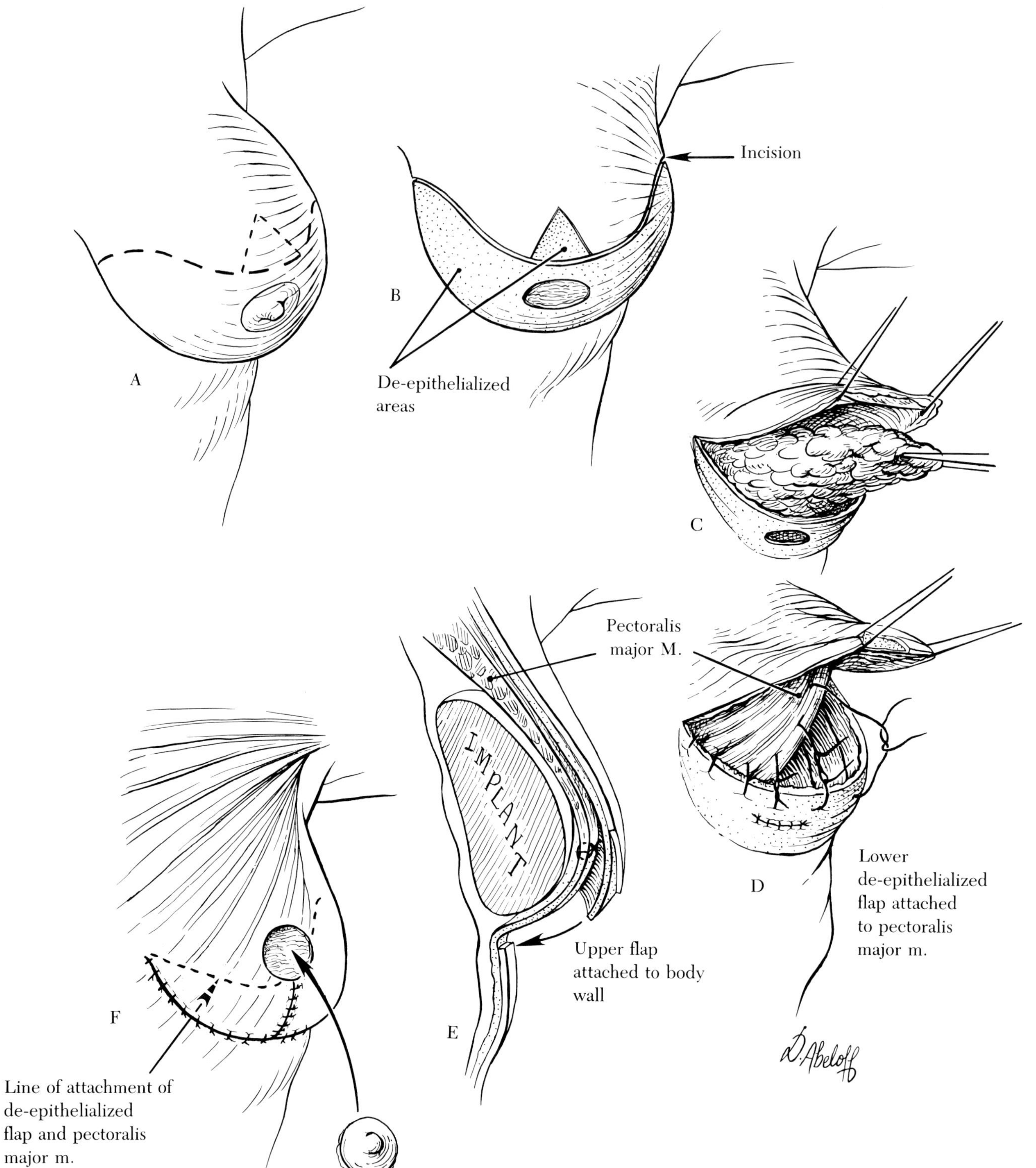

Figure 10.14. Subcutaneous mastectomy of a large ptotic breast, with immediate reconstruction. The deepithelialized lower part of the breast skin flap is sutured to the lower edge of the raised pectoralis muscle to form a submuscular dermal pocket for the implant. The upper breast skin flaps are brought down over the breast mound to form a skin brassiere. The nipple-areola is then applied as a graft or can be stored for future use if there is any doubt about the viability of the skin flap.

is excised and a transverse incision made laterally. This gives good access to the breast tissue, including the axillary tail. Part of the lower flap may be deepithelialized if there is redundancy of skin. The pectoral muscle may then be split directly through the line of its fibers and a submuscular space developed for the implant. Alternatively, the submuscular space may be approached laterally, and the serratus and pectoralis muscles can be elevated separately (Figure 10.20).

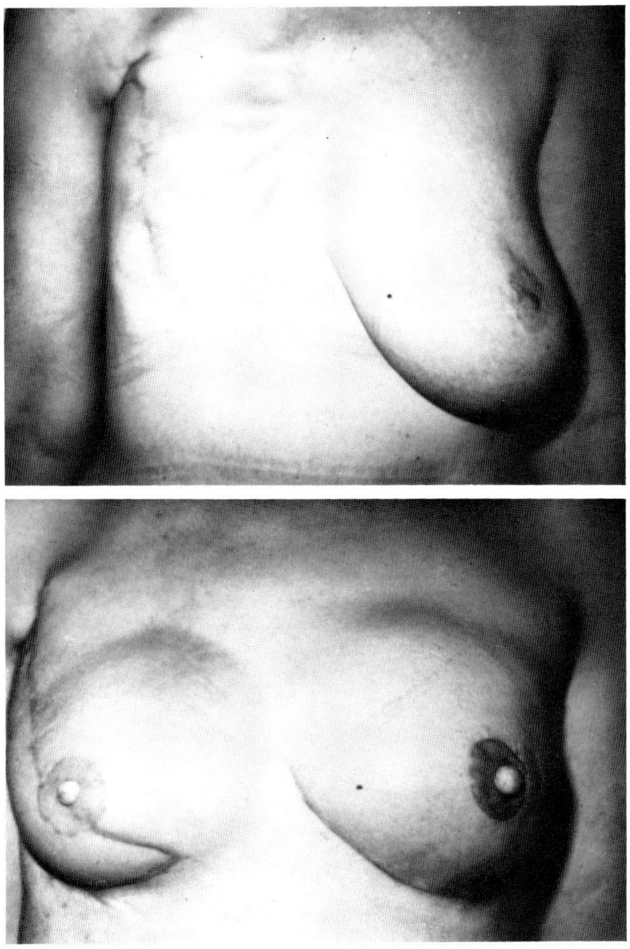

Figure 10.15. **Top:** Right radical mastectomy defect with an enlarged and ptotic left breast, AP view. **Bottom:** Right breast reconstruction using a latissimus dorsi musculocutaneous flap and a 250-cc bilumen implant. Three months later a left subcutaneous mastectomy and immediate reconstruction were done using a submuscular dermal pocket with a 250-cc bilumen implant. The right areola was formed from upper thigh skin, and local quadrapod flaps were used to form the nipple. The left areola was the original areola reapplied as a doughnut-shaped free graft. The nipple was formed from local quadrapod flaps.

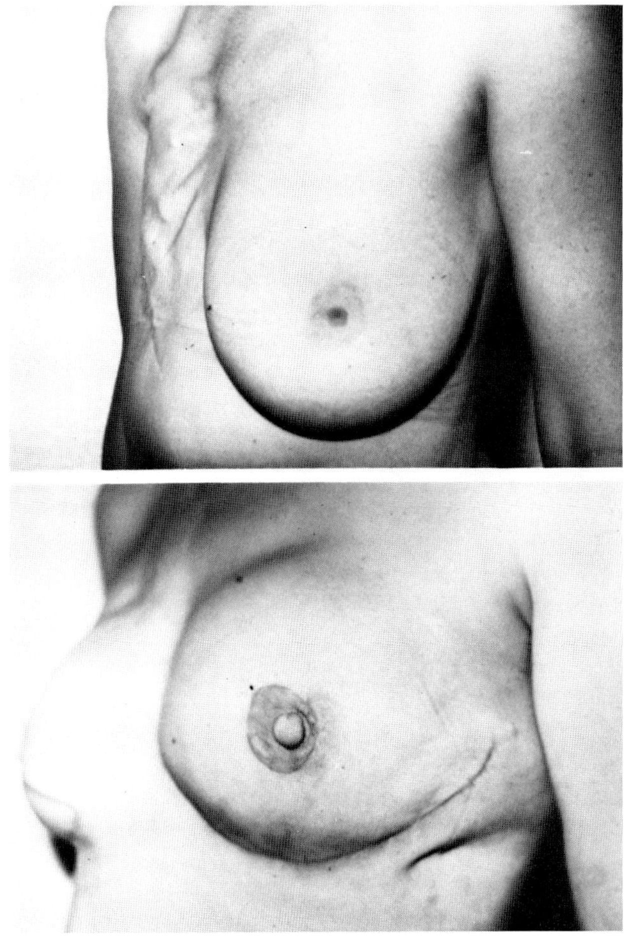

Figure 10.16. **Top:** Left oblique view showing a ptotic left breast. **Bottom:** Left oblique view after subcutaneous mastectomy and reconstruction.

Larger breasts require a greater amount of the lower flap to be deepithelialized, and the incisions may have to extend more medially than the nipple to avoid skin redundancy and "dog ear" deformity (Figures 10.21–10.23).

Techniques for Achieving Symmetry

If the contralateral breast tissue is to remain intact, the ultimate aim in breast reconstruction is to obtain symmetry that is apparent without clothing. In the ideal situation, the contralateral breast is of normal shape and size for the height and build of the woman, and no interference is necessary. All too often, however, the contralateral breast is less than perfect in regard to the bodily configuration and age of the patient. In this situation the reconstructed breast mound is made to conform as nearly as possible to the shape and size proportionate to each woman. At a second stage, when the nipple-areola complex is made, a procedure can then be performed on the contralateral side, if the patient wishes, in an attempt to produce symmetry. However, a woman often accepts minor degrees of asymmetry so long as the breasts are volumetrically equal when wearing a brassiere.

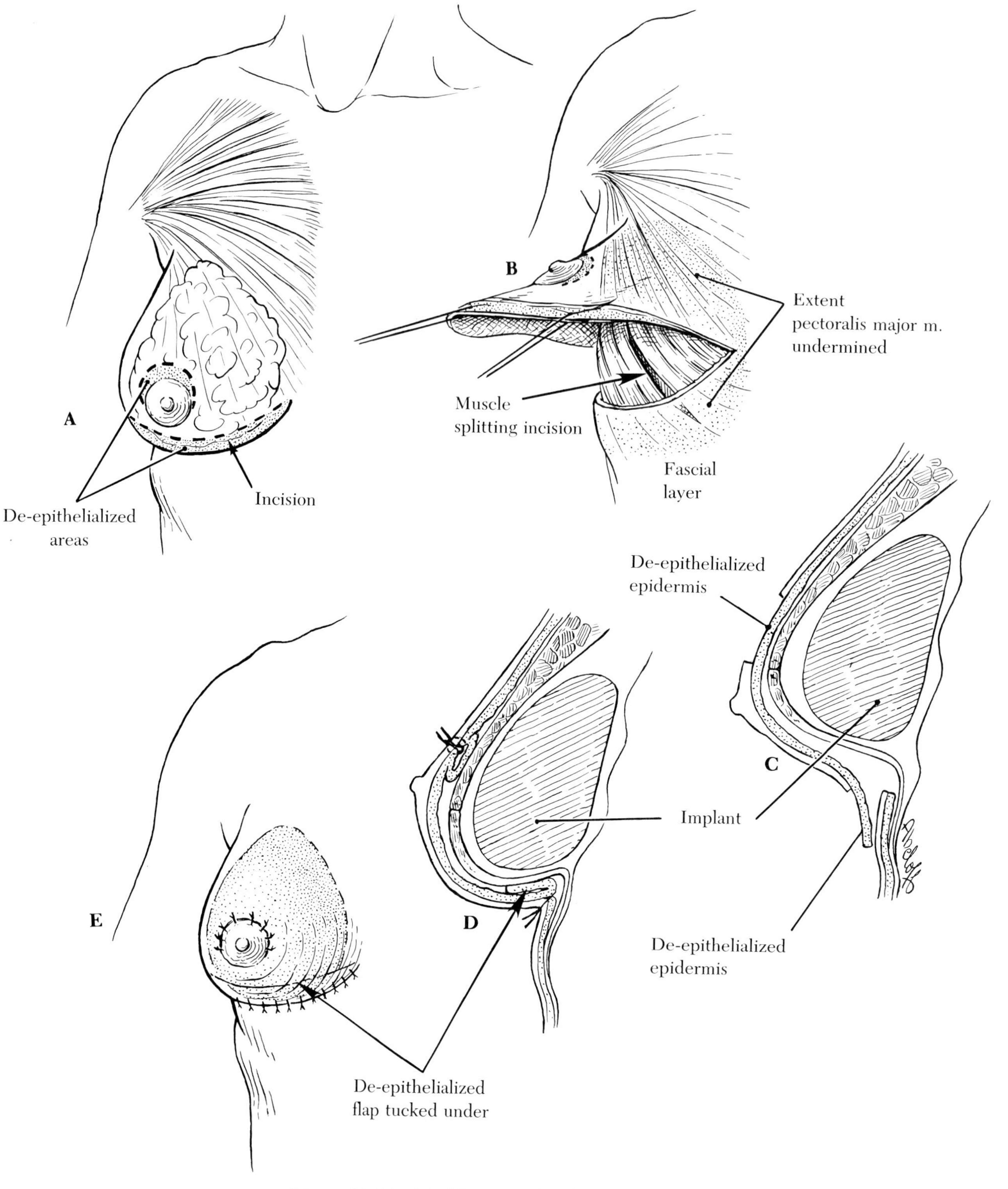

Figure 10.17. Modification of Rubin's "cushion augmentation" following a subcutaneous mastectomy.

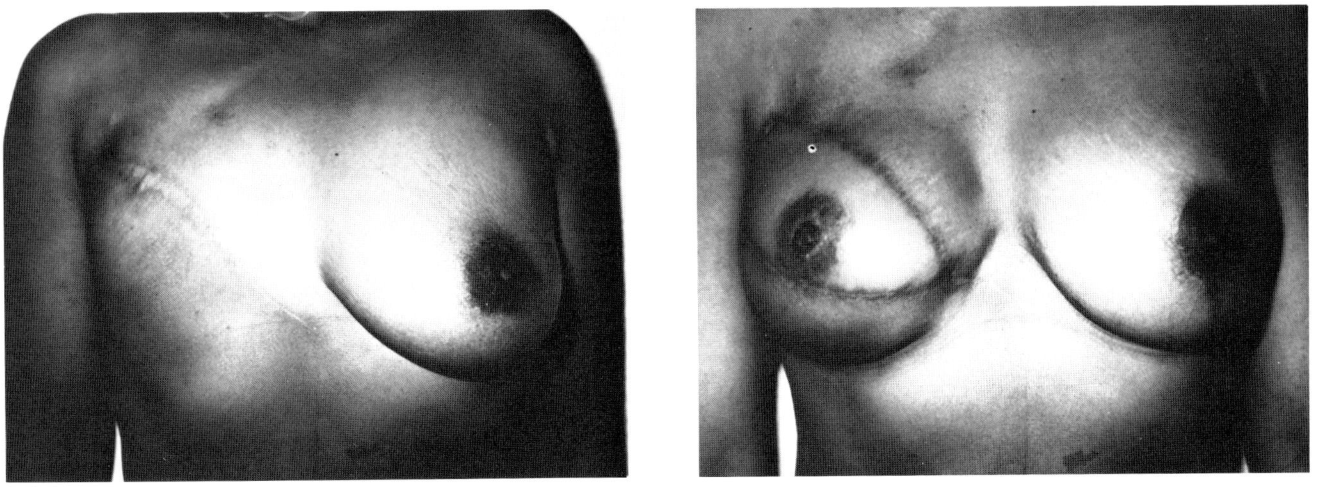

A B

Figure 10.18. **A:** Postoperative right radical mastectomy, AP view. Left breast has had a biopsy excision. **B:** Postoperative right latissimus dorsi musculocutaneous flap with implant. Some weeks later a left subcutaneous mastectomy through an inframammary incision and nipple repositioning by upward advancement were performed. The mild ptosis was corrected by infolding the deepithelialized lower part of the flap. A further area below the nipple was deepithelialized and infolded vertically to produce the T-scar. The right areola was formed from upper thigh skin and the nipple from labial tissue.

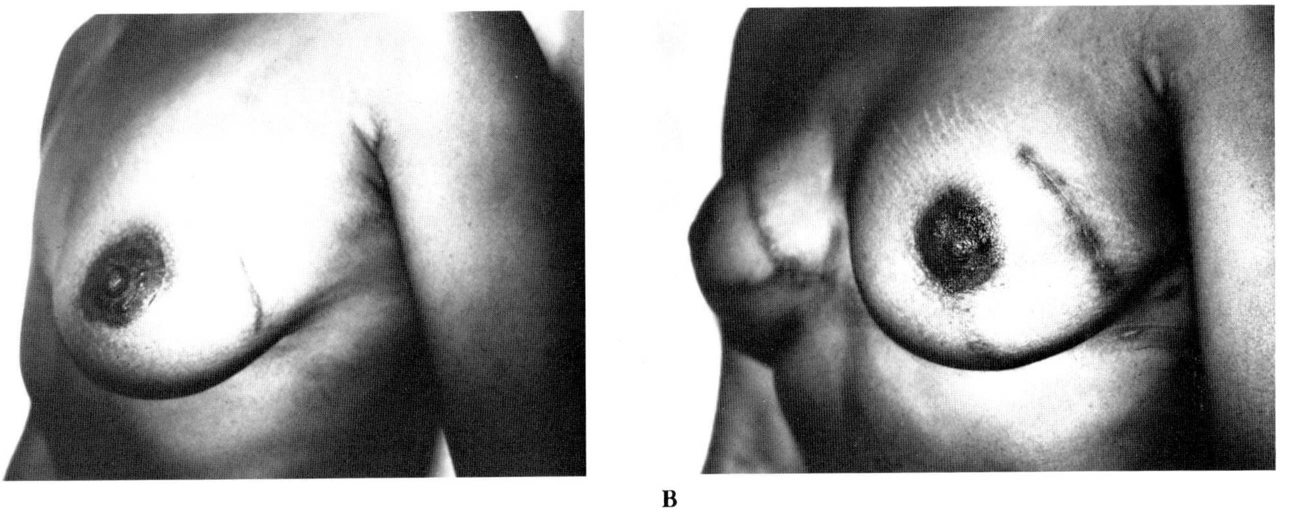

A B

Figure 10.19. **A:** Oblique preoperative view showing a biopsy excision scar. **B:** Postoperative subcutaneous mastectomy result.

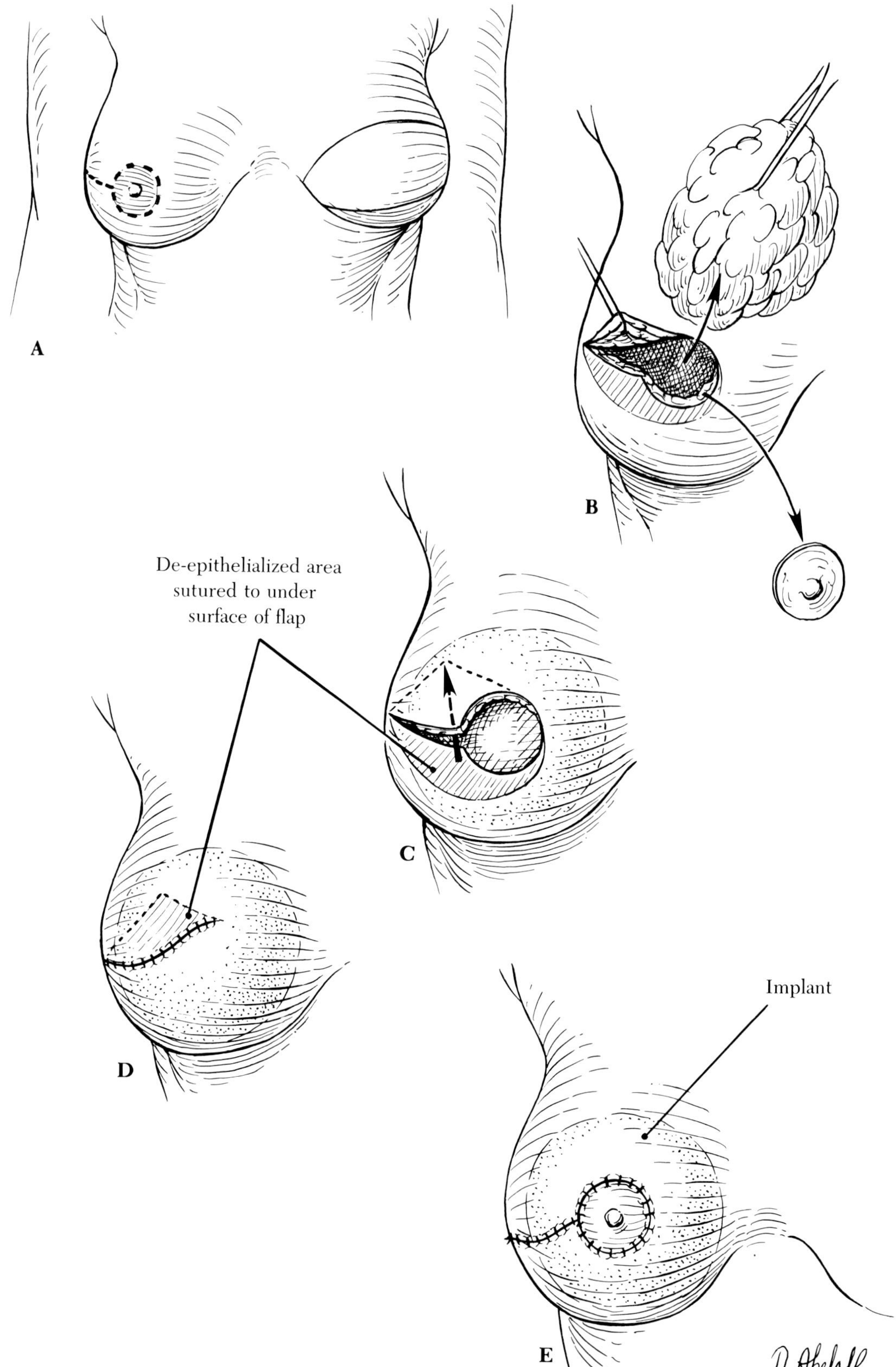

Figure 10.20. Simple mastectomy technique for small breasts, keeping the incision laterally.

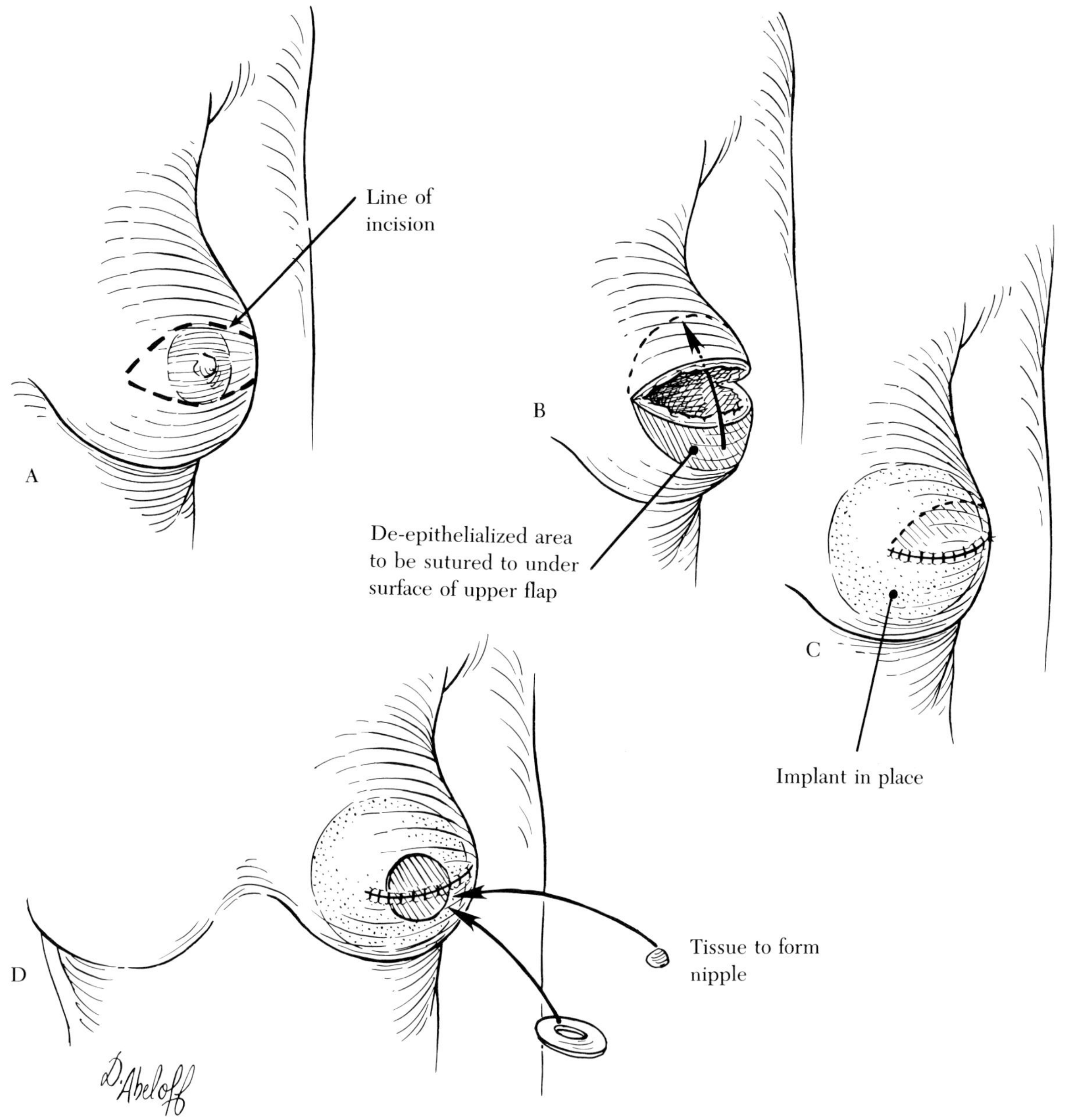

Figure 10.21. Simple mastectomy technique for large breasts, with the incision extending more medially.

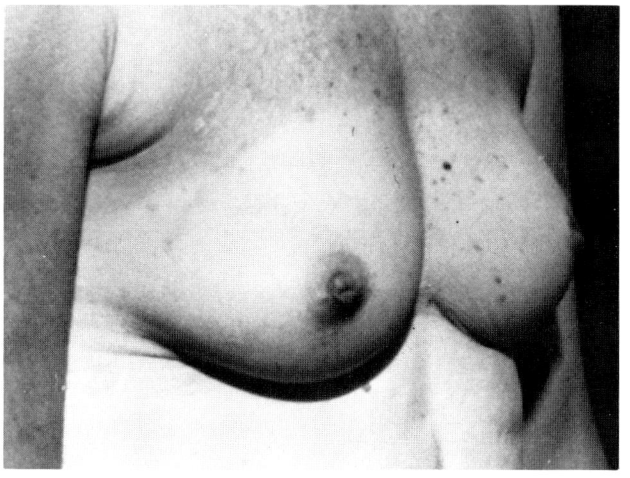

Figure 10.22. Right oblique preoperative view. Patient had a small carcinoma in the right breast and was treated by a simple mastectomy; a simultaneous simple mastectomy was done prophylactically to the left breast. Immediate bilateral reconstruction was done.

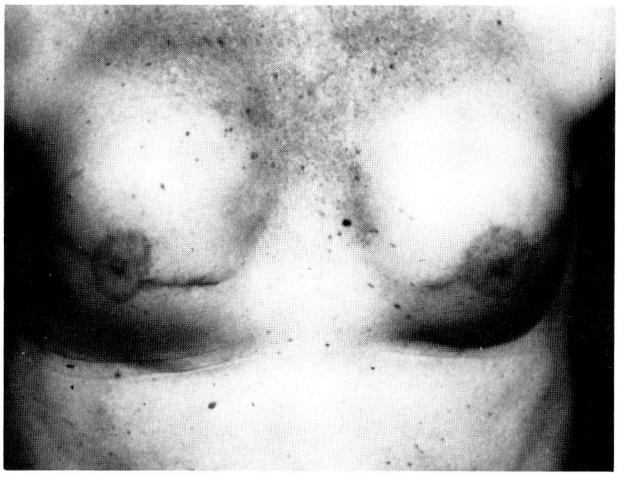

Figure 10.23. AP postoperative view of the patient in Figure 10.22. (Photographs in Figures 10.22 and 10.23 were kindly supplied by Dr. C. E. Horton.)

Augmentation

Occasionally, a woman who has had a mastectomy for carcinoma decides that if she is going to have breast reconstruction she would like an augmentation to her remaining breast (2,15). This is frequently the case if she has some degree of hypoplasia of the normal side. In this situation the reconstructed breast is made as close as possible to the size that she desires, and a subpectoral implantation is performed on the contralateral side at a second stage (Figures 10.24–10.27) (3).

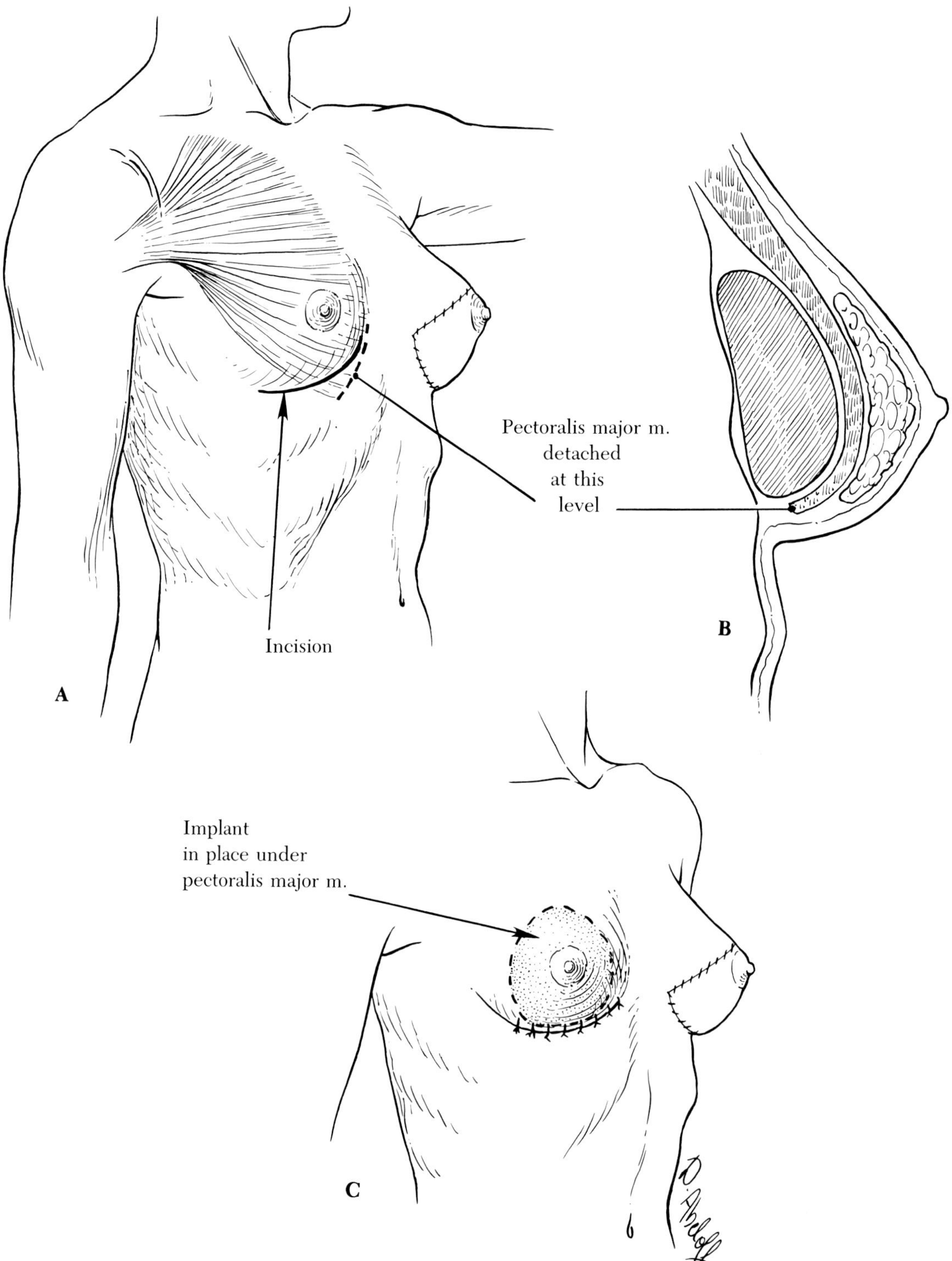

Figure 10.24. Submuscular augmentation technique with detachment of the pectoralis muscle from the lower sternum and costal region through an inframammary incision.

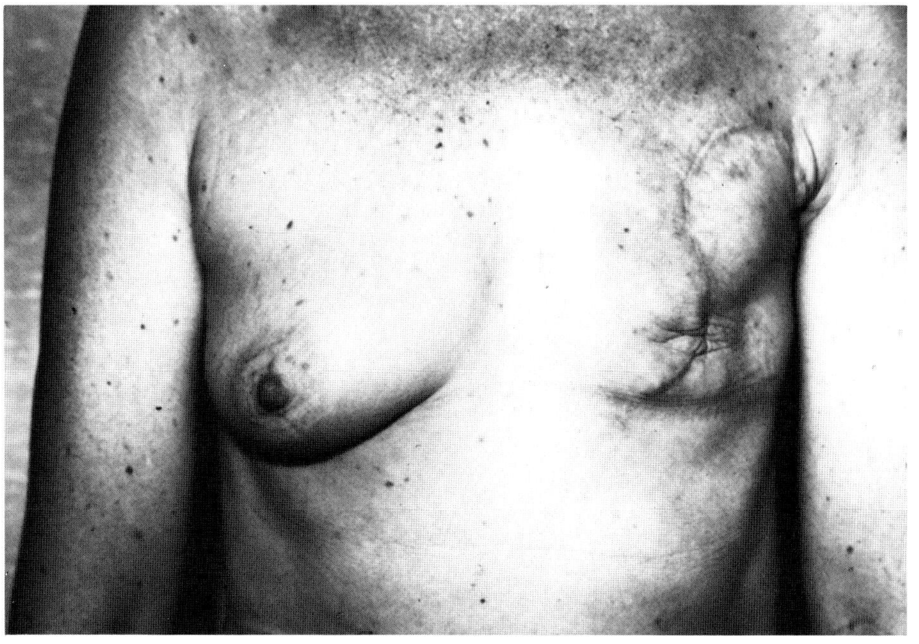

Figure 10.25. Preoperative left modified radical mastectomy defect.

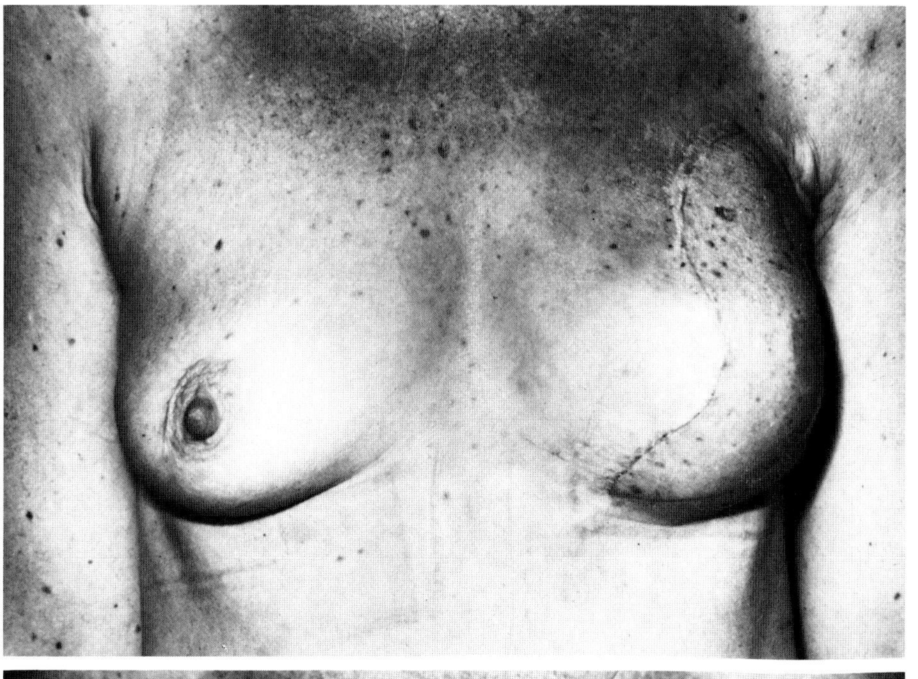

Figure 10.26. Postoperative left latissimus dorsi musculocutaneous flap with implant.

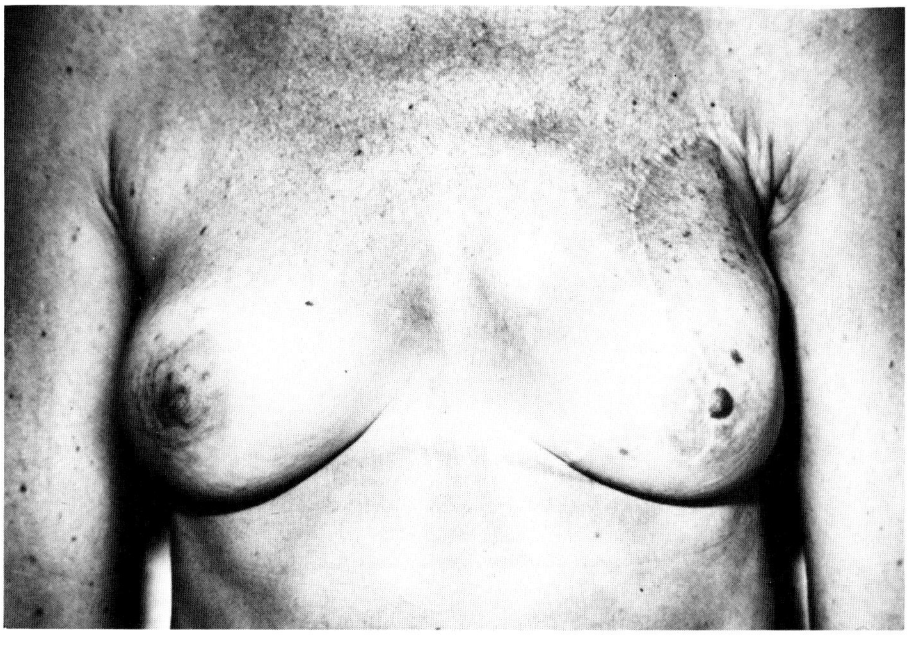

Figure 10.27. Postoperative right submuscular augmentation with a 150-cc implant for symmetry. The left areola came from postauricular skin, and the nipple from the left ear lobule.

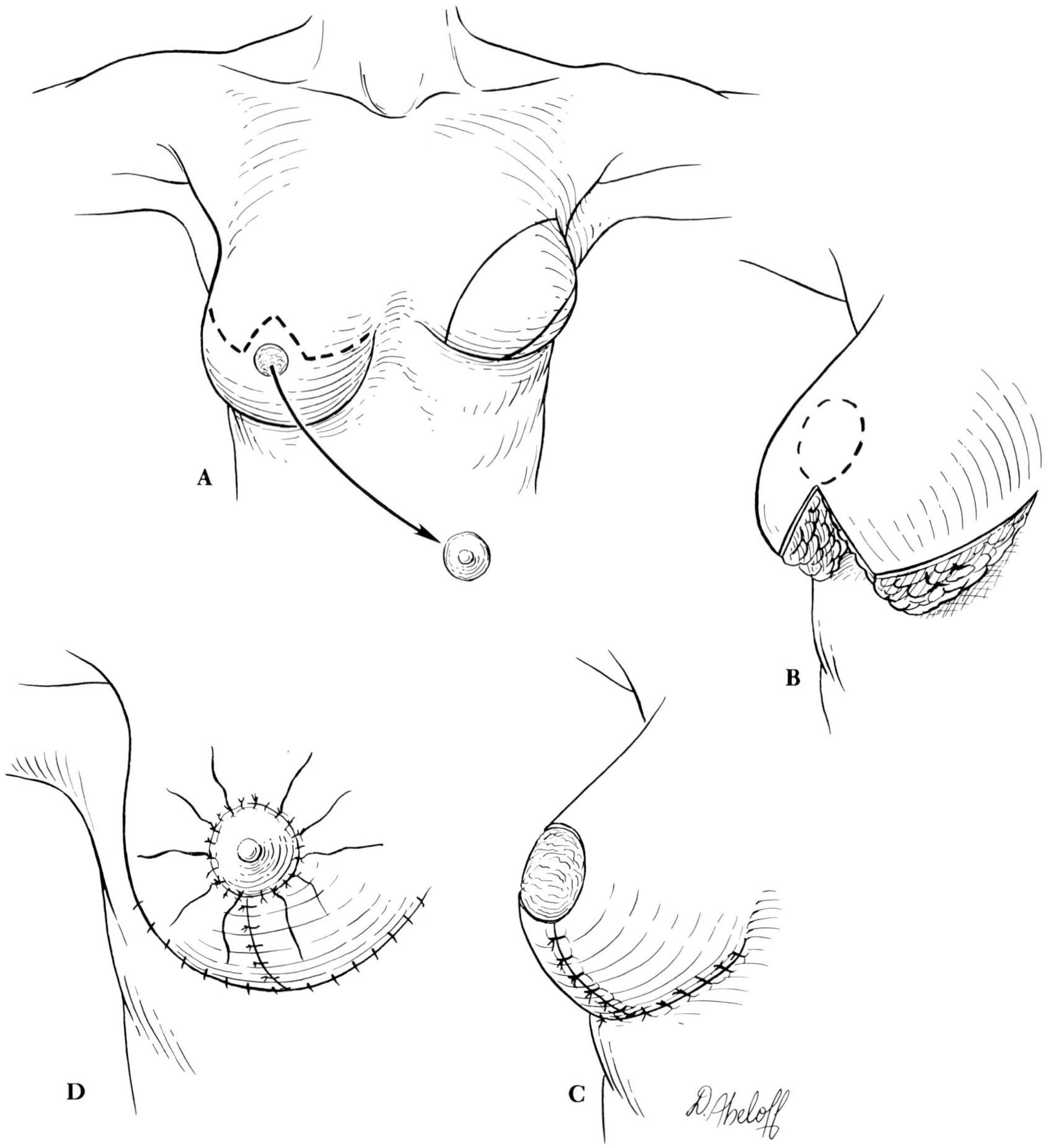

Figure 10.28. Reduction mammoplasty technique in overly large breast.

Reduction Mammoplasty

Often the contralateral breast is overly large, excessively ptotic, or both in regard to the patient's age, height, and build. In these instances it is undesirable and impractical to mimic the "normal" breast with the reconstructed side. Again, as in augmentation, the reconstructed breast is made as near as possible to the size and shape the patient wishes. On the contralateral side, a reduction mammoplasty or a mastopexy is performed, usually at the time of the nipple-areola reconstruction. If the nipple-areola complex is very large on the normal side, a "sharing" technique can be utilized, as described in Chapter 11.

When a reduction mammoplasty is needed for an excessively large breast, it is easier to obtain symmetry by using a free nipple graft technique. The breast mound can be "sculptured," and when a satisfactory size and shape are achieved, the defatted nipple-areola is applied as a full-thickness graft (Figures 10.28 and 10.29). As an alternative, the areola alone may be applied as a full-thickness doughnut-shaped graft after the nipple has been reconstructed using the Little method (Figure 10.30) (17). Avoidance of the Strombeck (27) and McKissock (18) dermal pedicle techniques during reduction of the large breast is recommended. It is more difficult to obtain symmetry with this method, and, more importantly, the method may make diagnosis in subse-

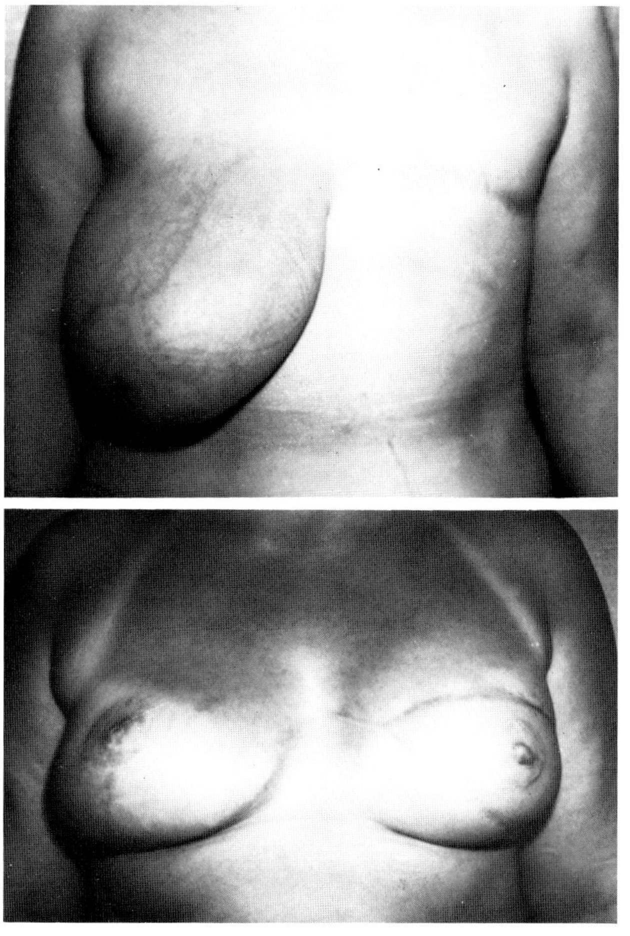

Figure 10.29. **Top:** Left modified radical mastectomy through a transverse Stewart incision with gross hypertrophy of the right breast. **Bottom:** Postoperative left latissimus dorsi musculocutaneous flap reconstruction with a 300-cc bilumen implant. Two months later a right reduction mammoplasty with free nipple areola graft was done. The left nipple-areola was reconstructed at the same time by the spiral sharing technique from the right side.

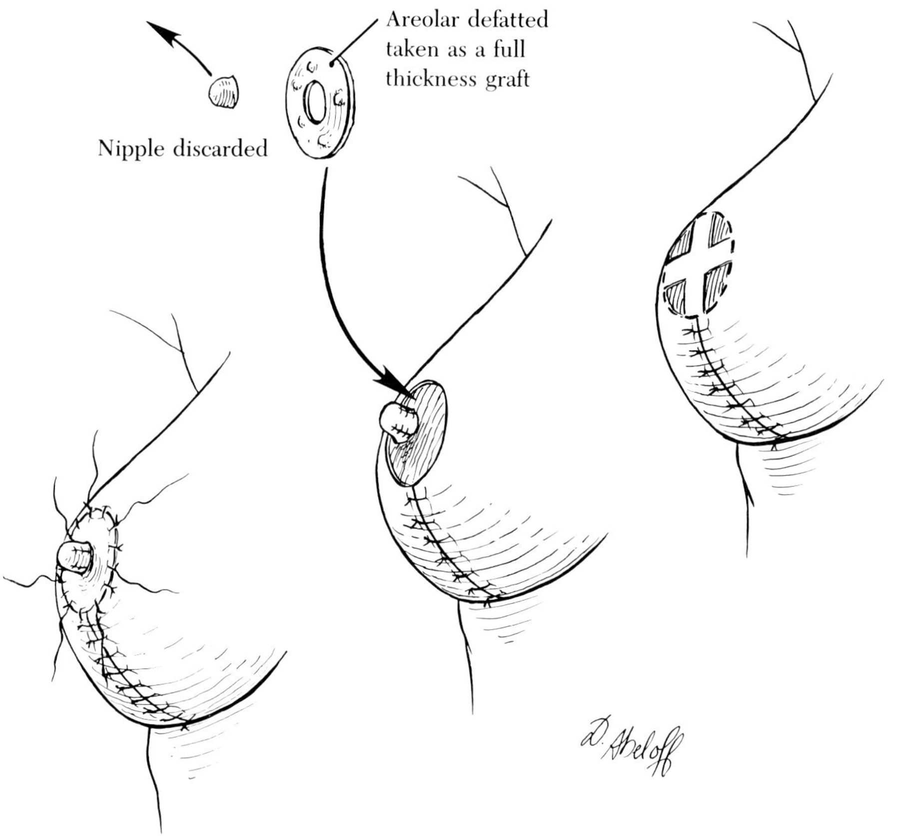

Figure 10.30. Alternative technique for nipple-areola reconstruction when reduction mammoplasty with a free graft is used. Because of a frequently poor take, the nipple is excised and discarded. The areola is saved and is used as a doughnut-shaped graft. The nipple shape is formed from local tissue using quadrapod flaps.

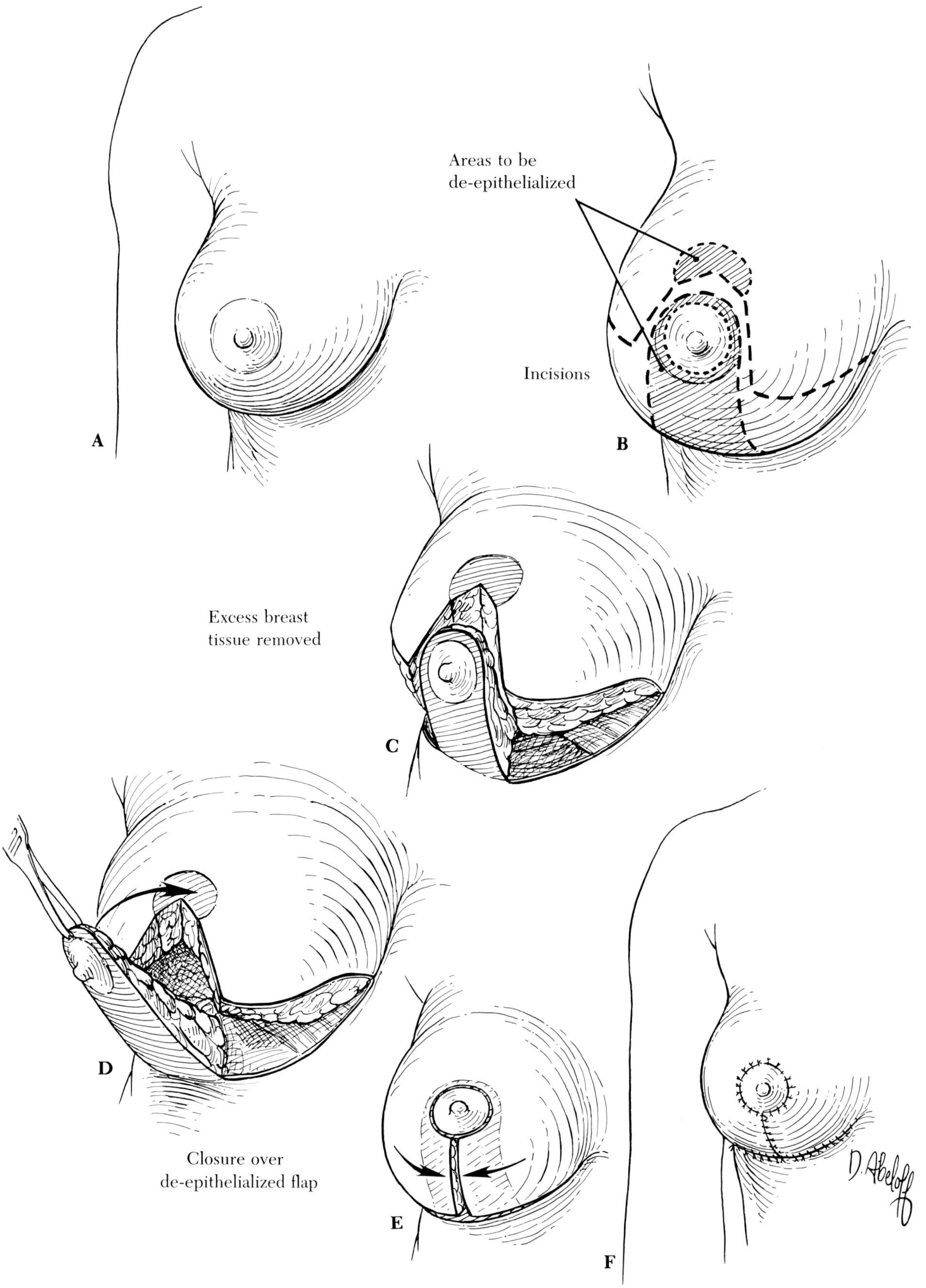

Figure 10.31. Technique of the inferior pedicle reduction mammoplasty.

quent mammograms difficult because of infolded dermal elements distorting the architecture (23).

In the moderately enlarged breast, the single-pedicle techniques may be utilized successfully. Courtiss (1) recommends the inferior pedicle technique (Figures 10.31–10.35) (7,22). Alternatively, the superior pedicle technique, advocated by Weiner (28), may be utilized (Figures 10.36 and 10.37).

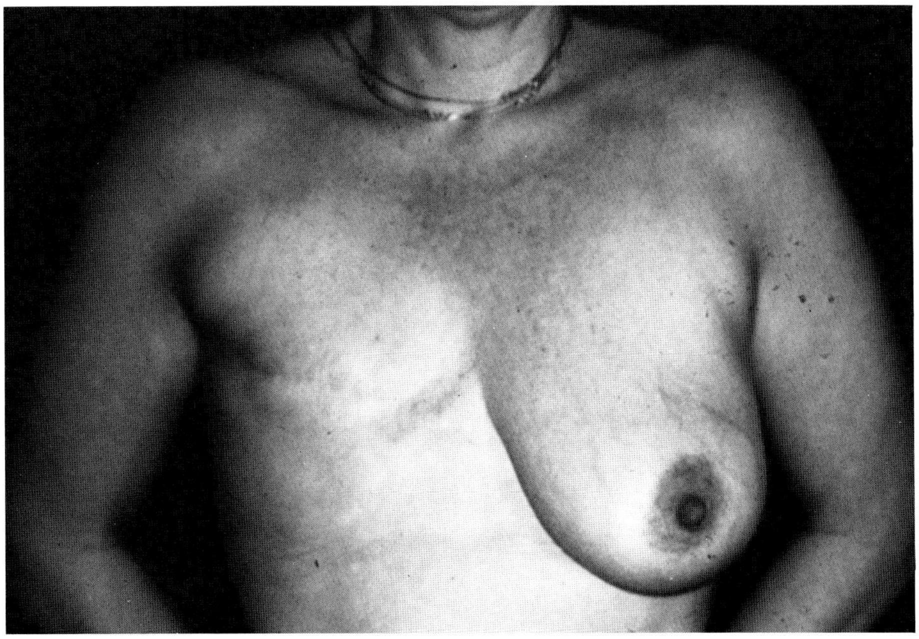

Figure 10.32. Right modified mastectomy defect with a moderately enlarged and ptotic left breast, AP view.

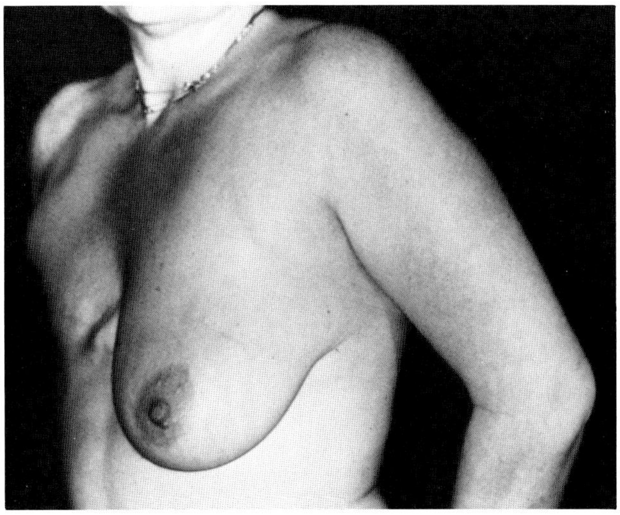

Figure 10.33. Oblique view of the patient in Figure 10.32 showing the enlarged left breast.

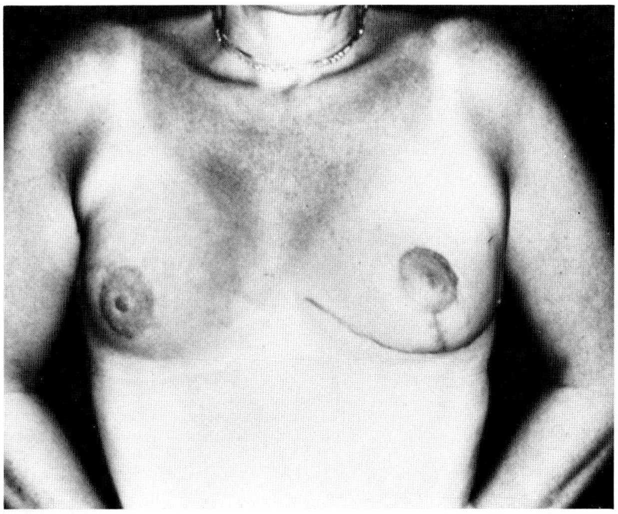

Figure 10.34. After right breast reconstruction and left reduction mammoplasty using the inferior pedicle technique, AP view.

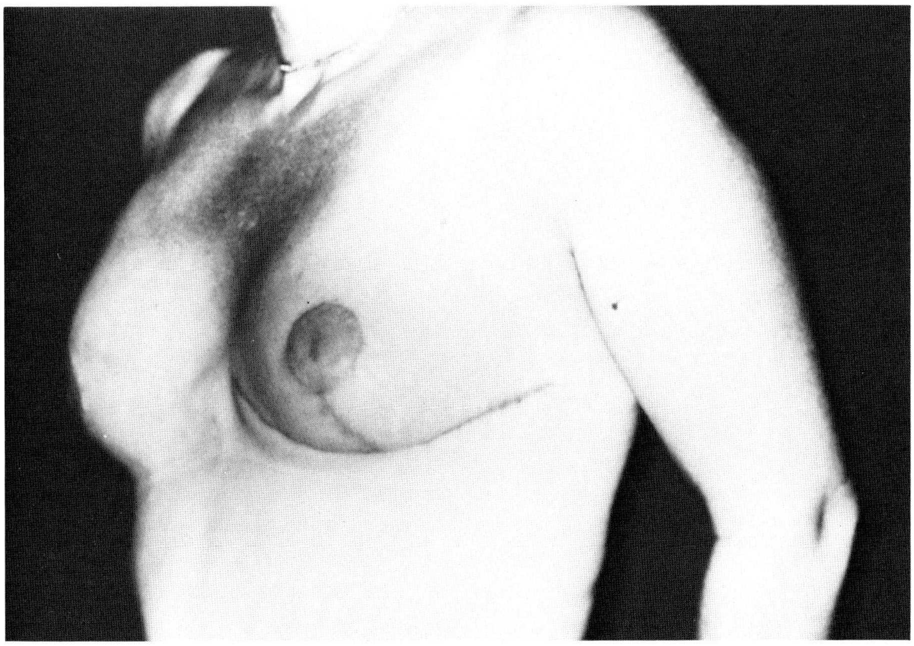

Figure 10.35. Oblique view of the patient in Figure 10.34 showing a left reduction mammoplasty. (Photographs in Figures 10.32–10.35 were kindly supplied by Dr. E. H. Courtiss.)

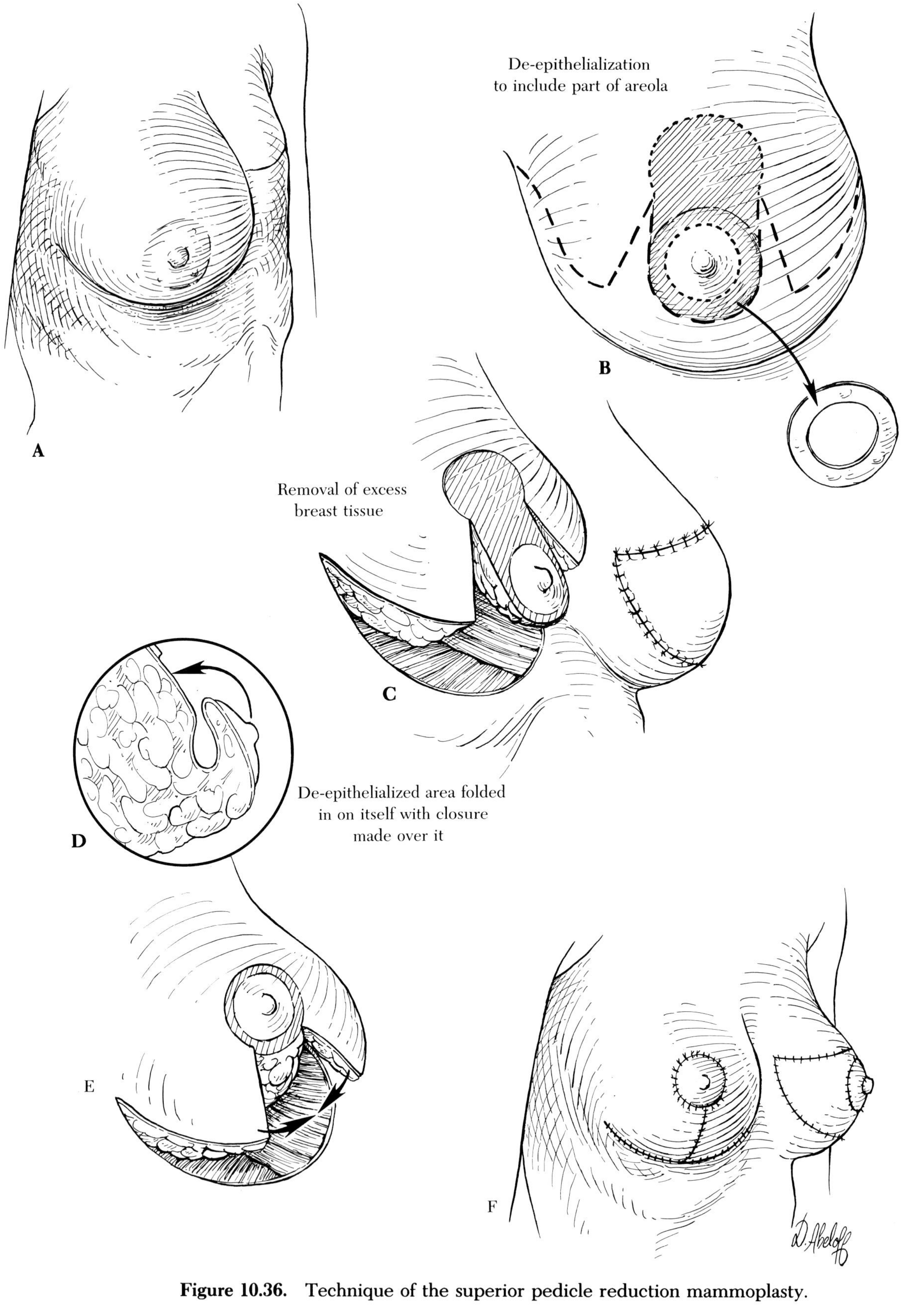

Figure 10.36. Technique of the superior pedicle reduction mammoplasty.

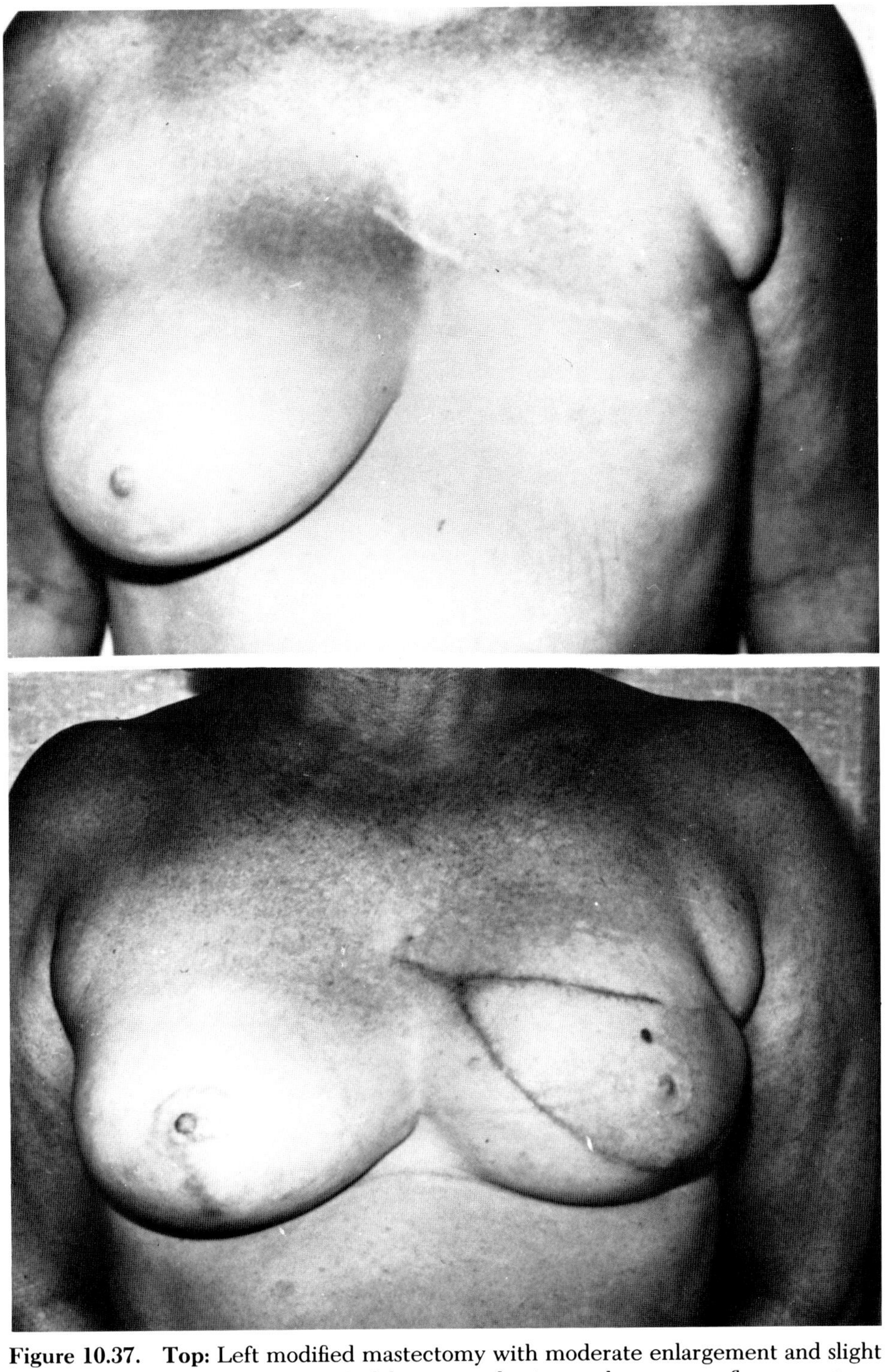

Figure 10.37. **Top:** Left modified mastectomy with moderate enlargement and slight ptosis of the right breast. **Bottom:** Left latissimus dorsimusculocutaneous flap reconstruction with implant and right reduction mammoplasty using the superior pedicle technique. The left areola was formed from part of the right areola discarded at the time of reduction mammoplasty. The left nipple was reconstructed from half of the right side.

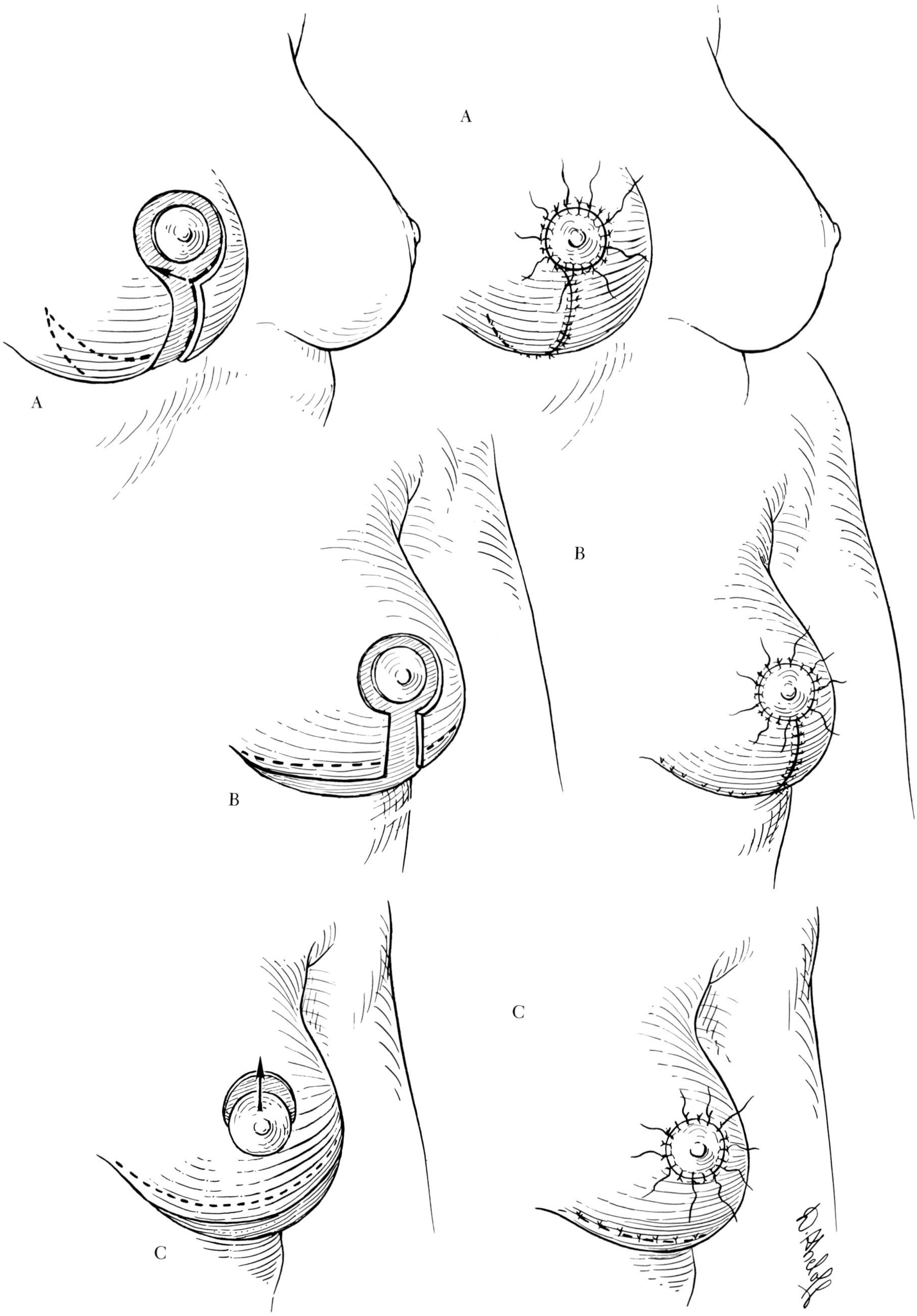

Figure 10.38. Various mastopexy techniques.

Mastopexy

If the contralateral breast is only ptotic and the patient does not desire a reduction, a mastopexy is performed. A variety of methods have been described (4,8,9,16,20,21), three of which are shown in Figure 10.38.

References

1. Courtiss EH, 1977: Reduction mammoplasty by the inferior pedicle technique, an alternative to free nipple and areola grafting for severe macromastia or extensive ptosis. Plast Reconstr Surg 59:500–507.
2. Cronin TD, Gerow FJ, 1964: Augmentation mammoplasty: a new "natural feel" prosthesis. In: Transactions of Third International Congress of Plastic Surgery, pp 41–49. Excerpta Medica, Amsterdam.
3. Dempsey WC, Latham WD, 1968: Subpectoral implants in augmentation mammoplasty—preliminary report. Plast Reconstr Surg 42:515–521.
4. Erol OO, Spira M, 1980: A mastopexy technique for mild to moderate ptosis. Plast Reconstr Surg 65:603–609.
5. Freeman BS, 1975: Subcutaneous mastectomy for the treatment of pre-malignant disease of the breast. In: Controversial Opinions, ICS No. 377, edited by JM Greep, pp 213–218. Excerpta Medica, Amsterdam.
6. Freeman BS, 1980: Subcutaneous mastectomy for benign breast lesions with immediate or delayed prosthetic replacement. Plast Reconstr Surg 65:371–372.
7. Georgiade NG, Serafin D, Morris R, et al, 1979: Reduction mammoplasty utilizing an inferior pedicle nipple-areola flap. Ann Plast Surg 3:211.
8. Goulian D, 1971: Dermal mastopexy. Plast Reconstr Surg 45:105.
9. Gruber RP, Jones HW, 1980: The "doughnut" mastopexy: indications and complications. Plast Reconstr Surg 65:34–38.
10. Hoffman S, Simon BE, Kahn S, 1979: Alternatives to subcutaneous mastectomy. Plast Reconstr Surg 64:214–220.
11. Horton CE, et al, 1974: Simple mastectomy with immediate reconstruction. Plast Reconstr Surg 53:42–47.
12. Horton CE, Rosato FA, McCraw JB, et al, 1979: Immediate reconstruction following mastectomy for cancer. Clin Plast Surg 6:37–46.
13. Jarrett JR, Cutler RG, Teal DF, 1978: Subcutaneous mastectomy in small, large and ptotic breasts with immediate submuscular placement of implants. Plast Reconstr Surg 62:702–705.
14. Lejour M, Gregoire JP, 1980: Management of the remaining breast in breast reconstruction. Acta Chir Belg 79:145–146.
15. Lewis JR Jr, 1965: The augmentation mammoplasty with special reference to alloplastic materials. Plast Reconstr Surg 35:51–59.
16. Lewis JR Jr, 1972: Classification and surgical correction of ptosis of the breasts. In: Symposium on Aesthetic Surgery of the Face, Eyelid and Breast, edited by FW Masters, JR Lewis Jr, pp 183–191. Mosby, St. Louis.
17. Little JW III, Munisifi T, McCullock DT, 1983: One-stage reconstruction of a projecting nipple: the quadrapod flap. Plast Reconstr Surg 71:126–132.
18. McKissock PK, 1972: Reduction mammoplasty with vertical dermal pedicle. Plast Reconstr Surg 49:245.
19. Randall P, Dabb R, Loc N, 1979: "Apple coring" the nipple in subcutaneous mastectomy. Plast Reconstr Surg 64:800–803.
20. Reginault P, 1974: Reduction mammoplasty by the "B" technique. Plast Reconstr Surg 53:19–24.
21. Reginault P, 1980: Breast reduction "B" technique. Plast Reconstr Surg 65:840–845.
22. Robbins TH, 1977: A reduction mammoplasty with the areola-nipple based on an inferior dermal pedicle. Plast Reconstr Surg 59:64.
23. Robertson JLA, 1977: Changed appearance of mammograms following breast reduction. Plast Reconstr Surg 59:347–351.
24. Rubin LR, 1976: The cushioned augmentation repair after a subcutaneous mastectomy. Plast Reconstr Surg 57:23–29.
25. Rubin LR, 1979: A preventative mastectomy with immediate reconstruction for the high risk breast cancer patient. Clin Plast Surg 6:107–119.
26. Spira M, 1976: Subcutaneous mastectomy in the large ptotic breast. Plast Reconstr Surg 59:200–205.
27. Strombeck JO, 1960: Mammoplasty: report of a new technique based on the two pedicle procedure. Br J Plast Surg 13:79–90.
28. Weiner DL, 1976: Reduction mammoplasty with a single superior dermapedicle. In: Plastic and Reconstructive Surgery of the Breast, edited by RM Goldwyn, p 257. Little Brown, Boston.

11

Reconstruction of the Nipple-Areola Complex

Raymond F. Morgan

Reconstruction of the nipple-areola complex is usually the last step in breast reconstruction after mastectomy. Many new techniques have been described, and the methods most commonly used are presented here.

Most authors prefer to allow the reconstructed breast mound to become stable in its position on the chest wall for some weeks before attempting nipple-areola reconstruction. Accurate placement on the breast mound is then easier. Measurements for the positioning of the new complex should be done with the patient in the upright position because the areola of the normal side contracts somewhat when the patient is lying supine on the operating table. The distances from two fixed points, e.g., the suprasternal notch and the tip of the xiphoid process to the normal nipple, are measured. These distances can then be duplicated on the reconstructed breast. Because the breast mounds are not identical, some minor adjustments in positioning are usually necessary. The proposed position of the areola and nipple can be drawn on the breast mound to see if it meets with the patient's approval (Figure 11.1).

The objective of nipple-areola reconstruction should be symmetry between the two nipple-areola complexes. The color, size, texture, and positioning on the breast mound are also critical.

The characteristics of the available donor tissue can be evaluated and used to advantage to match the normal nipple-areola complex. For example, the labia have long been accepted donor sites in areola reconstruction. However, hyperpigmentation, peeling, and desquamation have made these areas less popular (1). Many combinations of the various procedures may be used to obtain the most symmetrical result for an individual patient.

The banked nipple-areola graft has been advocated for reconstruction. At the time of ablative surgery, the graft is transferred to the groin and later used on the reconstructed breast mound (15). There are, however, disadvantages and risks to this procedure. Depigmentation of the areola may occur because of the two transfers required. More importantly, tumor cells may be inadvertently transferred with the graft to a distant site, an unfortunate

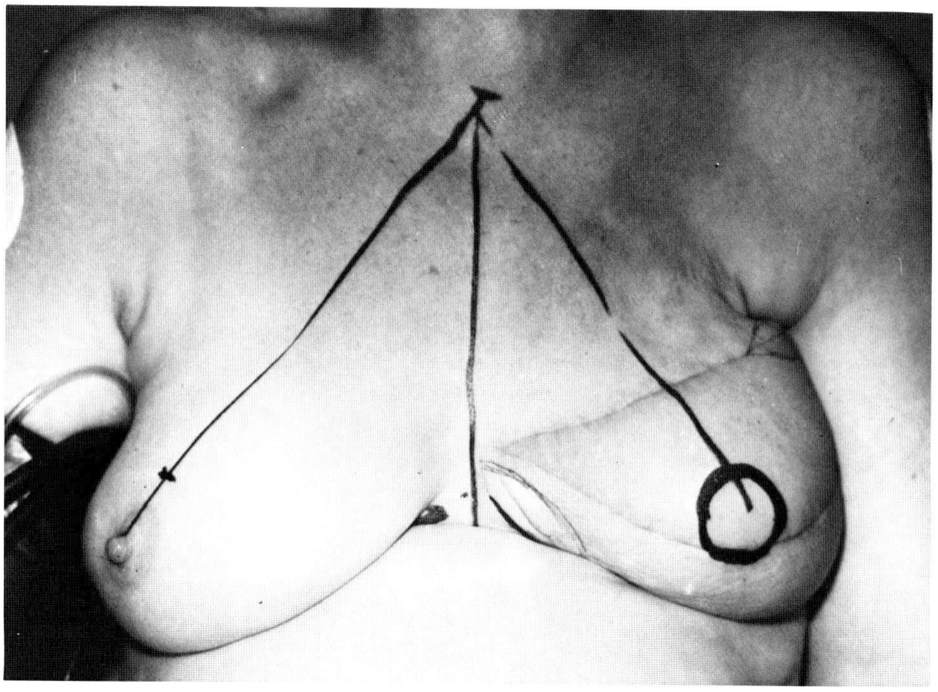

Figure 11.1. With the patient sitting, the location of the nipple-areolar site on the reconstructed left breast is marked. On the right side a mastopexy is planned.

sequela which has been reported (2). If the nipple-areola complex is preserved, multiple frozen sections at the base of the complex must be meticulously examined by the pathologist before transfer. Only patients with small tumors located away from the complex should be considered.

Areola Reconstruction

Full-Thickness Grafts

If the normal contralateral areola is sufficiently large, it often provides the best result when "shared" with the reconstructed breast. If a reduction mammoplasty or a ptosis procedure is planned for the normal breast, the excess outer areola, which is normally discarded, can be used as a full-thickness areolar graft. The width necessary for two areolae of approximately equal size can be calculated (16). The areolar graft is rotated in a circular fasion on the deepithelialized bed of the reconstructed breast. The inner margins are sutured with 5–0 absorbable interrupted sutures. The periphery is also closed with 5–0 silk sutures, which are left several inches long. After the nipple graft is placed, the ends of the sutures are tied over a bolus dressing, which remains in place 7–10 days (Figure 11.2A).

Full-thickness skin grafts from the upper inner thigh are suitable for areolar reconstruction (4). More melanin pigment is present in this area than in the skin of the breast. After the position is determined, an ellipse is designed to incorporate the circular graft (Figure 11.2B). The inconspicuous donor site can then be closed primarily. The defatted full-thickness graft is transferred to the reconstructed breast and secured with 5–0 silk sutures. The center is removed for a nipple graft, and a bolus dressing is then applied.

Retroauricular full-thickness skin may be used if a light pink areola is desired. This donor area is also inconspicuous and may be closed primarily. Both retroauricular areas may be used if the amount of tissue available from one side is insufficient. An ellipse is designed in the sulcus between the ear and the scalp, and the graft is taken from the center of the ellipse. The donor area can be closed with a continuous pull-out or running 4–0 nylon suture (Figure 11.2C). A cutaneous ring at the junction of the new nipple and areola which measures 1.0–1.5 mm serves to separate the two tissues, provides contrast, and facilitates attachment of the nipple (3) (Figures 11.2A and 11.3).

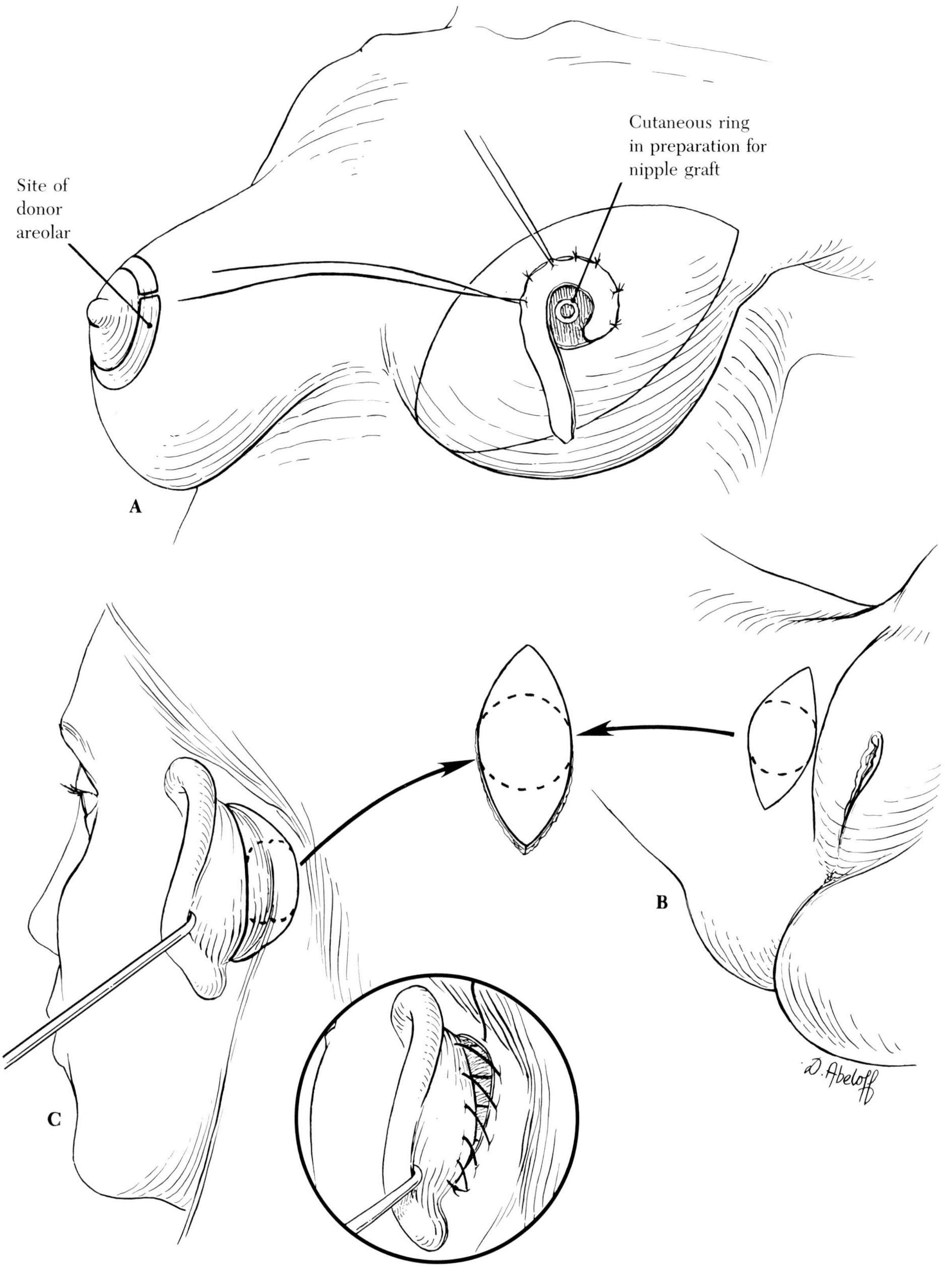

Figure 11.2. **A:** "Shared" areolar full-thickness graft, showing the cutaneous ring at the junction of the new nipple and areola. **B:** Full-thickness graft from the upper thigh. **C:** Retroauricular full-thickness graft.

Split-Thickness Grafts

In 1950 the skin grafting of a burned arm for which the chest was used as a donor site was reported, with a nipple-areola graft inadvertently transferred to the arm (9). Some years later in another case, a dermatome set at 0.010 inch was used to reconstruct the nipple-areola complex of a male patient (11).

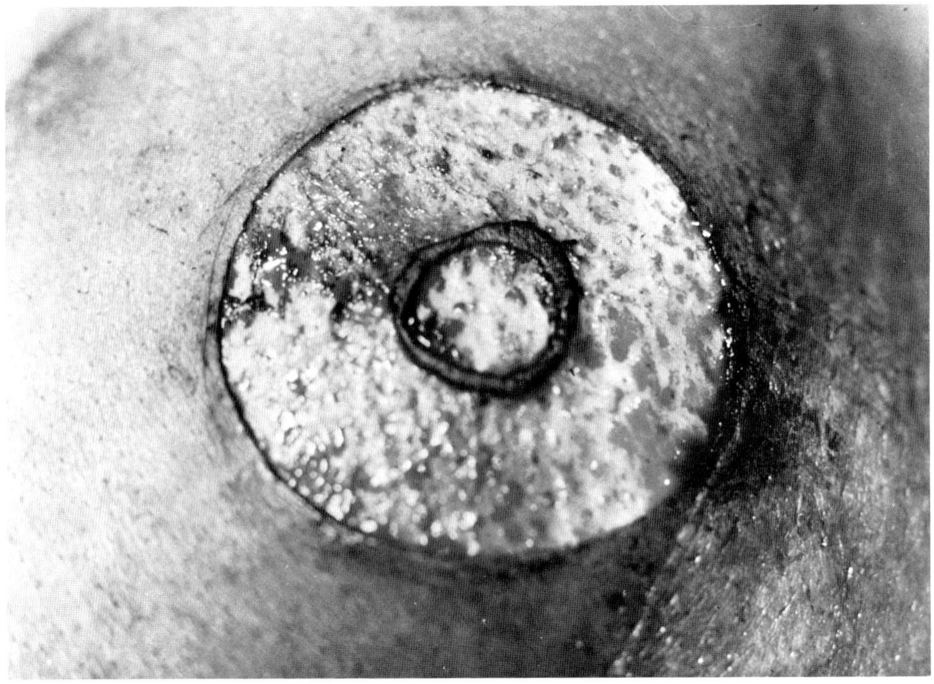

Figure 11.3. Cutaneous ring.

A split-thickness areolar graft may be taken using a drum dermatome (Reese). The dermatome cement is carefully applied only to the areola and not to the surrounding skin or nipple. While the assistant firmly holds the breast, the dermatome tape is elevated from the adjacent skin. The nipple retracts downward, and a doughnut-shaped graft is obtained. The donor areola is then dressed similar to a skin graft donor area. The thickness of the graft is critical. If it is too thin, the graft will not have enough pigmentation; however, if it is removed at too deep a level, the donor areola will depigment. The light, thin-skinned areola may be taken at 0.012–0.014 inch, and the dark, thick-skinned areola may be taken at 0.014–0.016 inch (Figure 11.4A).

The split-thickness areolar graft may also be obtained using a free-hand knife (Weck, Goulian, or Silver dermatome that holds a standard razor blade). Even the scalpel blade has been described as being suitable for taking a thick split-thickness graft (Figure 11.4B) (14). The split-thickness areolar graft is secured in place with 5–0 silk sutures. After the nipple graft is placed, a bolus dressing is applied.

Nipple Reconstruction

Composite Grafts

Nipple-sharing techniques have been used most frequently to provide a composite nipple graft. A simple technique which provides an aesthetically pleasing result is to simply amputate the distal one-third to one-half of the normal nipple (8). This portion is then transferred to the deepithelialized recipient site in the center of the reconstructed areola, sutured in place with 5–0 absorbable sutures, and firmly secured under the bolus dressing used for the areola graft. The donor defect is allowed to epithelialize. In another simple technique credited to Obi, a vertical incision is made in the nipple, the nipple is transferred to the recipient breast, and the donor defect is closed primarily (5) (Figure 11.5A).

In cases where the donor site deformity or the possible sensory changes associated with a contralateral nipple-sharing technique are not acceptable, other tissue may be used (3,10). A composite earlobe graft can be taken in the form of a wedge. The donor area is carefully closed with 6–0 nylon sutures. A circular "nipple" is taken from the center of the wedge and applied to

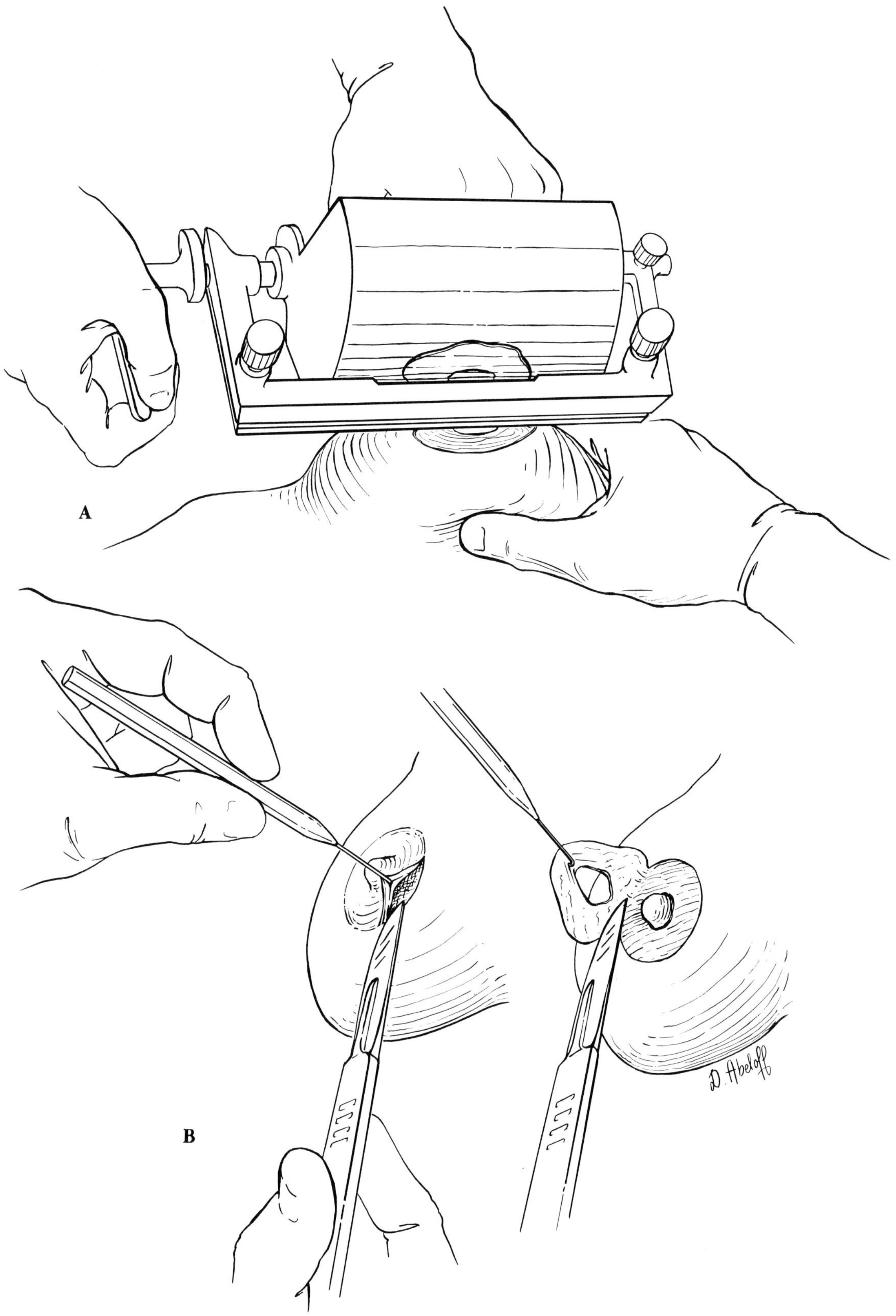

Figure 11.4. **A:** Split-thickness areola graft taken using a drum dermatome. **B:** Split-thickness areolar graft taken using a free-hand knife.

the deepithelialized bed in the center of the areolar graft. The "nipple" graft is usually light pink in color (Figure 11.5B).

As mentioned earlier, the free labial graft is a time-honored method of nipple reconstruction (1). Any area around the labia minora may be used. A wedge is excised and the resulting defect is closed primarily with 5–0 absorbable sutures. The composite graft is then trimmed appropriately and applied to the deepithelialized recipient breast. The nipple graft provided is usually brown and is very useful in bilateral reconstructions (Figure 11.5C).

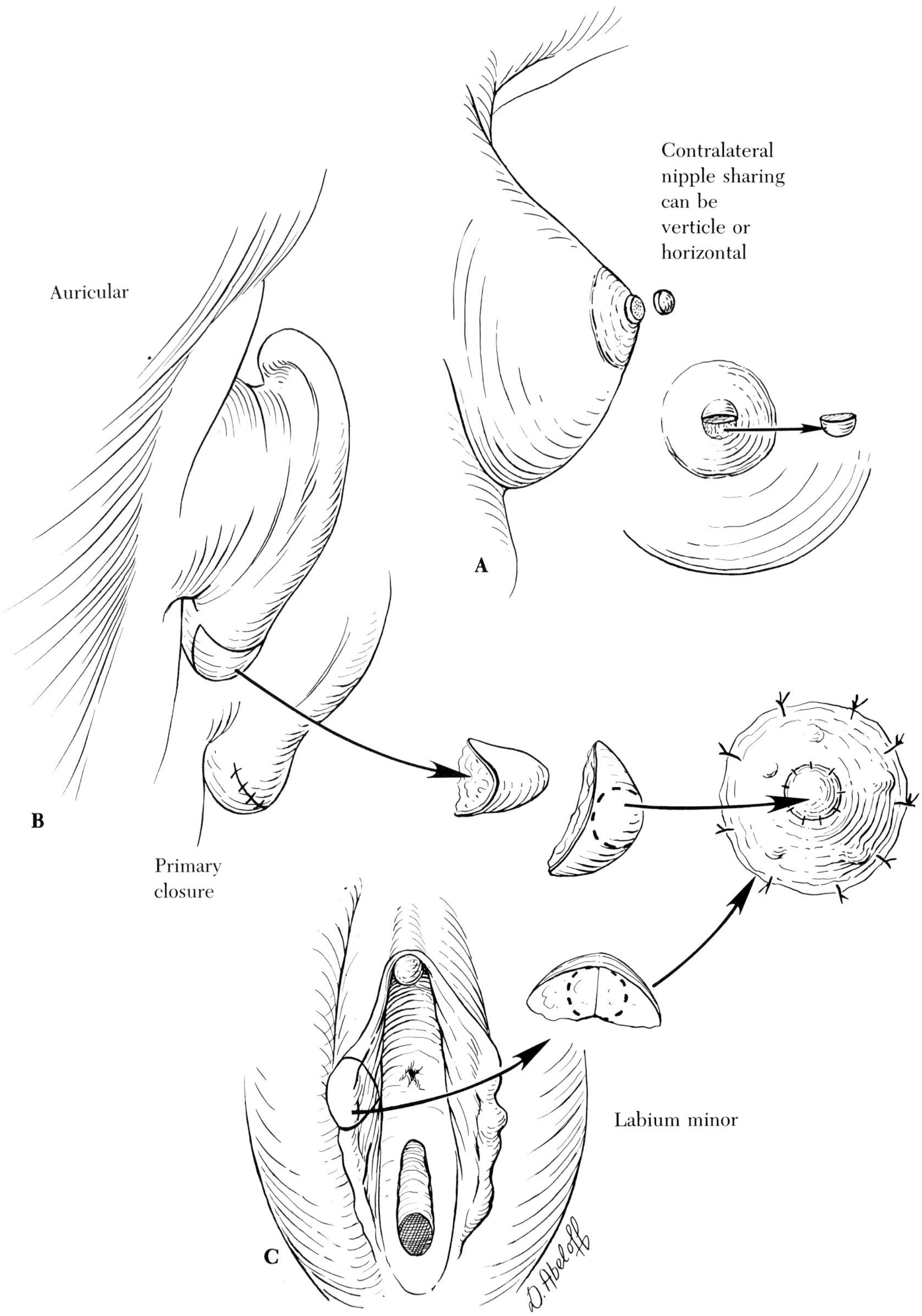

Figure 11.5. **A:** Composite nipple graft from the normal nipple. **B:** Composite earlobe graft. **C:** Labial graft.

Local Flap Technique

A well-formed projecting nipple shape can be produced by the technique of Little et al. (13). The site of the areola is circumscribed with a No. 15 blade. The shaded areas are deepithelialized (Figure 11.6A). The remaining tetrapod flaps are elevated, starting peripherally at a deeper plane, taking all of the dermis. When the central area is reached, the knife blade is turned at right angles to the surface, and a circular core is cut into the subcutaneous tissue (Figure 11.6B). Gentle traction with a skin hook elevates the core (Figure 11.6C). The flaps are then folded down and sewn to each other to maintain

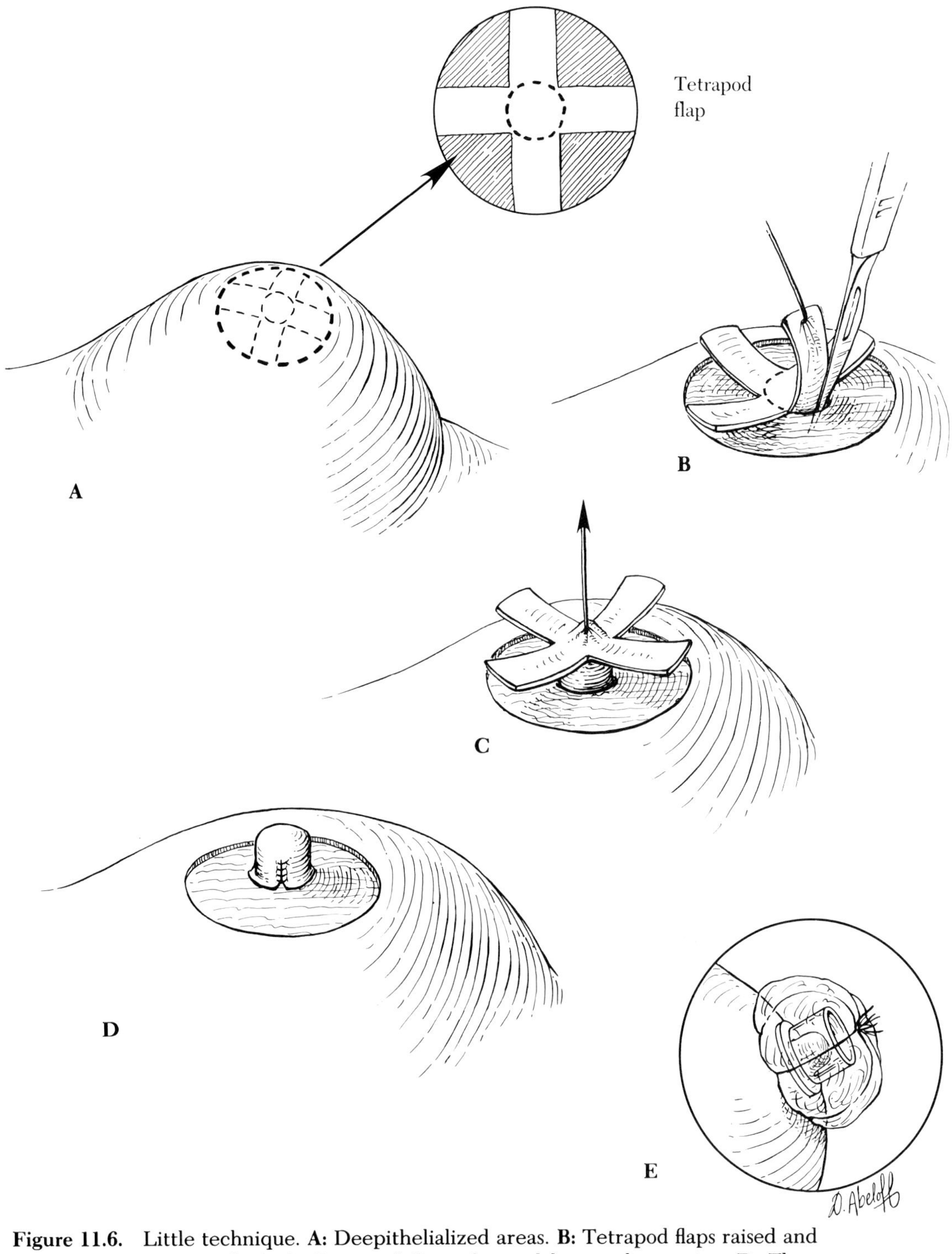

Figure 11.6. Little technique. **A:** Deepithelialized areas. **B:** Tetrapod flaps raised and central core circumscribed. **C:** Core and flaps elevated by gentle traction. **D:** Flaps sutured together to produce projection. **E:** Cut end of syringe barrel used in the dressing to protect the nipple.

the projection of the elevated "nipple" (Figure 11.6D). A full-thickness skin graft from the contralateral areola or from the inner thigh is then applied to the surrounding raw area. When applying the tie-over stent dressing, the flanged end is cut from a plastic syringe barrel and is placed over the protruding nipple like a sleeve. This protects it from pressure exerted by the tie-over dressing (Figures 11.6E, 11.7–11.11).

Combined Nipple-Areola Reconstruction

The conjoined spiral technique uses the entire nipple-areola complex as a full-thickness skin graft (5). The comma-shaped graft is removed, and the spiral is closed on itself on the recipient bed. Each complex has an area of 50% of

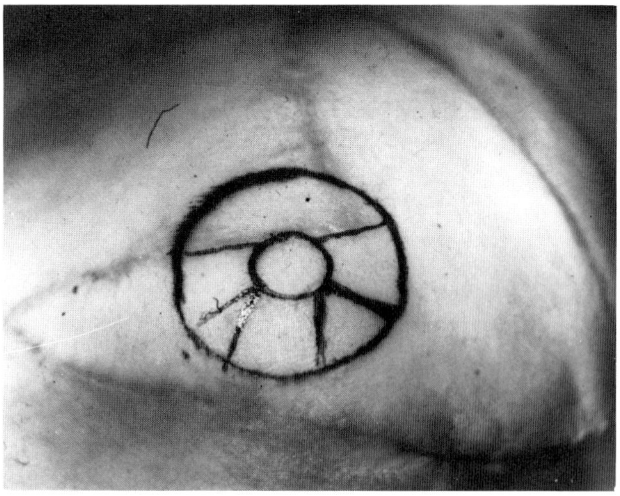

Figure 11.7. Little technique. Tripod flap outlined (the presence of a scar at the flap edge prevented the tetrapod design being used).

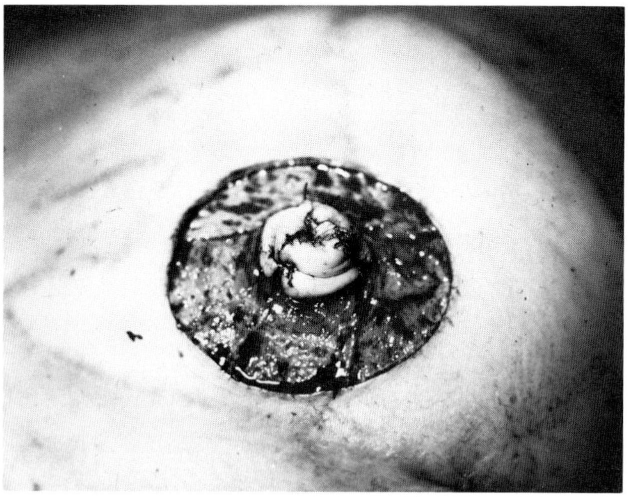

Figure 11.8. Tripod flaps sutured together to produce the "nipple" protrusion.

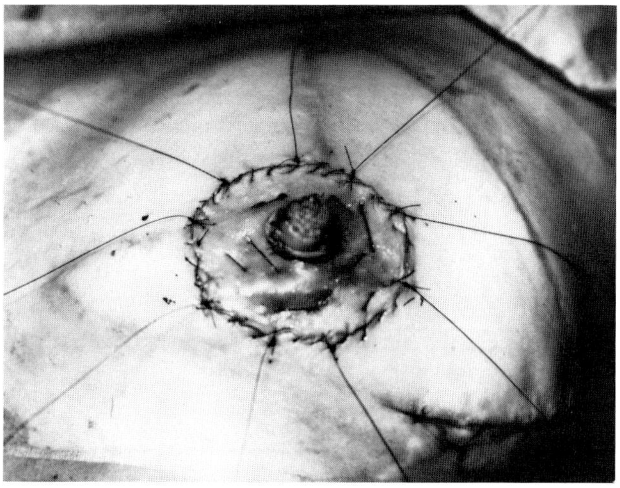

Figure 11.9. Full-thickness inner thigh graft sutured in position.

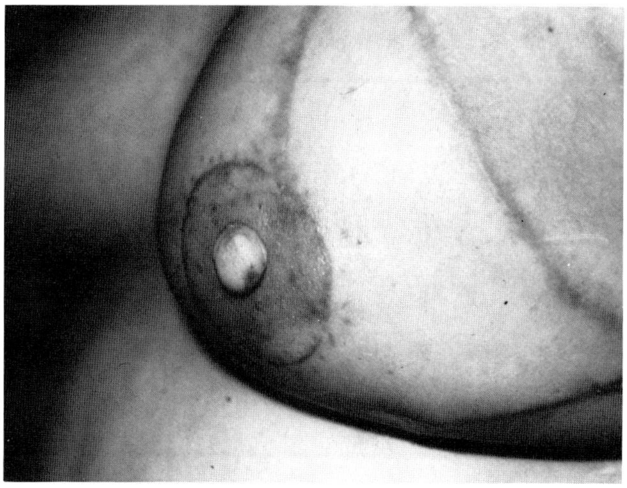

Figure 11.10. Postoperative result in the patient in Figures 11.7–11.9.

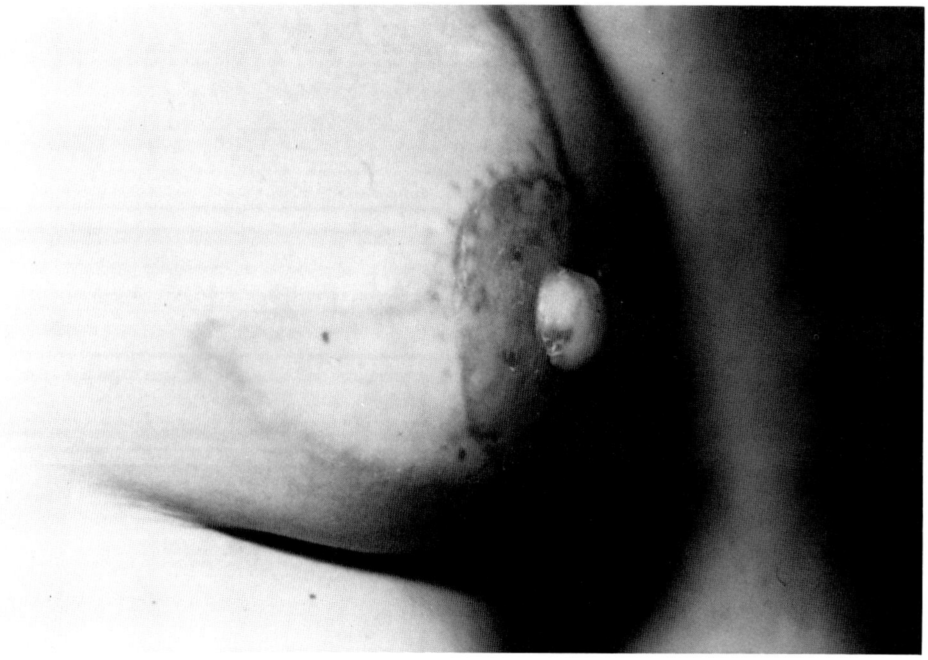

Figure 11.11. Postoperative result, showing good projection in the patient in Figure 11.7–11.10.

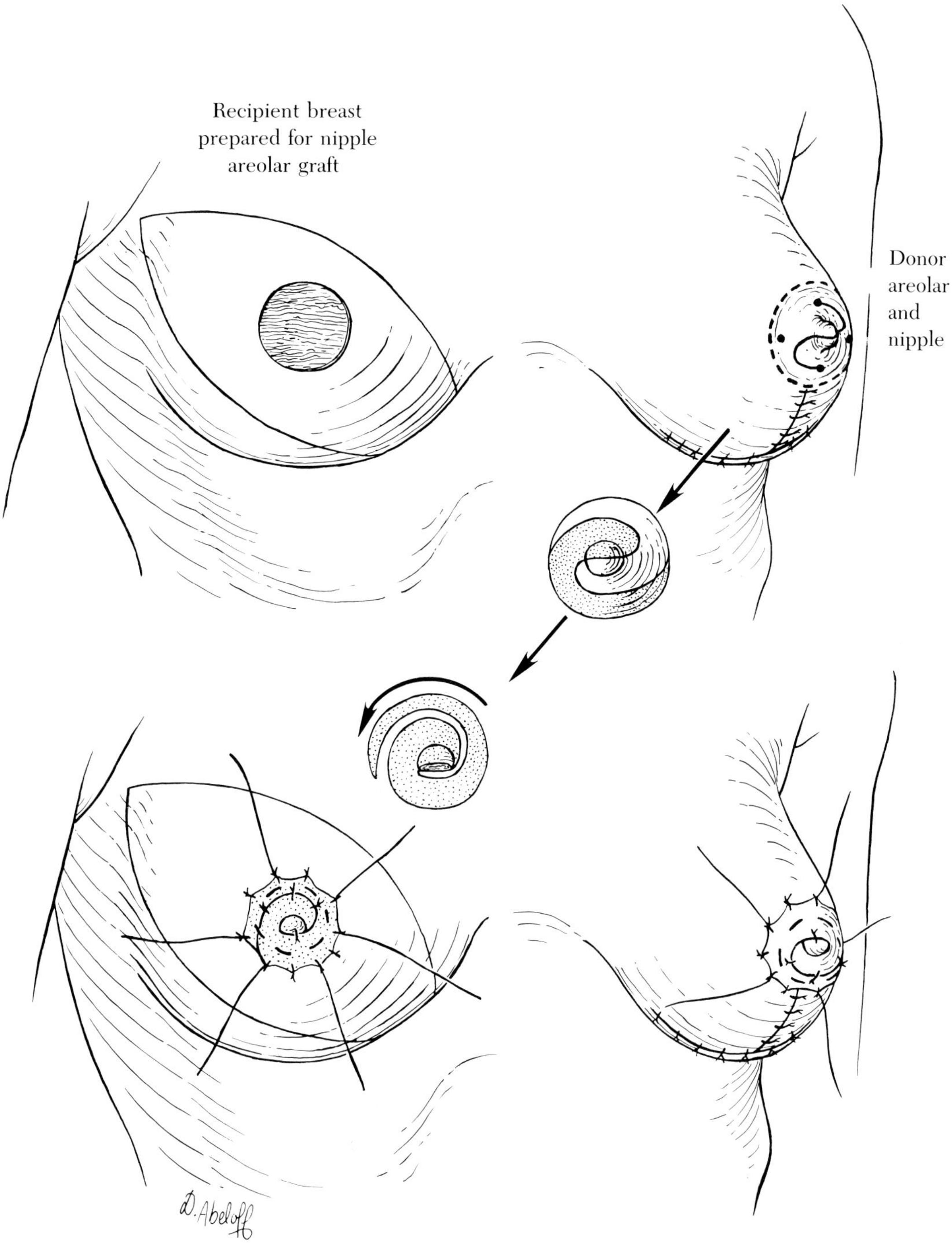

Figure 11.12. Conjoined spiral technique.

the donor complex. No tissue is wasted. To minimize anesthesia of the normal nipple, the nipple part of the graft may be left attached to the breast (6). If the donor complex is very small, a rim of normal breast skin may be incorporated into the spiral (Figures 11.12 and 11.13).

Ancillary Techniques

Montgomery glands can be simulated within the newly reconstructed areola (3). A small strip of conchal cartilage may be obtained and cut into small chips. These are then placed under the areola graft at the time of initial surgery (Figures 11.15A and 11.14).

In order to provide better approximation of the areola graft to the deepithelialized recipient bed, a continuous 5–0 nylon "tacking" suture may be used. A bolus dressing is then applied (Figures 11.15B and 11.16).

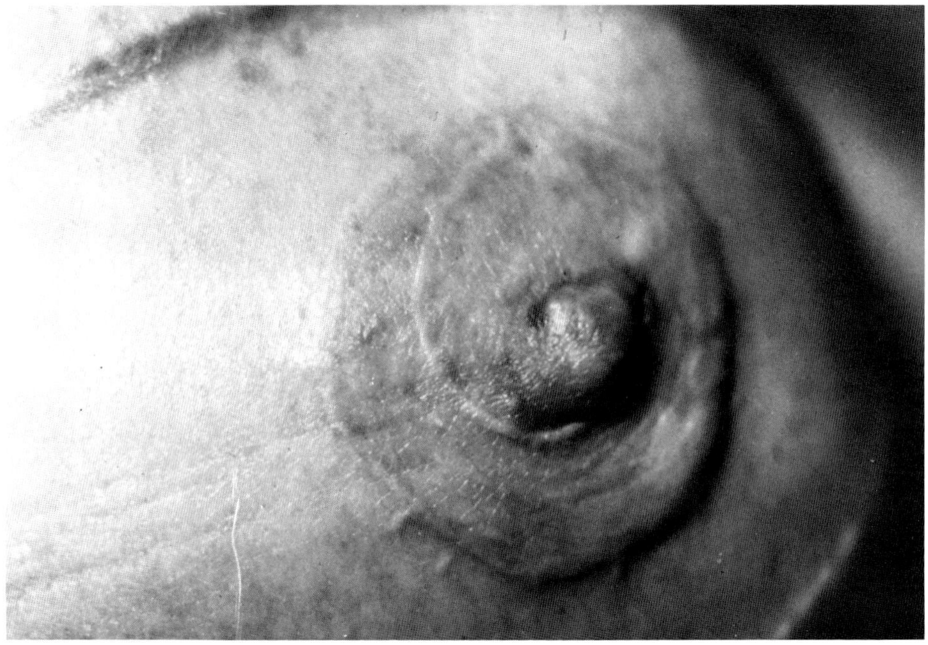

Figure 11.13. Reconstructed nipple using the conjoined spiral technique.

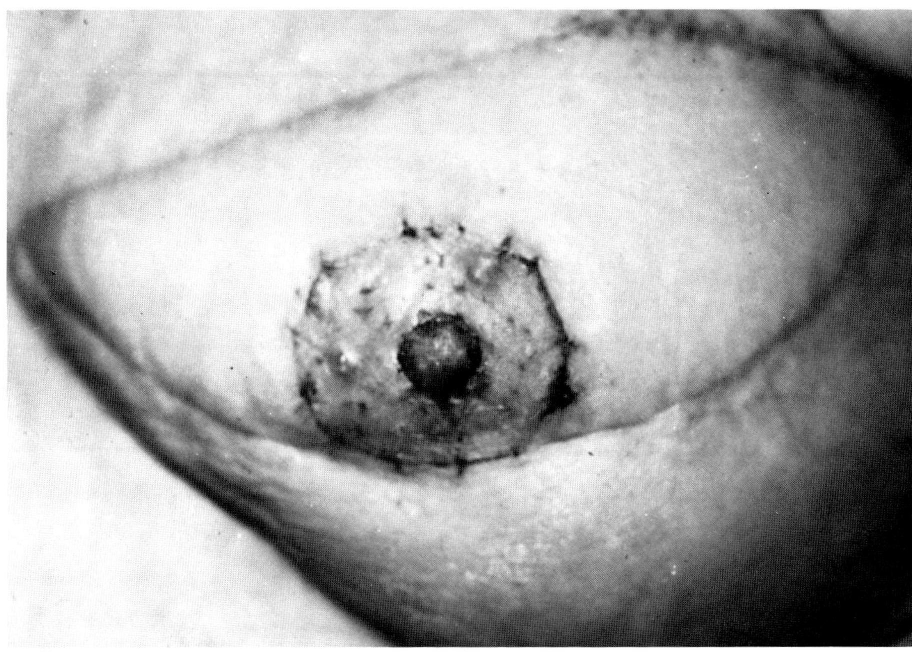

Figure 11.14. Postoperative result showing simulated Montgomery tubercles.

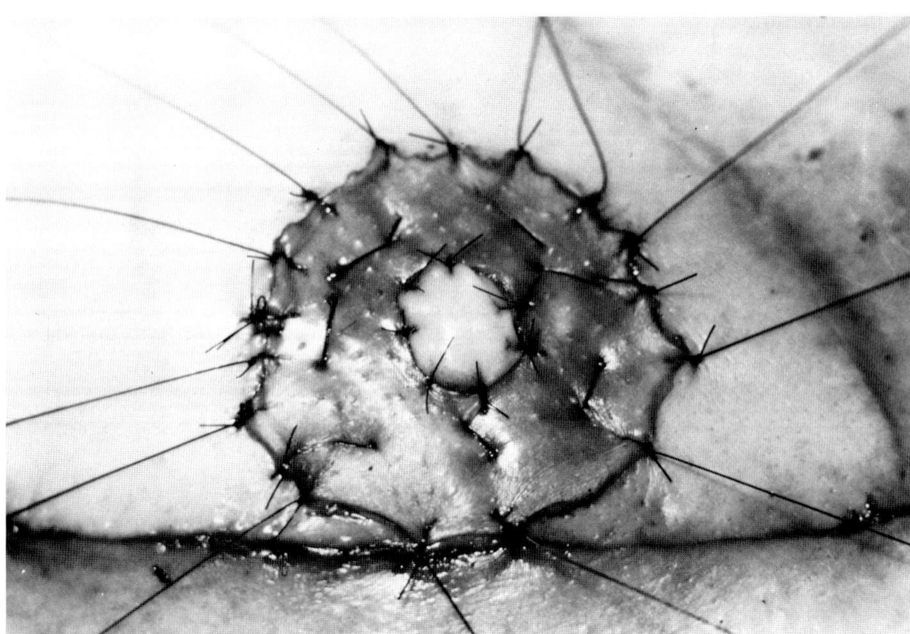

Figure 11.16. Tacking sutures hold diced cartilage in position and help get good contact between the areola graft and the deepithelialized recipient bed.

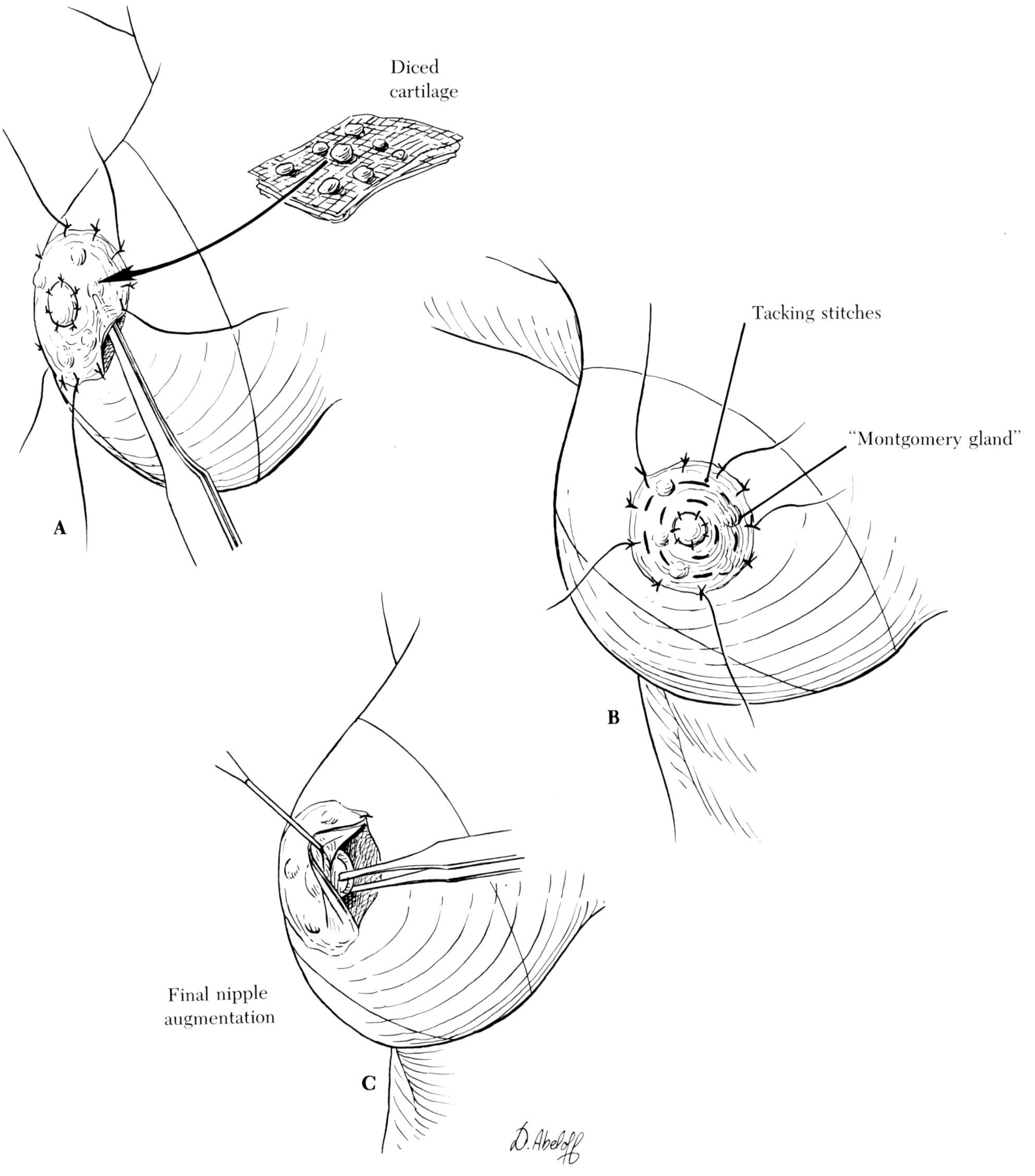

Figure 11.15. **A:** Simulated Montgomery tubercles using diced cartilage. **B:** "Tacking suture" stabilizes the diced cartilage under the areolar graft and ensures good approximation to the recipient bed. **C:** Improving nipple projection using a disc of cartilage.

If nipple projection is found to be inadequate after the reconstruction, silicone, cartilage, or dermis may be placed under the nipple as a secondary procedure. A biopsy punch may also be used to obtain a disc of conchal cartilage (3). This graft cannot be placed at the time of initial surgery because it would interfere with the vascularization of the nipple graft (Figure 11.15C). As an alternative to a skin graft, the areola may be simulated by a tattoo. The selected color should be darker than the other side because the color tends to fade with time (12).

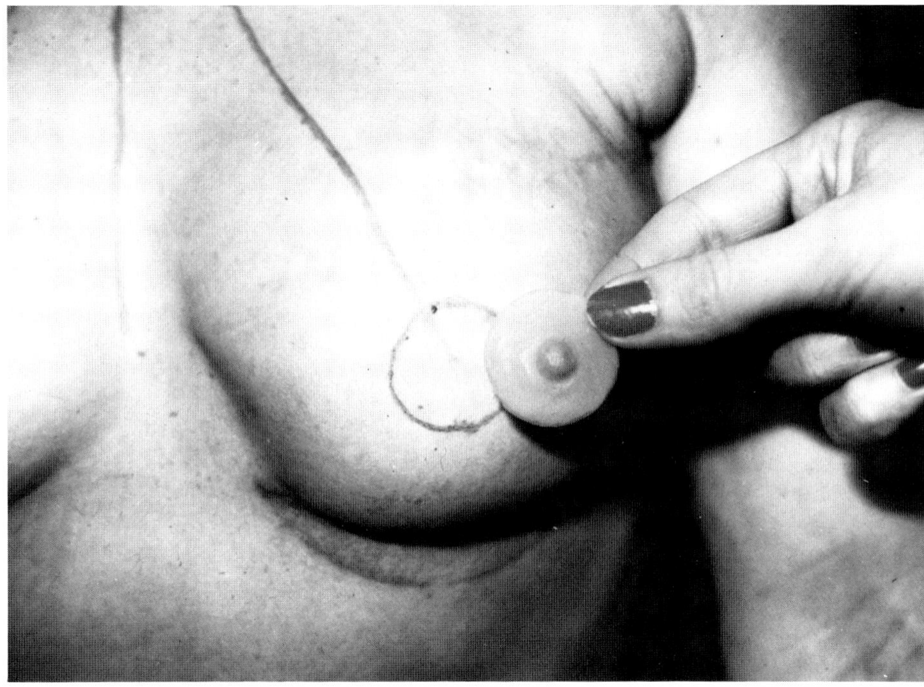

Figure 11.17. Synthetic nipple-areola.

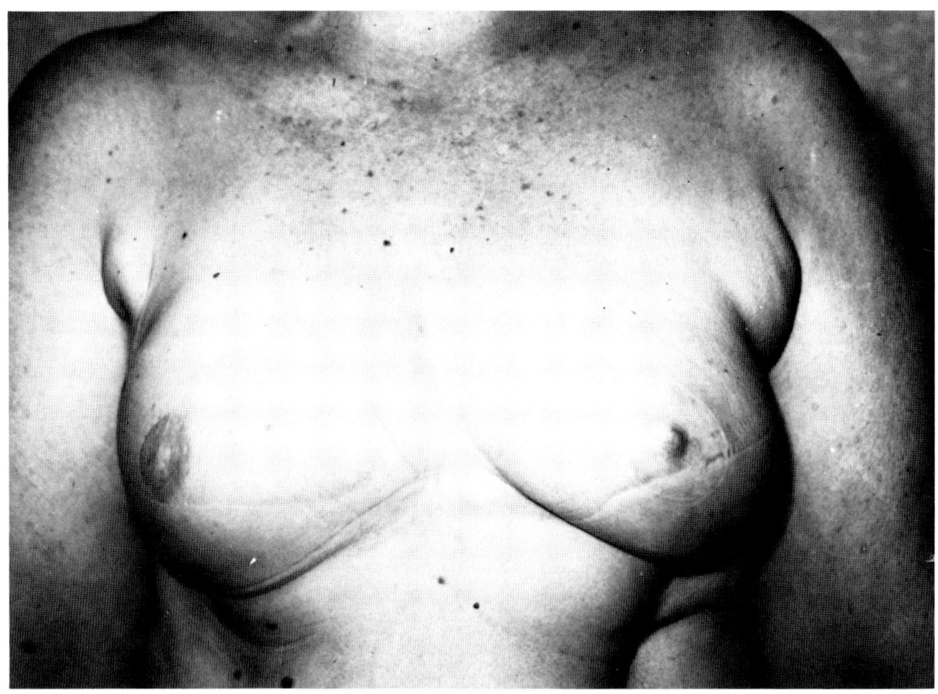

Figure 11.18. The areola was reconstructed from labial skin and became hyperpigmented. The size and position were estimated with the patient in the supine position. The size was too small and the placement too lateral.

Synthetic Nipple-Areola

Occasionally, a patient is unwilling or unable to go through surgical reconstruction of the nipple-areola complex and yet is anxious to have the projection to fill out her brassiere. For this situation a synthetic rubber nipple-areola (Brescare, Inc., S. Miami, Florida 33143) can be matched in size and color to the normal side and applied with adhesive. This can be worn in the shower, and the adhesive is replenished approximately every 7 days (Figure 11.17).

Complications and Errors

Complete loss of the nipple-areola graft is rare, although partial loss is not uncommon. Most cases can be left to heal by second intention.

The commonest errors that occur are related to size and placement of the areola. In the supine position the normal areola tends to contract, and so the size of the reconstructed side should be determined with the patient upright. There is a tendency to place the areola too laterally unless the position is marked with the patient in the upright position (Figure 11.18) (7).

References

1. Adams WM, 1949: Labial transplant for correction of the nipple. Plast Reconstr Surg 4:295–298.
2. Allison AB, Holworth MB, 1978: Carcinoma in a nipple preserved by heterotopic auto-implantation. N Engl J Med 298:1132.
3. Brent B, Bostwick J, 1977: Nipple-areola reconstruction with auricular tissues. Plast Reconstr Surg 60:353–361.
4. Broadbent TR, Woolf RH, Metz PS, 1977: Restoring the mammary areola by a skin graft from the upper inner thigh. Br J Plast Surg 30:220–222.
5. Cocke WM Jr, 1977: Nipple areola complex. In: Breast Reconstruction Following Mastectomy for Carcinoma. Little Brown, Boston.
6. Cronin TD, Upton J, McDonough MJ, 1977: Reconstruction of the breast after mastectomy. Plast Reconstr Surg 59:1–14.
7. Eder H, Lejour M, 1980: Reconstruction of the nipple-areola complex after radical mastectomy. Acta Chir Belg 2:146–153.
8. Gruber RP, 1979: Nipple-areola reconstruction: a review of techniques. Clin Plast Surg 6:71–83.
9. Kiskadden WS, 1950: Case report on split grafting of the nipple. Plast Reconstr Surg 5:184–185.
10. Klatsky SA, Manson PN, 1981: Toe pulp free grafts in nipple reconstruction. Plast Reconstr Surg 68:254–258.
11. Klein D, 1952: Correction of loss of the areola mammae. Plast Reconstr Surg 10:469–472.
12. Lemperle G, Spitalmy H, 1980: Reconstruction of the nipple and areola after radical mastectomy. Acta Chir Belg 2:155–157.
13. Little WJ, Munasifi T, McCulloch DT, 1983: One-stage reconstruction of a projecting nipple: the quadrapod flap. Plast Reconstr Surg 126–132.
14. Millard DR, 1972: Nipple and areola reconstruction by split skin graft from the normal side. Plast Reconstr Surg 50:350–353.
15. Millard DR, Devine J, Warren WD, 1971: Breast reconstruction: a plea for saving the uninvolved nipple. Am J Surg 122:763–764.
16. Schwartz AW, 1976: Reconstruction of the nipple and areola. Br J Plast Surg 29:230–233.

Index